D1408130

Imaging of Lung Cancer

Guest Editors

BASKARAN SUNDARAM, MBBS, MRCP, FRCR
ELLA A. KAZEROONI, MD, MS

RADIOLOGIC CLINICS OF NORTH AMERICA

www.radiologic.theclinics.com

Consulting Editor
FRANK H. MILLER, MD

September 2012 • Volume 50 • Number 5

SAUNDERS an imprint of ELSEVIER, Inc.

W.B. SAUNDERS COMPANY
A Division of Elsevier Inc.

1600 John F. Kennedy Boulevard ● Suite 1800 ● Philadelphia, Pennsylvania 19103-2899

http://www.theclinics.com

RADIOLOGIC CLINICS OF NORTH AMERICA Volume 50, Number 5
September 2012 ISSN 0033-8389, ISBN 13: 978-1-4557-3930-1

Editor: Sarah Barth
Developmental Editor: Donald Mumford

© **2012 Elsevier Inc. All rights reserved.**

This journal and the individual contributions contained in it are protected under copyright by Elsevier, and the following terms and conditions apply to their use:

Photocopying
Single photocopies of single articles may be made for personal use as allowed by national copyright laws. Permission of the Publisher and payment of a fee is required for all other photocopying, including multiple or systematic copying, copying for advertising or promotional purposes, resale, and all forms of document delivery. Special rates are available for educational institutions that wish to make photocopies for non-profit educational classroom use. For information on how to seek permission visit www.elsevier.com/permissions or call: (+44) 1865 843830 (UK)/(+1) 215 239 3804 (USA).

Derivative Works
Subscribers may reproduce tables of contents or prepare lists of articles including abstracts for internal circulation within their institutions. Permission of the Publisher is required for resale or distribution outside the institution. Permission of the Publisher is required for all other derivative works, including compilations and translations (please consult www.elsevier.com/permissions).

Electronic Storage or Usage
Permission of the Publisher is required to store or use electronically any material contained in this journal, including any article or part of an article (please consult www.elsevier.com/permissions). Except as outlined above, no part of this publication may be reproduced, stored in a retrieval system or transmitted in any form or by any means, electronic, mechanical, photocopying, recording or otherwise, without prior written permission of the Publisher.

Notice
No responsibility is assumed by the Publisher for any injury and/or damage to persons or property as a matter of products liability, negligence or otherwise, or from any use or operation of any methods, products, instructions or ideas contained in the material herein. Because of rapid advances in the medical sciences, in particular, independent verification of diagnoses and drug dosages should be made.

Although all advertising material is expected to conform to ethical (medical) standards, inclusion in this publication does not constitute a guarantee or endorsement of the quality or value of such product or of the claims made of it by its manufacturer.

Radiologic Clinics of North America (ISSN 0033-8389) is published bimonthly by Elsevier Inc., 360 Park Avenue South, New York, NY 10010-1710. Months of issue are January, March, May, July, September, and November. Periodicals postage paid at New York, NY and additional mailing offices. Subscription prices are USD 421 per year for US individuals, USD 659 per year for US institutions, USD 202 per year for US students and residents, USD 491 per year for Canadian individuals, USD 827 per year for Canadian institutions, USD 606 per year for international individuals, USD 827 per year for international institutions, and USD 290 per year for Canadian and foreign students/residents. To receive student and resident rate, orders must be accompanied by name of affiliated institution, date of term and the signature of program/residency coordinatior on institution letterhead. Orders will be billed at individual rate until proof of status is received. Foreign air speed delivery is included in all *Clinics* subscription prices. All prices are subject to change without notice. **POSTMASTER:** Send address changes to *Radiologic Clinics of North America*, Elsevier Health Sciences Division, Subscription Customer Service, 3251 Riverport Lane, Maryland Heights, MO63043. **Customer Service: Telephone: 1-800-654-2452** (U.S. and Canada); **1-314-447-8871** (outside U.S. and Canada). **Fax: 1-314-447-8029. E-mail: journalscustomerservice-usa@ elsevier.com** (for print support); **journalsonlinesupport-usa@elsevier.com** (for online support).

Reprints. For copies of 100 or more of articles in this publication, please contact the Commercial Reprints Department, Elsevier Inc., 360 Park Avenue South, New York, New York 10010-1710. Tel.: (+1) 212-633-3812; Fax: (+1) 212-462-1935; E-mail: reprints@elsevier.com.

Radiologic Clinics of North America also published in Greek Paschalidis Medical Publications, Athens, Greece.

Radiologic Clinics of North America is covered in *MEDLINE/PubMed (Index Medicus), EMBASE/Excerpta Medica, Current Contents/Life Sciences, Current Contents/Clinical Medicine, RSNA Index to Imaging Literature, BIOSIS, Science Citation Index,* and *ISI/BIOMED*.

Printed in the United States of America.

Contributors

CONSULTING EDITOR

FRANK H. MILLER, MD
Professor of Radiology; Chief, Body Imaging
Section and Fellowship Program and GI
Radiology; Medical Director MRI, Department
of Radiology, Northwestern University
Feinberg School of Medicine, Chicago, Illinois

GUEST EDITORS

BASKARAN SUNDARAM, MBBS, MRCP, FRCR
Associate Professor, Department of Radiology,
University of Michigan Health System,
Ann Arbor, Michigan

ELLA A. KAZEROONI, MD, MS, FACR
Professor, Director, Cardiothoracic Radiology
Division, University of Michigan Health System,
Ann Arbor, Michigan

AUTHORS

FEREIDOUN ABTIN, MD
Assistant Professor, Department of Radiology,
UCLA Medical Center, Los Angeles, California

DOUGLAS A. ARENBERG, MD
Associate Professor of Medicine, Pulmonary &
Critical Care Medicine, Ann Arbor, Michigan

SANJEEV BHALLA, MD
Professor of Diagnostic Radiology, Section
Chief of Cardiothoracic Imaging Section,
Mallinckrodt Institute of Radiology at
Washington University-St Louis, St Louis,
Missouri

ANDREW C. CHANG, MD
John Alexander Distinguished Professor,
Associate Professor and Head, Section of
Thoracic Surgery, University of Michigan,
Ann Arbor, Michigan

JARED D. CHRISTENSEN, MD
Assistant Professor of Radiology, Department
of Radiology, Duke University Medical Center,
Durham, North Carolina

PATRICIA DE GROOT, MD
Division of Diagnostic Imaging, Department
of Diagnostic Radiology, The University of
Texas M.D. Anderson Cancer Center,
Houston, Texas

SHIRISH M. GADGEEL, MD
Associate Professor, Department of
Hematology and Oncology, Karmanos Cancer
Institute, Wayne State University, Detroit,
Michigan

PHILIP A. HODNETT, MD
Thoracic Imaging, Department of Radiology,
New York University Langone Medical Center,
New York, New York

GREGORY P. KALEMKERIAN, MD
Professor, Division of Hematology/Oncology,
University of Michigan, Ann Arbor, Michigan

ELLA A. KAZEROONI, MD, MS, FACR
Professor, Department of Radiology,
University of Michigan Health System,
Ann Arbor, Michigan

JANE P. KO, MD
Thoracic Imaging, Department of Radiology,
New York University School of Medicine,
New York University Langone Medical Center,
New York, New York

SEBASTIAN LEY, MD
Cardiothoracic Radiologist, University Health
Network, Mount Sinai and Women's College
Hospital, University of Toronto, Ontario, Canada

UR METSER, MD
Abdominal Radiologist, University Health
Network, Mount Sinai and Women's College
Hospital, University of Toronto, Ontario,
Canada

REGINALD F. MUNDEN, MD, DMD, MBA
Division of Diagnostic Imaging, Department
of Diagnostic Radiology, The University of
Texas M.D. Anderson Cancer Center,
Houston, Texas

EDWARD F. PATZ JR, MD
James and Alice Chen Professor of Radiology,
Department of Radiology; Professor in
Pharmacology and Cancer Biology,
Department of Pharmacology and Cancer
Biology, Duke University Medical Center,
Durham, North Carolina

NARINDER S. PAUL, MD
Division Chief of Cardiothoracic Radiology,
University Health Network, Mount Sinai and
Women's College Hospital, University of
Toronto, Ontario, Canada

SURESH S. RAMALINGAM, MD
Professor, Department of Hematology
and Medical Oncology, Winship Cancer
Institute, Emory University, Atlanta,
Georgia

CONSTANTINE A. RAPTIS, MD
Assistant Professor of Diagnostic Radiology,
Cardiothoracic Imaging Section, Mallinckrodt
Institute of Radiology at Washington
University-St Louis, St Louis, Missouri

ERIC J. SCHMIDLIN, MD
Lecturer, Department of Radiology, University
of Michigan Health System, Ann Arbor,
Michigan; University of Mass Memorial Medical
Center-University campus, Worcester,
Massachusetts

AMITA SHARMA, MD
Assistant Professor of Radiology, Harvard
Medical School; Department of Radiology,
Massachusetts General Hospital, Boston,
Massachusetts

JO-ANNE O. SHEPARD, MD
Professor of Radiology, Harvard Medical
School; Department of Radiology,
Massachusetts General Hospital, Boston,
Massachusetts

**BASKARAN SUNDARAM, MBBS, MRCP,
FRCR**
Associate Professor, Department of Radiology,
University of Michigan Health System,
Ann Arbor, Michigan

Contents

> The greatest risk by far for developing lung cancer is cigarette smoking, but age, radon exposure, environmental pollution, occupational exposures, gender, race, and pre-existing lung disease also are important contributors. However, not all people with these risk factors develop lung cancer, and some without any known risk factor do, indicating the importance of genetic influences. Future advances in understanding and treating lung cancer will be based on genetic analysis. The most effective preventive measure is to never start or to stop cigarette smoking.

> 1. Screening with low-dose computed tomography reduces mortality from lung cancer in high-risk patients. 2. Lung cancer screening with chest radiography alone or in combination with sputum analysis is currently not recommended. 3. The feasibility and impact of screening in patients with a low or moderate risk for primary lung cancer are currently not known. 4. A standardized framework for testing and management in a multidisciplinary fashion is necessary to provide lung cancer screening. 5. The National Comprehensive Cancer Network and the American Lung Association have recently issued guidelines for lung cancer screening with computed tomography in high-risk patients.

> The radiologic evaluation and management of the indeterminate solitary pulmonary nodule provide common diagnostic dilemma. With continued technologic advancements in multidetector computed tomography leading to higher spatial resolution and greater overall sensitivity of computed tomography scanners, increasing numbers of indeterminate solitary pulmonary nodules are being detected. Malignant and benign solitary pulmonary nodules have similar imaging features. Clinical management of these incidental nodules relies not only on imaging characteristics but also on malignancy risk factors, along with the risks and benefits of further investigation.

> Today lung cancer remains the leading cause of cancer-related death in the United States, accounting for 28% of all cases. Radiologists play an important role in the assessment of this large number of patients. Given the important role imaging plays in the care of patients with lung cancer, it is incumbent on the radiologist to have

a firm understanding of the TNM (tumor-node-metastasis) staging system used to describe the distribution of disease in lung cancer. This article reviews the 7th Edition of the TNM staging system for lung cancer and important changes from the 6th Edition.

Chest radiography, the most commonly performed imaging technique for the detection of lung disease, is limited in accurately detecting early lung cancer. The main imaging modality for the staging of lung cancer is computed tomography (CT), supplemented by positron emission tomography (PET), usually as a hybrid technique in conjunction with CT (PET/CT). Magnetic resonance (MR) imaging is a useful diagnostic tool for specific indications and has the advantage of not using ionizing radiation. This article discusses the optimal imaging protocols for lung cancer staging using CT, PET (PET/CT), and MR imaging, and the role of imaging in patient management.

Diagnostic confirmation through tissue sampling plays a central role in managing patients with suspected lung malignancy. Tissue samples may be obtained in various ways using bronchoscopy, computed tomography guidance, or surgery. Multidisciplinary discussion between members of the lung cancer care team is helpful in assessing the appropriateness of sampling and the best place to sample that would establish both the diagnosis and the correct stage of the disease in a safe manner.

Lung cancer is a heterogenous disease with 2 main subtypes: non–small cell lung cancer (NSCLC) and small cell lung cancer (SCLC). Early-stage NSCLC is managed primarily by surgical resection, with adjuvant chemotherapy for selected. Locally advanced stage III NSCLC is usually treated with combined modality therapy. For advanced NSCLC, newer molecularly targeted agents can improve survival in selected patients. Limited-stage SCLC is treated with chemoradiotherapy with curative intent, while extensive-stage SCLC remains an incurable disease. Further advances will rely on improvements in understanding of the molecular events driving the malignant phenotype and the development of novel, targeted therapeutic strategies.

Lung cancer is the commonest cause of cancer death in adults. Although the treatment of choice is surgical resection with lobectomy, many patients are nonsurgical candidates because of medical comorbidities. Patients may also have recurrent disease after resection or radiotherapy and some patients refuse surgical options. Image-guided ablation has been recently introduced as a safe, alternative treatment of localized disease in carefully selected patients. This article discusses the principles, technique, and follow-up of the 3 main ablative therapies currently used in the lung, radiofrequency ablation, microwave ablation, and percutaneous cryotherapy.

Jared D. Christensen and Edward F. Patz Jr

Imaging continues to play an essential role in evaluating patients with lung cancer. Improvement in radiologic techniques will produce more accurate diagnostic information, but complementing conventional studies with molecular diagnostics will likely have an even greater impact on patient management. Integration of imaging studies and biomarkers into the diagnostic evaluation of patients with lung cancer provides an opportunity to more efficiently guide diagnosis, staging, treatment, and follow-up.

GOAL STATEMENT

The goal of the *Radiologic Clinics of North America* is to keep practicing radiologists and radiology residents up to date with current clinical practice in radiology by providing timely articles reviewing the state of the art in patient care.

ACCREDITATION

The *Radiologic Clinics of North America* is planned and implemented in accordance with the Essential Areas and Policies of the Accreditation Council for Continuing Medical Education (ACCME) through the joint sponsorship of the University of Virginia School of Medicine and Elsevier. The University of Virginia School of Medicine is accredited by the ACCME to provide continuing medical education for physicians.

The University of Virginia School of Medicine designates this enduring material activity for a maximum of 15 *AMA PRA Category 1 Credit*(s)™ for each issue, 90 credits per year. Physicians should only claim credit commensurate with the extent of their participation in the activity.

The American Medical Association has determined that physicians not licensed in the US who participate in this CME enduring material activity are eligible for a maximum of 15 *AMA PRA Category 1 Credit*(s)™ for each issue, 90 credits per year.

Credit can be earned by reading the text material, taking the CME examination online at http://www.theclinics.com/home/cme, and completing the evaluation. After taking the test, you will be required to review any and all incorrect answers. Following completion of the test and evaluation, your credit will be awarded and you may print your certificate.

FACULTY DISCLOSURE/CONFLICT OF INTEREST

The University of Virginia School of Medicine, as an ACCME accredited provider, endorses and strives to comply with the Accreditation Council for Continuing Medical Education (ACCME) Standards of Commercial Support, Commonwealth of Virginia statutes, University of Virginia policies and procedures, and associated federal and private regulations and guidelines on the need for disclosure and monitoring of proprietary and financial interests that may affect the scientific integrity and balance of content delivered in continuing medical education activities under our auspices.

The University of Virginia School of Medicine requires that all CME activities accredited through this institution be developed independently and be scientifically rigorous, balanced and objective in the presentation/discussion of its content, theories and practices.

All authors/editors participating in an accredited CME activity are expected to disclose to the readers relevant financial relationships with commercial entities occurring within the past 12 months (such as grants or research support, employee, consultant, stock holder, member of speakers bureau, etc.). The University of Virginia School of Medicine will employ appropriate mechanisms to resolve potential conflicts of interest to maintain the standards of fair and balanced education to the reader. Questions about specific strategies can be directed to the Office of Continuing Medical Education, University of Virginia School of Medicine, Charlottesville, Virginia.

The faculty and staff of the University of Virginia Office of Continuing Medical Education have no financial affiliations to disclose.

The authors/editors listed below have identified no financial or professional relationships for themselves or their spouse/partner:

Fereidoun Abtin, MD; Douglas A. Arenberg, MD; Sanjeev Bhalla, MD; Adrianne Brigido, (Acquisitions Editor); Andrew C. Chang, MD; Jared D. Christensen, MD; Patricia de Groot, MD; Philip A. Hodnett, MD; Ella A. Kazerooni, MD, MS (Guest Editor); Jane P. Ko, MD; Sebastian Ley, MD; Ur Metser, MD; Frank H. Miller, MD (Consulting Editor); Reginald F. Munden, MD, DMD, MBA; Eric J. Schmidlin, MD; Amita Sharma, MD; Jo-Anne O. Shepard, MD; and Baskaran Sundaram, MBBS, MRCP, FRCR (Guest Editor).

The authors/editors listed below have identified the following financial or professional relationships for themselves or their spouse/partner:

Shirish M. Gadgeel, MD is on the Speakers' Bureau for Pfizer, Genetech, and Eli Lilly; is on the Advisory Board for Boehringer-Ingelheim and Methylgene; and receives research support from Clovis, Pfizer, Inc., Novartis, GSK, Chugai, Genentech, and Abbot.
Klaus D. Hagspiel, MD (Test Author) is an industry funded research/investigator for Siemens Medical Solutions.
Gregory P. Kalemkerian, MD is an industry funded research/investigator for Eli Lilly.
Edward F. Patz, Jr., MD receives research funding from LabCorp.
Narinder S. Paul, MD receives research support from Toshiba Medical Systems.
Suresh S. Ramalingam, MD is on the Advisory Board for Genentech, Pfizer, Inc., Astellus, AVEO, Lilly, Boehringer Ingelheim, and Abbott.
Constantine A. Raptis, MD receives research funding from and is on the Speakers' Bureau for Lantheus Medical Imaging.

__Disclosure of Discussion of Non-FDA Approved Uses for Pharmaceutical Products and/or Medical Devices.__
The University of Virginia School of Medicine, as an ACCME provider, requires that all faculty presenters identify and disclose any off-label uses for pharmaceutical and medical device products. The University of Virginia School of Medicine recommends that each physician fully review all the available data on new products or procedures prior to clinical use.

TO ENROLL

To enroll in the Radiologic Clinics of North America Continuing Medical Education program, call customer service at 1-800-654-2452 or sign up online at http://www.theclinics.com/home/cme. The CME program is available to subscribers for an additional annual fee USD 245.

RADIOLOGIC CLINICS OF NORTH AMERICA

RELATED INTERESTS

Magnetic Resonance Imaging Clinics, Vol. 16, No. 4 (November 2008)
Chest MR
Michael B. Gotway, MD

PET Clinics, Vol. 1, No. 4 (October 2006)
Lung Cancer
James W. Fletcher, MD

**DOWNLOAD
Free App!**

Review Articles
THE CLINICS

NOW AVAILABLE FOR YOUR iPhone and iPad

Preface

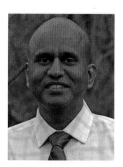

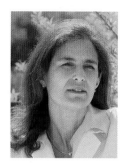

Baskaran Sundaram, MBBS, MRCP, FRCR   Ella A. Kazerooni, MD, MS
Guest Editors

As the leading cause of cancer mortality in both men and women, lung cancer is an important public health care issue. Our understanding of lung cancer biology and management of lung cancer patients continues to evolve. Over the last decade, there were many advances in the study of lung cancer. Notable events pertaining specifically to radiology include the advances in low-dose CT screening culminating in the publication of the National Lung Screening Trial, the revised TNM staging system, widespread acceptance of PET in lung cancer staging, a revised classification scheme for adenocarcinomas, and image-guided local ablation therapy. Together with disciplines of pulmonary medicine, thoracic oncology, and thoracic surgery, radiology plays a key role in the detection, diagnosis, and management of lung cancer. Hence, it is timely that the *Radiologic Clinics of North America* chose lung cancer for a focused edition.

We are extremely grateful to all the contributing authors for their willingness to share their expertise. In these outstanding articles, leading experts in this field from major institutions in North America have held the magnifying glass over the relevant issues on lung cancer. This issue begins with lung cancer epidemiology, risk factors, and prevention by Drs Groot and Munden, followed by screening for lung cancer by Drs Schmidlin, Sundaram, and Kazerooni, and the evaluation and the management of indeterminate pulmonary nodules by Drs Hodnett and Ko. These follow with a series of topics on the staging and management of lung cancer, including the revised TNM lung cancer staging system by Drs Raptis and Bhalla, optimal imaging protocols for lung cancer staging by Drs Paul, Metser, and Ley, a multidisciplinary approach to lung cancer tissue sampling by Drs Chang, Sundaram, and Arenberg, lung cancer treatment by Drs Gadgeel, Ramalingam, and Kalemkerian, and image-guided ablative therapies for lung cancer by Drs Sharma, Abtin, and Shepard. The final article is forward-thinking, covering future trends in lung cancer diagnosis and staging, genetics, novel biomarkers for lung cancer detection by Drs Christensen and Patz.

We also thank Dr Frank H. Miller and Elsevier publishers for the opportunity to compile the current knowledge on lung cancer. Last, we would like to acknowledge and appreciate the unconditional love and support from our family members, enabling us to bring this project to fruition.

Baskaran Sundaram, MBBS, MRCP, FRCR
Division of Cardiothoracic Radiology
Department of Radiology
University of Michigan Health System
CVC-Room 5481, 1500 East Medical Center Drive
Ann Arbor, MI 48109, USA

Ella A. Kazerooni, MD, MS
Division of Cardiothoracic Radiology
Department of Radiology
University of Michigan Health System
CVC-Room 5482, 1500 East Medical Center Drive
Ann Arbor, MI 48109, USA

E-mail addresses:
sundbask@med.umich.edu (B. Sundaram)
ellakaz@med.umich.edu (E.A. Kazerooni)

Radiol Clin N Am 50 (2012) xi
http://dx.doi.org/10.1016/j.rcl.2012.06.009
0033-8389/12/$ – see front matter © 2012 Elsevier Inc. All rights reserved.

Lung Cancer Epidemiology, Risk Factors, and Prevention

Patricia de Groot, MD*, Reginald F. Munden, MD, DMD, MBA

KEYWORDS

- Lung cancer • Epidemiology • Risk factors • Prevention

KEY POINTS

- All types of lung cancer are directly correlated with cigarette smoking. Adenocarcinoma rates have increased significantly over the last 30 years.
- Environmental tobacco smoke is a major contributor to morbidity and mortality worldwide. There is no safe level of second-hand smoke.
- Pollution, occupational exposures, and environmental radon are additional risk factors for developing lung cancer.
- Genetic factors contribute to development of lung cancer. Future progress in understanding and treating lung cancer will be based on genetic analysis.

EPIDEMIOLOGY

Carcinoma of the lung is currently the leading cause worldwide of death due to cancer. The disease has become an epidemic as incidence rates and lung cancer deaths have risen dramatically over the last century, correlating with an increase in cigarette consumption. The magnitude of the impact on mortality is indicated by comparing changes over time. More than 1.5 million new cases of lung cancer are now diagnosed annually worldwide,[1,2] with incidence in the United States projected to be 221,130 cases in 2011,[3] compared with 1974, when new cases of lung cancer were estimated at 83,000 worldwide, with an expected 75,400 deaths that year.[4] Even more dramatically, in 1927 cancers of the lungs and pleura were implicated in just 2012 deaths in the United States[5] and before the turn of the twentieth century, lung cancer was considered an extremely rare malignancy.[6]

Trends in Incidence and Mortality

In 2011 in the United States there were 115,060 new cases of lung cancer in men and 106,070 new cases in women. The number of deaths in 2011 caused by lung and bronchus cancers was an estimated 156,940: 84,600 in men and 71,340 in women. In men, this represents a continuing decline in incidence and mortality after a peak in the 1980s. Between 1990 and 2007, male mortality from lung cancer in the United States decreased by almost 28%.[3] In women, however, lung cancer rates began to increase in 1965, and only in the last few years since 2000 has there been a slight decline of about 2%. Overall, female lung cancer mortality is increased by 6.31% in comparison with 1990.[3]

Within the United States there is geographic diversity in cases of lung cancer, with Kentucky having the highest number at a rate 3 times that of Utah, the state with the lowest incidence. California, Florida, and Texas lead the nation in age-standardized death rates from lung cancer, whereas Alaska, Wyoming, and North Dakota have some of the lowest annual death rates.[3]

Age, racial and ethnic, and socioeconomic disparities also exist. Cancer is a disease of aging, with 60% of cancers diagnosed in persons older than 65 years and 70% of cancer deaths belonging

Division of Diagnostic Imaging, Department of Diagnostic Radiology, The University of Texas M.D. Anderson Cancer Center, 1515 Holcombe Boulevard, Unit 1478, Houston, TX 77030, USA
* Corresponding author.
E-mail address: pdegroot@mdanderson.org

Radiol Clin N Am 50 (2012) 863–876
http://dx.doi.org/10.1016/j.rcl.2012.06.006
0033-8389/12/$ – see front matter © 2012 Elsevier Inc. All rights reserved.

to the same age cohort.[7] The incidence and death rates from lung cancer are higher for Caucasian and African American populations in the United States than for other ethnic and racial groups, including Asian Americans and Pacific Islanders, Native Americans, and Hispanic people. Education levels, as a proxy for socioeconomic status, show a striking inverse correlation with death rates from lung cancer.[3] Survival rates for lung cancer remain abysmal, with a 5-year survival of approximately 15%, unchanged for decades despite advances in medical knowledge.[3]

Incidence of and mortality from lung cancer are higher in Caucasians and African Americans than in other ethnic groups in the United States. Age and geographic location also are important.

Histopathology of Lung Cancer

The major cell types of cancer are small cell lung cancer (SCLC) and non–small cell lung cancer (NSCLC), with the latter category comprising several histologic subtypes, the major ones being squamous cell cancer, adenocarcinoma, and large cell cancer. The cell types with the strongest association to cigarette smoking are SCLC and squamous cell lung cancer, but there is growing evidence that adenocarcinoma also is strongly associated with smoking.[8] In 1979, squamous cell lung carcinoma was significantly more common than adenocarcinoma, at a ratio of approximately 17:1. In the last 30 years, there has been a relative increase in the number of lung adenocarcinomas, bringing that ratio to 1.4:1.[9,10] Adenocarcinoma is the most common type of lung cancer in North America, whereas squamous cell carcinoma remains more prevalent in Europe and Australia.[11]

In recent years new techniques in immunohistochemistry have allowed for more accurate identification of cell type, and testing is available for detecting specific genetic mutations that have prognostic and treatment implications, such as epidermal growth factor receptor (EGFR) mutations in adenocarcinomas of nonsmokers.

All subtypes of lung cancer are related to cigarette smoking. Adenocarcinoma rates have increased significantly over the last 30 years.

Lung Cancer in Never-Smokers

A growing number of incident lung carcinomas are occurring in never-smokers, defined by many as individuals who have smoked fewer than 100 cigarettes in a lifetime. This group comprises 15% to 25% of the lung cancer population, with 300,000 deaths resulting annually.[12,13] This subset of patients with lung cancer is more likely to be female, and the cancer cell type is more likely to be adenocarcinoma.[14] Although lung cancer in nonsmokers occurs worldwide, geographic variation is striking, with 30% to 40% of Asian patients with lung cancer being never-smokers, compared with 10% to 20% of Caucasians.[12,13] In the United States, nonsmoking African Americans have greater incidence and mortality rates of lung cancer compared with nonsmoking whites.[12]

Lung cancer in never-smokers (LCINS) is linked with environmental factors, including secondhand tobacco smoke, outdoor and indoor air pollution, and radon. In addition, human papillomavirus infection is seen frequently in nonsmoking Chinese women with lung cancer.[13] However, no single risk factor appears to be dominant.

Specific genetic mutations associated with LCINS are not common in the lung cancers of smokers, suggesting a different biological disease, with implications for chemotherapeutic response. For instance, EGFR gene mutation and the EML4-ALK fusion gene are more common in never-smokers, whereas epigenetic changes such as promoter gene methylation are less common in nonsmokers.[13] Although women are disproportionately affected by LCINS, as a group their survival is better than that of nonsmoking men who develop lung cancer.[12,14]

RISK FACTORS

The hallmarks of tumorigenesis are acquired capabilities of individual cells or groups of cells that enable transformation to a malignant entity. These requisite acquired abilities of cells have been described by Hanahan and Weinberg[15] as (1) self-sufficiency in growth signals; (2) insensitivity to antigrowth signals; (3) evasion of apoptosis; (4) limitless replication potential; (5) sustained angiogenesis; and (6) tissue invasion and metastasis. The underlying mechanism that allows these changes to occur is instability of the genome; in particular, breakdown of DNA repair capacity.[15] This process is influenced by a complex interplay of genetic, behavioral, and environmental factors, which can increase the risk of an individual developing lung cancer.

Genetic Factors

Individual organisms respond to environmental challenges in different ways. For instance, although the vast majority of lung cancers (up to 90%) occur in smokers, only 15% of smokers will develop lung cancer.[16] Variation in genetic makeup is an important survival mechanism in the face of disease.

Heredity and genetic susceptibility

Certain families possess an inherited susceptibility to malignancies, primarily in the context of uncommon germ-line mutations in tumor suppressor genes p53 and RB or RB1 (retinoblastoma),[17] and in other unusual autosomal recessive disorders such as Bloom syndrome and Werner syndrome.[18] In the absence of a genetic syndrome, the published literature on risk of lung cancer within families suggests a twofold increased risk in smoking individuals with a positive family history of cancer, and this risk is additionally elevated if a family member was diagnosed at an early age and/or if multiple relatives have been affected.[19] In nonsmoking families, a positive family history for lung cancer is associated with a 1.5-fold increased odds ratio of developing the disease.[12]

Variant alleles of several genes are associated with increased susceptibility to lung cancer. Some of these genes encode proteins that are involved in the metabolism of tobacco carcinogens, such as the cytochrome P450 enzyme (CYP1A1 gene) and the glutathione-S-transferases (GSTM1, GSTT1). Other genes are those responsible for DNA damage repair, including XRCC1, XPA, XPC, and XPD, which encode nucleotide excision repair proteins.[20]

Genome-wide association (GWA) studies have attempted to identify other polymorphisms that engender susceptibility or predisposition to lung cancer. Several chromosomal regions have been proposed, including 5p15.33, 6q21, and a locus on the long arm of chromosome 15, 15q24-25.[17] The 5p15.33 region encodes the gene for telomerase reverse transcriptase (TERT), which is involved in cell replication and is linked with a wide variety of cancers. In lung cancer it is associated with adenocarcinomas, including in never-smokers, but not with squamous cell carcinoma or SCLC.[20,21] 6q21 encodes a regulator of the G-protein signaling family. Never-smokers with this variant have a 4.7-fold greater risk of lung cancer than those without the haplotype.[20]

The 15q24-25 region of chromosome 15 contains the genes for several cholinergic nicotinic receptor subunits, CHRNA5, CHRNA3, and CHRNB4. Studies have shown an increased risk of lung cancer independent of smoking status associated with this variant.[20,22,23] In addition, it confers greater susceptibility to nicotine dependence.[24] Among smokers, carriers of this polymorphism smoke more and may find it harder to quit.[24]

This risk haplotype is found more frequently in people of European descent; it is less common in Asians and is not present in Africans.[22,25]

Genomic instability Tumors also exhibit acquired genetic mutations and amplifications, which require the breakdown of multiple regulatory steps and safeguards in the cellular processes of replication, repair, and apoptosis. Most of the best studied driver mutations in lung cancer involve signaling pathways within the cell. The ErbB family (EGFR/HER1, HER2, HER3, and HER4) and the c-MET gene (a proto-oncogene encoding the Hepatocyte Growth Factor Receptor [HGFR] protein) code for tyrosine kinase receptors in cell membranes; mutations or amplifications of these receptors can constitutively activate intracellular signaling cascades involved in cell division and proliferation.[17,26] Other oncogenic mutations, such as that of GTPase K-Ras, activate proteins downstream in the signaling pathways. Still other mutations, deletions, or epigenetic changes are responsible for inactivation of tumor suppressor genes p53, p16, and PTEN. Some mutations are more associated with adenocarcinomas, such as EGFR mutation, LKB1 mutation, and the EML4-ALK fusion gene.[17] Others are linked with squamous cell carcinomas, including phosphatidylinositol-3-kinase (PI3K), PTEN, focal fibroblast growth factor receptor 1 (FGFR1) amplification,[27] and discoidin domain receptor family, member 2 (DDR2) mutation.[28] Mutations in the same signaling pathway appear to be mutually exclusive, including HER2, EGFR, and K-Ras.[26]

The mechanisms of genome instability include both genetic and epigenetic changes to DNA. Genetic variation is normal and occurs constantly throughout the genome. However, changes that are positionally or functionally clustered in critical regions of the genome are associated with malignancy, including lung cancer. Single nucleotide polymorphisms (SNPs) are substitutions of one nucleotide for another in a DNA sequence, and depending on their location can cause functional changes in the gene product. Copy number alterations (CNAs) indicate either repetition or deletion of segments of DNA, which can result in multiple copies of a gene or its absence. Normally, CNAs are much more likely to occur outside gene-encoding regions. In lung-tumor tissue, CNAs tend to be gains rather than losses, are more frequent in later-stage tumors, and have an equal chance of being located within a gene sequence.[29] The formation of DNA adducts from tobacco-specific and other carcinogens that covalently bind to sections of DNA can result in miscoding and permanent mutations. Methylation is an example of an epigenetic mechanism that may cause constitutive activation or deactivation of a gene without an actual change in the encoded DNA.

Age

Lung cancer is partly a disease of senescence, with continual shortening of telomeres during repeated cell replication cycles, and greater chances of DNA damage as a factor of time.[4] Although lung cancer does manifest in persons younger than 55 years, it continues to be uncommon in that age group.[3] At present the median age at diagnosis is older than 70 years.[30] In 2006, 14% of all patients with lung cancer and 24% of all deaths attributable to lung cancer were in persons older than 80 years. The number of patients older than 85 years with lung cancer is expected to quadruple by the middle of this century,[30] at least in part because of the aging of the population in the Western world. There is decreased survival from lung cancer in the octogenarian group compared with the 70- to 79-year-old and the younger than 70-year age groups.[30,31]

Gender

Although men historically have had a much higher incidence of lung cancer than women, rates in men declined fairly dramatically in the late twentieth century in tandem with a proportional decrease in the male smoking population. Conversely, rates of lung cancer in women have been increasing since 1965, with a very modest reduction beginning only in the year 2000.[3] Cigarette smoking remains prevalent, especially in younger women.[32] In addition, nonsmoking women are more likely than men to be subject to second-hand smoke from a smoking spouse (**Figs. 1** and **2**).

Multiple large cohort studies have found no association between sex and risk of lung cancer.[32] Nonetheless, lung cancer may be a biologically different disease in women. Women are more likely to develop adenocarcinoma than squamous cell cancer; in particular, adenocarcinoma with lepidic predominant features is 2 to 4 times more common in women than in men. In addition, women with lung cancer have improved survival compared with male counterparts.[32,33]

These differences may be explained by some genetic variations between the sexes. For instance, the CYP1A1 gene has increased expression in the lungs of women smokers in comparison with men, possibly induced by estrogen. The CYP1A1 enzyme metabolizes tobacco carcinogens such as polycyclic aromatic hydrocarbons (PAHs), with the resulting products able to form DNA adducts. Other potential sex-related differences in genotype or phenotype may involve the detoxification enzyme glutathione-S-transferase M1 (GSTM1), and the X-linked gene for gastrin-releasing peptide receptor (GRPR), which stimulates bronchial epithelial cell growth.[32]

On a molecular level, tobacco-related mutations in the p53 tumor suppressor gene are more common in women than in men. EGFR, and possibly K-Ras, mutations are more common in the resected NSCLC of women.[33] DNA repair capacity has been reported to be lower in women than in men.[32] Evidence suggests that endogenous and exogenous estrogens affect lung carcinogenesis. Estrogens can activate cellular proliferation pathways through estrogen receptors

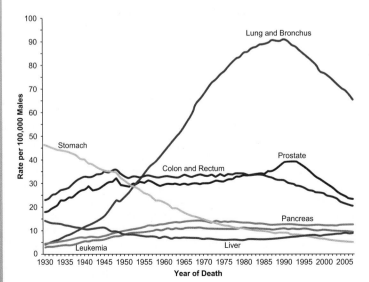

Fig. 1. Annual age-adjusted cancer death rates among males for selected cancers, United States, 1930 to 2007. Rates are age-adjusted to the 2000 US standard population. Because of changes in International Classification of Diseases (ICD) coding, numerator information has changed over time. Rates for cancers of the lung and bronchus, colon and rectum, and liver are affected by these changes. Source: US Mortality Volumes 1930 to 1959, US Mortality Data 1960 to 2007, National Center for Health Statistics, Centers for Disease Control and Prevention. (*Reprinted from* Siegel R, Ward E, Brawley O, et al. Cancer statistics, 2011. CA Cancer J Clin 2011;61:212–36; with permission.)

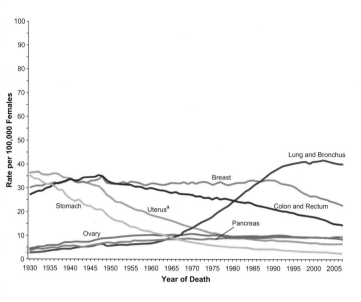

Fig. 2. Annual age-adjusted cancer death rates among females for selected cancers, United States, 1930 to 2007. Rates are age-adjusted to the 2000 US standard population. [a]Uterus indicates uterine cervix and uterine corpus. Because of changes in ICD coding, numerator information has changed over time. Rates for cancers of the uterus, ovary, lung and bronchus, and colon and rectum are affected by these changes. Source: US Mortality Volumes 1930 to 1959, US Mortality Data 1960 to 2007, National Center for Health Statistics, Centers for Disease Control and Prevention. (*Reprinted from* Siegel R, Ward E, Brawley O, et al. Cancer statistics, 2011. CA Cancer J Clin 2011;61:212–36; with permission.)

(ER), and the EGFR and ER pathways may have interactive elements.[33] Estrogen and its derivatives can also be metabolized to reactive intermediates that bind to DNA, producing adducts, or may cause oxidative damage.[32]

Race

Both incidence rates and mortality rates of lung cancer differ by racial and ethnic groups in the United States. African American men have markedly higher rates of lung cancer than non-Hispanic Caucasian white men, while both of those groups have a higher risk than do the other groups for which statistics are available: Native American, Asian American and Pacific Islander, and Hispanic. Death rates for lung cancer in African American men are 87.5 per 100,000 population, more than twice that of the lowest group, the Hispanic population, at 32.5 per 100,000 population. This figure has been linked with higher levels of smoking among African Americans.[3] For women, non-Hispanic Caucasian whites have a slightly higher rate of both incidence and mortality of lung cancer than the other groups, with African American women the next highest.

African Americans have poorer survival once diagnosed.[3] Minority populations are often diagnosed at a later stage of disease than Caucasian whites,[34] and in addition, the 5-year survival for African Americans is lower for every stage of diagnosis.[3] Education levels, socioeconomic status, medical insurance, access to health care, and receipt of good-quality health care all play roles in these inequalities. However, ethnicity was shown in a United States study to be a predictor of more advanced disease at diagnosis after controlling for insurance status, suggesting that other factors are present.[34]

Place of birth and cultural influences may also affect the risk of lung cancer within racial groups. Asians have a lower overall rate of lung cancers and have a relatively higher proportion of well-differentiated or minimally invasive adenocarcinoma, which carries a better prognosis. However, Asian men and women who are born in other countries have a 35% higher incidence of NSCLC than United States–born Asian Americans. High smoking rates among foreign-born Asian men may contribute to this difference.[35]

Behavioral Factors

Tobacco and smoking

Tobacco cigarette smoking is the predominant risk factor for lung cancer. There is a direct dose-response relationship between the number of cigarettes smoked and the risk of lung cancer.[5,36,37] Although the association had been proposed by clinicians and others in the first half of the twentieth century, it was not widely given credit. The 1950 publication of two landmark studies, in Britain[36] and the United States,[37] promoted recognition and acceptance of cigarette smoking as the cause of rising rates of lung cancer.

In retrospect, the correlation between consumption of cigarettes and rates of lung cancer is much more apparent than it likely was prospectively. Following its introduction to Europe from the New World in the sixteenth century, tobacco was used mainly in the forms of pipe-smoking, cigars, and snuff up until the late nineteenth century.[6] It was suspected by some observers that cancers of the mouth and lips were related to these practices.[6] Cigarettes were hand rolled and were smoked by relatively few people.

Several developments beginning in the 1880s dramatically changed the consumption of tobacco. A cigarette-rolling machine was patented, leading to mass production, a drop in prices, and wide availability.[38] A new method of curing tobacco, flue-curing, made the smoke smoother and more palatable.[6] Lastly, safety matches were invented, leading to increased convenience.[39] In 1880, the number of manufactured cigarettes consumed was almost zero.[6] By 1928, the consumption of so-called light cigarettes was 108 billion.[5] At present, more than 5.7 trillion cigarettes are produced annually.[40]

Composition of tobacco smoke Tobacco smoke contains some 4000 chemical substances, of which approximately 60 are known carcinogens. The most important molecules implicated in the development of lung cancer are PAHs, of which the most significant is benzo[a]pyrene (B[a]P); nitrates; and tobacco-specific *N*-nitrosamines (TSNAs), particularly 4-(methylnitrosamino)-1-(13-pyridyl-1-butanone) (NNK).[10,41] Polonium-210, an α-particle–emitting radon daughter element, is also present. Tobacco smoke has both a vapor phase, made up of molecules smaller than 0.1 μm that can pass through the cigarette filter, and a particulate phase. The concentration of free-radical production in these 2 phases is 10^{15} free radicals per gram and 10^{17} free radicals per gram, respectively.[42]

Cigarettes manufactured in the United States use a blend of different types of tobacco, including bright (flue-cured) and burley (air-cured) tobacco, with small fractions of Turkish (sun-cured) and Maryland (air-cured) tobacco. Over the last several decades there have been changes in the proportions of these constituents, as well as increased use of tobacco parts that were previously considered discard but which now make up about 30% of a cigarette.[9] These constituents include reconstituted tobacco, a homogenized tobacco sheet made from the pulp of mashed tobacco stems and sprayed with additives; expanded tobacco, made by freeze-drying saturated tobacco leaves to expand them; and the ribs and stems from tobacco plants. The filling weight of tobacco used in a cigarette has decreased from 1.2 g in the 1950s to approximately 0.7 to 0.8 mg today.[9]

These changes have significantly affected the composition of cigarette smoke. The introduction of filters has also changed the content of inhaled smoke. The amount of tar emissions from cigarette smoke has decreased from 38 mg to 12 mg. B[a]P concentration in smoke, which is linked with squamous cell lung cancer and coronary artery disease, has decreased by 62% since 1959.[9] Several other toxic elements in smoke have also lessened by about 60%.[9] However, nitrates and TSNAs have actually increased. NNK concentration in cigarettes is now 73% higher than it was in 1978.[9] Higher levels of TSNAs in cigarette smoke are associated with an increased risk of lung cancer, and NNK is implicated specifically with adenocarcinoma development in laboratory animals.[41,43] The mechanisms of tobacco carcinogenesis include free-radical damage and the formation of DNA adducts by tobacco carcinogens and their metabolites.[44]

Nicotine Nicotine levels in cigarettes blended in the United States have decreased, concomitant with other changes in the composition of cigarettes. In the 1950s, the average cigarette contained 2.7 mg of nicotine. At present, the nicotine yield is approximately 0.8 to 0.9 mg per cigarette.[9] It has been speculated that this decrease has led to changes in smoking behavior, including an increased number of cigarettes smoked, deeper inhalations, and smoking cigarettes to a shorter stump, to satisfy the smoker's programmed level of nicotine dependence.[10]

Nicotine binds to nicotinic acetylcholine receptors (NAChR) at the cell membrane, activating calcium and other ion channels. Nicotine addiction is caused by increased nicotinic receptor expression induced by long-term exposure.[42] The 15q25-26 susceptibility gene for lung cancer is positively linked to nicotine dependence.[24]

There is no evidence that nicotine itself induces tumorigenesis, but it is associated with progression of existing tumors, primarily lung, colon, and gastric cancers. Increasing data suggests a proangiogenic effect of nicotine, possibly through the activation of α7-NAChR but also by induction of proangiogenic signaling molecules including basic fibroblast growth factor, platelet-derived growth factor, and vascular endothelial growth factor.[42]

Cannabis sativa Limited evidence is available on a potential association between marijuana (*Cannabis sativa*) smoking and risk of lung cancer. Studies are difficult to undertake in many parts of the world because of legal restrictions on marijuana use. Confounding variables are also present, because tobacco use is concurrent with marijuana smoking in some users, and there is a practice of cutting hashish with tobacco in some parts of the world.[45–47] Nevertheless, several studies point to an increased risk of lung cancer among the heaviest one-third of marijuana smokers, after adjusting for confounders.[45] These patients tend to be in a younger age cohort. Several factors that may affect risk include the PAH concentration in marijuana cigarettes (twice that of tobacco), lack of a filter, and smoking habits that include deep inhalation.[45]

Socioeconomic status Studies of incidence of lung cancer relative to socioeconomic status have shown that there is an overall increased risk of lung cancer in persons of lower educational levels, lower income, and low occupational positions.[48] There is a striking correlation in the United States population between levels of educational achievement and lung cancer death rates. In men with more than 16 years of formal schooling, age-adjusted death rates for lung cancer are 10.35 per 100,000 population, whereas in men with less than a high school education, there are 51.63 deaths per 100,000 population, or 5 times the rate of the most educated group. Women with less education are 4 times more likely to die of lung cancer than the best educated.[3]

In some studies, the increased risk of lung cancer in lower socioeconomic groups has been linked with the greater prevalence of cigarette smoking in this population.[3,49] A recent British study of hardcore smokers, as defined by defensive and defiant attitudes regarding smoking, found that this group was overwhelmingly white, single, male, poor, poorly educated, and living in rented accommodation.[50] However, other studies that have focused on nonsmokers or have adjusted for smoking habits show a correlation between lower socioeconomic status and incidence of lung cancer apart from smoking.[48] Multiple factors, including occupational exposure to carcinogens, environmental tobacco smoke, suboptimal housing conditions, poor diet, and, in many parts of the world, unequal access to health care resources, likely play a part.[48,49]

Diet

The human diet contains both mutagenic and anti-mutagenic natural substances. The typical diet of the developed Western world, with processed foods containing high levels of fat and sodium, is promoting poor health in general and is estimated to be responsible for up to one-third of cancer deaths in Western countries.[51]

Macronutrients Some specific carcinogens associated with diet include heterocyclic amines (HCAs), which are produced by cooking meat and fish. Charring of protein causes particularly high levels of HCAs in the resulting crust. HCAs are broken down by the cytochrome P450s enzymes, chiefly CYP1A2. The derivatives of this process can form DNA adducts, leading to transcription changes in the genome. In rodent experiments, HCAs have produced mutations of H-Ras, K-Ras, and p53, among other cancer-linked genes. HCAs have been listed as a possible risk factor for carcinogenesis in humans by the International Agency for Research on Cancer.[52]

Excess calorie intake is also a risk factor for cancer. Elevated levels of dietary fat have been linked with breast and colon cancer in particular. Sodium chloride is associated with gastric cancer.[52,53] Saturated fatty acids from animal fat and polyunsaturated fatty acids found in some plant-derived oils (corn, safflower) have been shown to enhance cancer development in animal models. Conversely, homounsaturated fatty acids such as oleic acid in olive oil have no effect on cancer development.[52]

Micronutrients There have been contradictory data regarding vitamins as chemopreventive agents in lung cancer. The B vitamins are essential for DNA replication and repair of DNA damage. Several studies have found that folate (vitamin B_9) is associated with increased risk for lung cancer, both as a dietary supplement and in high dietary concentrations.[54,55] A more recent study, however, found no association between vitamin B supplementation and lung cancer, other than a possible weak connection of riboflavin (Vitamin B_2) with decreased risk in current smokers.[56]

Based on some early studies of vitamin A and its precursor β-carotene, which showed low levels of serum β-carotene in smokers and an increased risk for lung cancer at low serum levels, 2 large-scale studies looked at supplementation of this micronutrient.[57,58] Both showed higher than expected mortality from lung cancer in the β-carotene group, and those arms of the studies were terminated. A third study found neither harm nor benefit from β-carotene supplementation, although the dose was lower than in the other 2 trials.[59]

Preexisting lung disease Inflammatory processes are thought to play a role in lung carcinogenesis through increased genetic mutation, antiapoptotic signaling, and increased angiogenesis. Several preexisting lung conditions have been implicated to increase the risk for lung cancer. Emphysema and chronic obstructive pulmonary disease carry an elevated risk but have the confounding effect of being related to tobacco smoking. However, asthma and chronic bronchitis are associated with risk of lung cancer in nonsmokers.[60]

The presence of fibrosis in the lung parenchyma has been associated with an increased risk for lung cancer. Fibrosis includes idiopathic pulmonary fibrosis (IPF) as well as fibrosis related to systemic autoimmune diseases and to asbestos exposure. Focal scarring in the lung is also linked with the development of lung cancer at that site.[18] Several pulmonary and systemic infections are known to increase the risk for lung cancer.

Pneumonia and mycobacterial disease A history of pneumonia or of *Mycobacterium tuberculosis* infection is associated with odds ratios of developing lung cancer of 1.43 and 1.76, respectively. This ratio holds true independently of smoking status, with never-smokers having a similar increased risk.[61] It is not known whether the inflammatory processes related to infection increase the risk of tumorigenesis or whether there is a specific pathophysiology related to the disease. The increase in cancer risk is maintained over considerable latency periods following the diagnosis of infection, up to 20 years in some cases of tuberculosis.[61]

Human papillomavirus More than 50% of the world's population is infected during their lifetime with human papillomavirus (HPV). More than 100 serotypes of the virus are known; several of these (types 16, 18, 31, 33, and 35) are oncogenic, and have known causal relationships with anogenital malignancies in both sexes and with head and neck squamous cell carcinomas. Recent work has suggested a possible association of HPV with lung carcinoma, with traces of HPV DNA being found in 24.5% of lung cancers.[62] The overall association is not dependent on lung cancer cell type, although lung squamous cell cancer is reported to be more associated with the lower-risk HPV serotypes 6 and 11,[62] whereas HPV types 16 and 18 are seen in 56% of adenocarcinomas.[63] Geographic variations are present, with reported frequencies of HPV in tissue samples of lung cancer being lower in Europe (17%) and America (15%) than in Asia (35.7%–54.6%).[11,12,62,63]

The method of HPV transmission to the lungs is debated, because the historically validated mode of communication of this virus is direct mucosal contact. It is posited that HPV may pass to the oral cavity through sexual contact and from there directly into the upper aerodigestive tract and the lung. Alternatively, HPV DNA and mRNA has been found in the peripheral blood cells, plasma, and serum of patients with both cervical cancers and head and neck cancers, raising the possibility of hematogenous dissemination.[11]

The proposed mechanisms of carcinogenesis of HPV in studies thus far show a role for the E6 and E7 oncoproteins produced by the virus. E6 binds to tumor suppressor gene p53 and inactivates it, inhibiting cell apoptosis. E7 degrades the RB tumor suppressor and activates cell proliferation. The presence of HPV DNA in normal lung tissue as well as in tumor tissue raises questions about causality.[11] If a causal link between HPV and lung cancer can be proved, HPV infection will constitute the second most important risk factor for lung cancer, following tobacco smoking.[62]

Human immunodeficiency virus Lung cancer is the leading cause of death among the non–AIDS-defining malignancies (NADC) in the population infected by human immunodeficiency virus (HIV).[64,65] The incidence in this population has risen in the era of highly active antiretroviral therapy (HAART), as AIDS-defining cancers have decreased. Some studies suggest that the increased incidence is due to improved survival and the aging of the HIV-positive population.[64] A prospective study of HIV-infected women and at-risk but noninfected women found no difference in rates of lung cancer between these groups, and also no difference between the pre-HAART and post-HAART time periods.[66]

However, other work suggests that immunosuppression plays a role in the development of malignancy. HIV patients and organ-transplant patients have a similarly increased rate of cancer occurrence, 2 to 4 times that of the general population.[67] CD4 cell counts do not have a linear relationship with development of lung cancer, but may have an indirect association with cancer risk, as patients with CD4 levels higher than 500 cells/mL have incidence rates approaching those of the overall population. Declining CD4 counts increase the rate of lung cancer[68] and low CD4 counts are associated with advanced stage at diagnosis.[65,68] Viral loads have not been shown to have a correlation.[64]

The HIV-infected population has a higher prevalence of smoking than does the general population; however, this alone does not explain the increased risk. Lung cancer affects younger patients in the HIV population; in one study, the median age was 52 years.[64] The latency from diagnosis of HIV to lung cancer is shorter for women than for men.[64] A mechanism of oncogenesis has not been established for the HIV virus itself, although proteins involved in viral replication could affect the expression of genes that control the cell cycle in the host.[65]

Environmental Factors

Second-hand tobacco smoke
Environmental exposure to second-hand tobacco smoke, also known as passive or involuntary smoking, has been recognized as a major contributor to worldwide morbidity and mortality.[40,69,70] Much of the epidemiologic data regarding the risk of lung cancer from environmental tobacco smoke (ETS) has focused on nonsmokers,

especially women, who have smoking spouses, because exposure in workplaces and social settings is more difficult to quantify.[18,71] Multiple studies have shown that nonsmoking spouses of smokers have an approximately 20% to 30% increased risk of lung cancer, with remarkable agreement between almost all studies.[71,72] A dose-response relationship between lung cancer and ETS has been confirmed; there is no safe level of second-hand tobacco exposure.[70]

Side-stream smoke from the burning end of a cigarette is unfiltered and can contain increased concentrations of proven carcinogens, including PAHs, nitrosamines, and aromatic amines. B[a]P levels are up to 4 times higher in side-stream smoke than in the mainstream smoke inhaled by the active smoker.[71] Both nicotine and its metabolite cotinine, which are specific to tobacco smoking, can be detected in the body fluids of exposed nonsmokers.[71,73] Overall, lung function is affected adversely in workers exposed to tobacco smoke in the workplace.[73] DNA adducts from tobacco carcinogens have also been found in the urine of nonsmokers with second-hand exposure to ETS.[71]

There is evidence that exposure to second-hand cigarette smoke varies according to ethnicity, gender, and socioeconomic status.[70] Certain workplaces are also disproportionately affected, particularly in the entertainment and hospitality industries.[70]

Other environmental pollutants

It was suggested as early as 1927 that pollution in the ambient environment could be linked to lung cancer.[74] Acceptable levels of air pollutants began to be legislated in the 1950s, following thousands of deaths during the London "great smog" of 1952.[18] Studies showing unexpected adverse health effects at low levels of air-particulate concentrations motivated the US Environmental Protection Agency in 1997 to revise its air quality standards, imposing regulatory limits on fine particles less than 2.5 μm in diameter ($PM_{2.5}$).[75] Studies have shown a robust association between risk of lung cancer and levels of fine-particulate pollution regardless of smoking status, though strongest in nonsmokers. Each 10-μg/m^3 increase in the average long-term $PM_{2.5}$ concentration is associated with an 8% increased risk of death by lung cancer. Risk is not differentiated based on age or sex, but a higher risk is strongly linked with a lower level of education.[75] Of the gaseous pollutants from fossil-fuel combustion, sulfur dioxide is associated with increased risk of mortality from lung cancer. Other gases and coarse-particulate fractions in the atmosphere are not consistently linked

with mortality.[75] Diesel engine exhaust, however, contains known and suspected carcinogens, and occupational exposures in the trucking industry are associated with a 30% to 50% increase in the relative risk of lung cancer.[18]

Indoor air pollution from cooking-oil fumes and the burning of solid fuels such as coal are also implicated in the development of lung cancer in some parts of the world, including Asia.[12,13] Air pollution as a risk factor for lung cancer is potentiated in combination with other risk factors.

Radon

Radon (^{222}Rn) is recognized as the second leading cause of lung cancer, with approximately 10% of all deaths from lung cancer attributed to radon exposure in homes.[60] Designated a carcinogen in 1988 by the International Agency for Research on Cancer, radon is omnipresent in the earth's crust, including rocks, soil, and water.[76] An inert gas formed by the decay of uranium (^{238}Ur), radon produces radioactive polonium daughters. Both radon and its daughter elements are α-particle emitters. Most of the data involving the cancer risk of radon have been acquired through epidemiologic studies of miners, who experience significantly higher levels of radon underground compared with the average residential exposure.[60,77] In the United States, levels of occupational radon exposure in underground workplaces are governed by legislation.[18]

The amount of radon in homes is variable, influenced by factors such as the local bedrock, the type of building foundation, and ventilation of the living areas within the home. Radon leakage into buildings tends to accumulate in basements and lower levels.[78] The average environmental radon concentration is 0.2 pCi/L.[18] A 1991 survey found that the mean indoor radon level in United States homes was 1.25 pCi/L, ranging from 0.2 pCi/L to 100 pCi/L.[18]

The mechanism whereby radon initiates tumor genesis is not completely known. The α particles in radon generate free radicals and oxidative stress, which can directly damage DNA in exposed cell nuclei. There is also evidence that adjacent cells may sustain damage via a "bystander effect," even if not directly radiated.[60] The risk of lung cancer from radon is increased in combination with cigarette use.[79]

Asbestos

Asbestos is a naturally occurring silicate mineral that has been used since the late nineteenth century in construction and insulation. It is therefore ubiquitous in the environment of industrialized countries. However, prolonged and heavy exposure to asbestos, such as in occupational settings, is required to trigger nonmalignant lung and pleural disease as well as increased risk for thoracic malignancies. There is some debate about whether asbestosis is a prerequisite for the development of lung carcinoma, or whether asbestos fibers themselves act as carcinogens in the absence of fibrosis. Asbestos fibers are of 2 types: the amphibole (amosite, crocidolite, trenolite, and others) and the serpentine (chrysotile). Chrysotile fibers are most closely linked with thoracic malignancies. Exposure to both asbestos and tobacco smoking has a synergistic effect; together, they confer a 15- to 50-fold increased risk of developing carcinoma of the lung over individuals without exposure to either.[18]

Other occupational exposures

Industries and occupations that are either known or suspected to be associated with lung cancer have been listed since 1982. List A contains those occupations known to increase the risk of pulmonary tumors and includes mining and quarrying; metal production industries, including smelting and refining; asbestos production; shipbuilding; and construction. List B enumerates occupations and industries suspected to be associated with risk of lung cancer, such as meat-production industries, leather working, wood working, rubber and glass manufacture, motor vehicle production, and the transport industry.[1] A recent study in France demonstrated that men who had ever worked in a List A occupation had an odds ratio for lung cancer twice that of men who had never been employed in a list A or B occupation. Former employment in a list B occupation also conferred increased risk.[1]

> The greatest risk for developing lung cancer is cigarette smoking, by a large margin. Age, radon exposure, environmental pollution, occupational exposures, gender, race, and lung disease also are important contributors. However, not all people with these risk factors develop lung cancer, and some without any known risk factors do, which indicates the importance of genetic factors in contributing to the development of lung cancer. Future developments in understanding and treating lung cancer will be based on genetic analysis.

PREVENTION

In 2011, the National Lung Cancer Screening Trial reported that low-dose computed tomography scanning of the lungs is effective in reducing lung cancer mortality, proving that screening can affect outcomes in high-risk patients.[80] Ongoing research efforts for ways to identify early markers of disease, such as volatile organic compounds (VOCs) that are found in the breath, blood, and urine, are undergoing intensive study.[81]

Although screening for cancer to identify it in its potentially curable stages is important, total prevention should be the preferred goal. There are several ways through which the incidence of lung cancer might be reduced.

Tobacco Cessation

As tobacco use is the premier cause of lung cancers, reduction in the number of smokers is the most important step. Epidemiologic data from the twentieth and twenty-first centuries has shown a decline in male deaths from lung cancer since 1990, directly related to the decreasing proportion of male smokers.[3] However, smoking prevalence has diminished while the absolute numbers of smokers and former smokers at risk for disease has remained static in the growing population. There are an estimated 54.9 million active smokers and 50 million former smokers in the United States, similar to 1960.[32]

Smoking cessation results in reduced risk of all histologic types of cancer, but particularly in SCLC and squamous cell types. The reduction in risk is most pronounced in heavier smokers, especially women.[82] Risk of lung cancer in former smokers is decreased by 50% within the first 15 years after quitting.[83]

The Affordable Health Care Act of March 2010 contains provisions for coverage of evidence-based tobacco-cessation programs, including pharmacologic therapy and counseling, for previously uninsured persons, and also for expanding Medicare coverage for these programs; in the past coverage has been limited to those with diagnosed tobacco-related illnesses.[84]

Tobacco-Control Legislation

The World Health Organization has made the Tobacco-Free Initiative a priority. Data have shown that tobacco-control legislation such as bans on smoking in workplaces has resulted in reductions in nonmalignant diseases related to tobacco use, such as cardiovascular disease, in as little as 1 year. Bans on tobacco smoking in the workplace and social settings reduce exposure for nonsmokers and also result in less smoking by active smokers.[40,72] Despite this, only 11% of the world's population resides in areas with some form of protection from ETS.[40] This number is higher in the United States, with approximately 23 states in addition to the District of Columbia and 2 United States territories having complete protection from second-hand smoke in workplaces, restaurants, and bars. In the rest of the country, however, local laws govern the extent of the ban.[84] In fact, the seventh largest metropolitan area in the United States, with a population of more than 1.3 million people, only recently enacted a smoking ban in restaurants and bars on August 19, 2011, which remained controversial.

Vaccination

At this time there is a proposed association between HPV and lung cancer, rather than a proven causal link. Nevertheless, HPV is implicated as a causative agent in other types of cancer, and a vaccine has been developed. Since 2006, the Centers for Disease Control and Prevention (CDC) has recommended that all preteen girls of 11 to 12 years of age be routinely vaccinated and that young women from age 13 through 26 also receive vaccination for HPV to prevent genital cancers. The CDC now recommends routine vaccination of all boys 11 to 12 years of age, plus vaccination of young men 13 through 21 years if not previously completed, and vaccination of high-risk men through age 26, based on the accumulating data that HPV and HPV-related disease is widespread.[85] If future research reveals a stronger and contributory relationship between HPV and lung cancer, the vaccination program may be very helpful, and similar strategies could be used in other nations with high HPV prevalence.

Radon Control

Radon testing kits are easily available, and the US Environmental Protection Agency has advised that houses with radon levels of 4 pCi/L or above should undergo interventions to reduce the radon level in living areas. There are well-established ventilation techniques, and foundation and other home repairs may also be beneficial.

Diet

A diet of moderation rich in fruits and vegetables is recommended as the healthiest alternative. The possibility of chemoprevention of cancer by dietary strategies has been informed by the study of molecules in common food sources that have antiangiogenic properties.[51] Angiogenesis is a critical process in the transformation of indolent precursor lesions into invasive and metastatic malignancies. Antiangiogenic pharmaceutical therapy is a validated treatment of already developed tumors.

Dietary sources with antiangiogenic properties include green tea and its catechols; the isoflavonoid genistein in soybeans; resveratrol, a polyphenol found in grapes, red and rosé wine, and peanuts; lycopene in tomatoes and papayas; ω-3 fatty acids from cold-water fish; and isothiocyanates and related compounds in cruciferous vegetables. Other compounds are quercetin in leafy greens and red onions, and anthocyanins and proanthocyanidins in berries, cocoa, and cinnamon. Apples and pears contain procyanidins as well as quercetin and catechols. Menaquinone, the fat-soluble vitamin K_2, is found in fermented dairy products such as yogurt and cheese. Curcumin is a flavonoid found in turmeric spice. Mechanisms of action of these molecules differ. Many of them have been shown in epidemiologic studies and clinical trials to significantly reduce the risk of lung cancer, among other malignancies.[51]

Proper diet, therefore, constitutes an important contribution to the prevention of lung cancer and offers a widely available way, through education, to reduce the risk of cancer in the general population.

SUMMARY

As the leading cause of cancer death in the world, lung cancer is a high priority for the health care community. Many of the most significant risk factors for lung cancer are preventable. Efforts in the twenty-first century should focus not just on early detection, but on eradication.

REFERENCES

1. Guida F, Papadopoulos A, Menvielle G, et al. Risk of lung cancer and occupational history: results of a French population-based case-control study, the ICARE study. J Occup Environ Med 2011;53:1068–77.
2. World Health Organization. World cancer report, 2008. Lyon (France): World Health Organization; 2008.
3. Siegel R, Ward E, Brawley O, et al. Cancer statistics, 2011: the impact of eliminating socioeconomic and racial disparities on premature cancer deaths. CA Cancer J Clin 2011;61:212–36.
4. Fraser RG. Diagnosis of diseases of the chest. 3rd edition. Philadelphia: Saunders; 1988.
5. Hoffman FL. Cancer and smoking habits. Ann Surg 1931;93:50–67.
6. Doll R. Evolution of knowledge of the smoking epidemic. In: Boyle P, Gray N, Henningfield JE, et al, editors. Tobacco: science, policy and public health. 2nd edition. New York: Oxford University Press; 2010. p. 1–12.
7. Center GWS. 2010 Update. 2010.
8. Yang P, Cerhan JR, Vierkant RA, et al. Adenocarcinoma of the lung is strongly associated with

cigarette smoking: further evidence from a prospective study of women. Am J Epidemiol 2002;156: 1114–22.

9. Hoffmann D, Djordjevic MV, Hoffmann I. The changing cigarette. Prev Med 1997;26:427–34.

10. Hoffmann I, Hoffmann D. The changing cigarette: chemical studies and bioassays. In: Boyle P, Gray N, Henningfield JE, et al, editors. Tobacco: science, policy and public health. New York: Oxford University Press; 2010. p. 93–126.

11. Li YJ, Tsai YC, Chen YC, et al. Human papilloma virus and female lung adenocarcinoma. Semin Oncol 2009;36:542–52.

12. Torok S, Hegedus B, Laszlo V, et al. Lung cancer in never smokers. Future Oncol 2011;7:1195–211.

13. Lee YJ, Kim JH, Kim SK, et al. Lung cancer in never smokers: change of a mindset in the molecular era. Lung Cancer 2011;72:9–15.

14. Wakelee HA, Chang ET, Gomez SL, et al. Lung cancer incidence in never smokers. J Clin Oncol 2007;25:472–8.

15. Hanahan D, Weinberg RA. The hallmarks of cancer. Cell 2000;100:57–70.

16. Spitz MR, Wei Q, Dong Q, et al. Genetic susceptibility to lung cancer: the role of DNA damage and repair. Cancer Epidemiol Biomarkers Prev 2003; 12:689–98.

17. Herbst RS, Heymach JV, Lippman SM. Lung cancer. N Engl J Med 2008;359:1367–80.

18. Dela Cruz CS, Tanoue LT, Matthany RA. Lung cancer: epidemiology and carcinogenesis. In: Shields TW, editor. General thoracic surgery. 7th edition. Philadelphia: Wolters Kluwer Health/Lippincott Williams & Wilkins; 2009. p. 1281–98.

19. Matakidou A, Eisen T, Houlston RS. Systematic review of the relationship between family history and lung cancer risk. Br J Cancer 2005;93:825–33.

20. Yokota J, Shiraishi K, Kohno T. Genetic basis for susceptibility to lung cancer: recent progress and future directions. Adv Cancer Res 2010;109: 51–72.

21. Landi MT, Chatterjee N, Yu K, et al. A genome-wide association study of lung cancer identifies a region of chromosome 5p15 associated with risk for adenocarcinoma. Am J Hum Genet 2009;85:679–91.

22. Hung RJ, McKay JD, Gaborieau V, et al. A susceptibility locus for lung cancer maps to nicotinic acetylcholine receptor subunit genes on 15q25. Nature 2008;452:633–7.

23. Kohno T, Kunitoh H, Mimaki S, et al. Contribution of the TP53, OGG1, CHRNA3, and HLA-DQA1 genes to the risk for lung squamous cell carcinoma. J Thorac Oncol 2011;6:813–7.

24. Thorgeirsson TE, Geller F, Sulem P, et al. A variant associated with nicotine dependence, lung cancer and peripheral arterial disease. Nature 2008;452: 638–42.

25. Wu C, Hu Z, Yu D, et al. Genetic variants on chromosome 15q25 associated with lung cancer risk in Chinese populations. Cancer Res 2009;69: 5065–72.

26. Kristeleit H, Enting D, Lai R. Basic science of lung cancer. Eur J Cancer 2011;47(Suppl 3):S319–21.

27. Weiss J, Sos ML, Seidel D, et al. Frequent and focal FGFR1 amplification associates with therapeutically tractable FGFR1 dependency in squamous cell lung cancer. Sci Transl Med 2010;2:62ra93.

28. Hammerman PS, Sos ML, Ramos AH, et al. Mutations in the DDR2 kinase gene identify a novel therapeutic target in squamous cell lung cancer. Cancer Discov 2011;1:78–89.

29. Huang YT, Lin X, Chirieac LR, et al. Impact on disease development, genomic location and biological function of copy number alterations in non-small cell lung cancer. PLoS One 2011;6:e22961.

30. Blanchard EM, Arnaoutakis K, Hesketh PJ. Lung cancer in octogenarians. J Thorac Oncol 2010;5: 909–16.

31. Blanchard EM, Moon J, Hesketh PJ, et al. Comparison of platinum-based chemotherapy in patients older and younger than 70 years: an analysis of Southwest Oncology Group Trials 9308 and 9509. J Thorac Oncol 2010;6:115–20.

32. Patel JD. Lung cancer in women. J Clin Oncol 2005; 23:3212–8.

33. Planchard D, Loriot Y, Goubar A, et al. Differential expression of biomarkers in men and women. Semin Oncol 2009;36:553–65.

34. Halpern MT, Ward EM, Pavluck AL, et al. Association of insurance status and ethnicity with cancer stage at diagnosis for 12 cancer sites: a retrospective analysis. Lancet Oncol 2008;9:222–31.

35. Raz DJ, Gomez SL, Chang ET, et al. Epidemiology of non-small cell lung cancer in Asian Americans: incidence patterns among six subgroups by nativity. J Thorac Oncol 2008;3:1391–7.

36. Doll R, Hill AB. Smoking and carcinoma of the lung; preliminary report. Br Med J 1950;2:739–48.

37. Wynder EL, Graham EA. Tobacco smoking as a possible etiologic factor in bronchiogenic carcinoma; a study of 684 proved cases. JAMA 1950; 143:329–36.

38. Doll R. Uncovering the effects of smoking: historical perspective. Stat Methods Med Res 1998;7:87–117.

39. Thun M, Henley SJ. The great studies of smoking and disease in the twentieth century. In: Boyle P, Gray N, Henningfield JE, et al, editors. Tobacco: science, policy and public health. New York: Oxford University Press; 2010. p. 13–30.

40. World Health Organization. Report on the global tobacco epidemic, 2011: warning about the dangers of tobacco. Geneva (Switzerland): World Health Organization; 2011.

41. Hecht SS. Biochemistry, biology, and carcinogenicity of tobacco-specific N-nitrosamines. Chem Res Toxicol 1998;11:559–603.

42. Costa F, Soares R. Nicotine: a pro-angiogenic factor. Life Sci 2009;84:785–90.

43. Stepanov I, Knezevich A, Zhang L, et al. Carcinogenic tobacco-specific N-nitrosamines in US cigarettes: three decades of remarkable neglect by the tobacco industry. Tob Control 2012;21(1): 44–8.

44. Hecht SS. Tobacco carcinogenesis: mechanisms and biomarkers. In: Boyle P, Gray N, Henningfield JE, et al, editors. Tobacco: science, policy and public health. New York: Oxford University Press; 2010. p. 127–54.

45. Aldington S, Harwood M, Cox B, et al. Cannabis use and risk of lung cancer: a case-control study. Eur Respir J 2008;31:280–6.

46. Berthiller J, Straif K, Boniol M, et al. Cannabis smoking and risk of lung cancer in men: a pooled analysis of three studies in Maghreb. J Thorac Oncol 2008;3:1398–403.

47. Voirin N, Berthiller J, Benhaim-Luzon V, et al. Risk of lung cancer and past use of cannabis in Tunisia. J Thorac Oncol 2006;1:577–9.

48. Sidorchuk A, Agardh EE, Aremu O, et al. Socioeconomic differences in lung cancer incidence: a systematic review and meta-analysis. Cancer Causes Control 2009;20:459–71.

49. Dalton SO, Frederiksen BL, Jacobsen E, et al. Socioeconomic position, stage of lung cancer and time between referral and diagnosis in Denmark, 2001-2008. Br J Cancer 2011;105:1042–8.

50. Jarvis MJ, Wardle J, Waller J, et al. Prevalence of hardcore smoking in England, and associated attitudes and beliefs: cross sectional study. BMJ 2003; 326:1061.

51. Li WW, Li VW, Hutnik M, et al. Tumor angiogenesis as a target for dietary cancer prevention. J Oncol 2011; 2012:879623.

52. Sugimura T. Nutrition and dietary carcinogens. Carcinogenesis 2000;21:387–95.

53. Ames BN. Dietary carcinogens and anticarcinogens. Oxygen radicals and degenerative diseases. Science 1983;221:1256–64.

54. Roswall N. Folate and lung cancer risk. Lung Cancer 2010;67:380–1.

55. Roswall N, Olsen A, Christensen J, et al. Source-specific effects of micronutrients in lung cancer prevention. Lung Cancer 2009;67:275–81.

56. Bassett JK, Hodge AM, English DR, et al. Dietary intake of B vitamins and methionine and risk of lung cancer. Eur J Clin Nutr 2012;66(2):182–7.

57. Omenn GS, Goodman GE, Thornquist MD, et al. Effects of a combination of beta carotene and vitamin A on lung cancer and cardiovascular disease. N Engl J Med 1996;334:1150–5.

58. The effect of vitamin E and beta carotene on the incidence of lung cancer and other cancers in male smokers. The Alpha-Tocopherol, Beta Carotene Cancer Prevention Study Group. N Engl J Med 1994;330:1029–35.

59. Hennekens CH, Buring JE, Manson JE, et al. Lack of effect of long-term supplementation with beta carotene on the incidence of malignant neoplasms and cardiovascular disease. N Engl J Med 1996;334: 1145–9.

60. Alavanja MC. Biologic damage resulting from exposure to tobacco smoke and from radon: implication for preventive interventions. Oncogene 2002;21: 7365–75.

61. Brenner DR, McLaughlin JR, Hung RJ. Previous lung diseases and lung cancer risk: a systematic review and meta-analysis. PLoS One 2011;6:e17479.

62. Klein F, Amin Kotb WF, Petersen I. Incidence of human papilloma virus in lung cancer. Lung Cancer 2009;65:13–8.

63. Chen YC, Chen JH, Richard K, et al. Lung adenocarcinoma and human papillomavirus infection. Cancer 2004;101:1428–36.

64. Pakkala S, Chen Z, Rimland D, et al. Human immunodeficiency virus-associated lung cancer in the era of highly active antiretroviral therapy. Cancer 2012;118(1):164–72.

65. Pakkala S, Ramalingam SS. Lung cancer in HIV-positive patients. J Thorac Oncol 2010;5:1864–71.

66. Levine AM, Seaberg EC, Hessol NA, et al. HIV as a risk factor for lung cancer in women: data from the Women's Interagency HIV Study. J Clin Oncol 2010;28:1514–9.

67. Grulich AE, van Leeuwen MT, Falster MO, et al. Incidence of cancers in people with HIV/AIDS compared with immunosuppressed transplant recipients: a meta-analysis. Lancet 2007;370:59–67.

68. Guiguet M, Boue F, Cadranel J, et al. Effect of immunodeficiency, HIV viral load, and antiretroviral therapy on the risk of individual malignancies (FHDH-ANRS CO4): a prospective cohort study. Lancet Oncol 2009;10:1152–9.

69. Tobacco smoke and involuntary smoking. IARC Monogr Eval Carcinog Risks Hum 2004;83:1–1438.

70. United States. Public Health Service. Office of the Surgeon General. The health consequences of involuntary exposure to tobacco smoke: a report of the Surgeon General. Atlanta (GA): U.S. Dept. of Health and Human Services, Public Health Service, Office of the Surgeon General; 2006.

71. Hackshaw AK. Lung cancer and passive smoking. Stat Methods Med Res 1998;7:119–36.

72. Oberg M, Jaakkola MS, Woodward A, et al. Worldwide burden of disease from exposure to second-hand smoke: a retrospective analysis of data from 192 countries. Lancet 2011;377:139–46.

73. Lai HK, Hedley AJ, Repace J, et al. Lung function and exposure to workplace second-hand smoke during exemptions from smoking ban legislation: an exposure-response relationship based on indoor PM2.5 and urinary cotinine levels. Thorax 2011;66: 615–23.

74. Tylecote F. Cancer of the lung. Lancet 1927;2:256–7.

75. Pope CA 3rd, Burnett RT, Thun MJ, et al. Lung cancer, cardiopulmonary mortality, and long-term exposure to fine particulate air pollution. JAMA 2002;287:1132–41.

76. Radon. IARC Monogr Eval Carcinog Risks Hum 1988;43:173–259.

77. Samet JM, Pathak DR, Morgan MV, et al. Lung cancer mortality and exposure to radon progeny in a cohort of New Mexico underground uranium miners. Health Phys 1991;61:745–52.

78. Turner MC, Krewski D, Chen Y, et al. Radon and COPD mortality in the American Cancer Society Cohort. Eur Respir J 2012;39(5):1113–9.

79. A citizen's guide to radon. United States Environmental Protection Agency. Available at: http://www.epa.gov/radon/pdfs/citizensguide.pdf. Accessed November 29, 2011.

80. Aberle DR, Adams AM, Berg CD, et al. Reduced lung-cancer mortality with low-dose computed tomographic screening. N Engl J Med 2011;365: 395–409.

81. Shirasu M, Touhara K. The scent of disease: volatile organic compounds of the human body related to disease and disorder. J Biochem 2011;150:257–66.

82. Khuder SA, Mutgi AB. Effect of smoking cessation on major histologic types of lung cancer. Chest 2001;120:1577–83.

83. Mong C, Garon EB, Fuller C, et al. High prevalence of lung cancer in a surgical cohort of lung cancer patients a decade after smoking cessation. J Cardiothorac Surg 2011;6:19.

84. American Cancer Society. Cancer prevention & early detection facts & figures 2011. American Cancer Society; 2011.

85. Human Papillomavirus (HPV) - Vaccines. 2012. Available at: http://www.cdc.gov/hpv/vaccine.html. Accessed June 7, 2012.

Computed Tomography Screening for Lung Cancer

Eric J. Schmidlin, MD[a], Baskaran Sundaram, MBBS, MRCP, FRCR[a],*,
Ella A. Kazerooni, MD, MS[b]

KEYWORDS

- Lung cancer • Screening • Chest radiography • CXR • Computed tomography • CT • NLST

KEY POINTS

- Screening with low-dose computed tomography reduces mortality from lung cancer in high-risk patients.
- Lung cancer screening with chest radiography alone or in combination with sputum analysis is currently not recommended.
- The feasibility and impact of screening in patients with a low or moderate risk for primary lung cancer are currently not known.
- A standardized framework for testing and management in a multidisciplinary fashion is necessary to provide lung cancer screening.
- The National Comprehensive Cancer Network and the American Lung Association have recently issued guidelines for lung cancer screening with computed tomography in highrisk patients.

INTRODUCTION

Lung cancer is the leading cause of cancer mortality for both men and women, responsible for more deaths than prostate, breast, and colorectal cancers combined.[1] Progress has been made toward reducing mortality from these cancers, largely attributed to the existence and use of screening tests that have been demonstrated to reduce mortality. Until recently, there has not been a screening test for lung cancer that has been proven to reduce mortality. Lung cancer is, therefore, diagnosed at a localized stage in only 15% of patients, whereas more than 50% of patients are diagnosed at an advanced stage, the latter having a 5-year relative survival of approximately 5% in patients with distant disease compared with 53% for localized stage disease and greater than 70% for stage 1A lung cancers.[1] The ability to detect lung cancer at a preclinical phase would allow the discovery of disease at an earlier stage when treatment is more likely to be curative. After a series of large single-arm cohort studies demonstrated improved survival using low-dose helical computed tomography (CT), the National Lung Screening Trial (NLST) demonstrated that this technique reduces both lung cancer–specific and all-cause mortality.[2] Professional societies have been developing guidelines for lung cancer screening with CT, and many lung cancer–screening programs are slowly increasing in number across the United States, although third-party payment is still largely unavailable to most.

Disclosures: The authors have nothing to disclose.

Dr. Eric J. Schmidlin is now with the University of Mass Memorial Medical Center-University campus, 55 Lake Avenue North, Worcester, MA 01655, USA

[a] Division of Cardiothoracic Radiology, Department of Radiology, University of Michigan Health System, 1500 East Medical Center Drive, Cardiovascular Center-Room 5481, Ann Arbor, MI 48109, USA; [b] Division of Cardiothoracic Radiology, Department of Radiology, University of Michigan Health System, 1500 East Medical Center Drive, Cardiovascular Center-Room 5480, Ann Arbor, MI 48109, USA

* Corresponding author.

E-mail address: sundbask@umich.edu

Radiol Clin N Am 50 (2012) 877–894

http://dx.doi.org/10.1016/j.rcl.2012.06.008
0033-8389/12/$ – see front matter © 2012 Elsevier Inc. All rights reserved.

BACKGROUND

The US Preventative Task Force uses analytic frameworks to map out specific linkages that must be present for a screening tool or preventative measure to be considered effective in reducing morbidity or mortality of a target condition.[3] Evidence must exist to support the analytic framework (**Fig. 1**) and the linkages and the linkages that evidence must support for a screening tool to be considered effective.[3] In some instances, a single body of evidence might directly link a screening tool to an improved health outcome. If direct evidence does not exist, linkages between 2 or more bodies of evidence must indirectly demonstrate this conclusion. In the case of lung cancer screening, disease-specific mortality is the most appropriate outcome measure. Studies must not only demonstrate that a screening tool leads to early diagnosis but also that treatment at an earlier stage leads to reduced morbidity and mortality (**Figs. 2–4**). A reduction in mortality must not occur in the setting of unacceptably high rates of adverse events that might occur during diagnosis and treatment.

Both randomized and nonrandomized trials have attempted to evaluate the effectiveness of screening tools, such as low-dose helical CT for the detection of lung cancer. Most trials performed have been single-arm prospective cohort studies that have reported a stage shift, compared with non–screen-detected cancers presenting themselves clinically, and improved survival. Although less costly and less time intensive than a randomized controlled trial (RCT), these studies cannot evaluate the impact of the screening test on lung cancer–specific mortality. Survival, as opposed to mortality, is not an appropriate measure of

a screening tool because 3 biases are known to impact this measure: lead-time bias, length bias, and overdiagnosis bias.

Lead-time bias occurs as a result of a screening test moving the time of disease diagnosis earlier in the time course of that cancer, without affecting the time of death. Although affected patients will live longer with the cancer diagnosis, their life expectancy may be unchanged. Lead-time bias can be adjusted for by subtracting the lead time from the screened cases but this is often not possible because the rate of disease progression is either not known or variable. Length bias occurs when a target disease has a variable rate of progression. For example, a screening test will likely detect cancers that are less aggressive. More-aggressive cancers are likely to present clinically between screening intervals. Cancer that is detected by a screening test is, therefore, likely to grow more slowly and have a higher chance of being detected by screening and, therefore, inherently associated with better outcomes, giving the appearance of improved survival. Overdiagnosis bias occurs when a screening test detects slower-growing cancers that would have remained silent during the patients' lifetime had the screening tool not been used. The cause of death in these cases is unrelated to the detected cancer, therefore, this is often referred to as *pseudodisease*. Slowly growing cancers are more likely to contribute to overdiagnosis and, in the case of lung cancer, this could include some adenocarcinomas previously classified as bronchioalveolar carcinoma.

SCREENING WITH CHEST RADIOGRAPHY

Case-control trials, RCTs, and nonrandomized controlled and nonrandomized uncontrolled trials

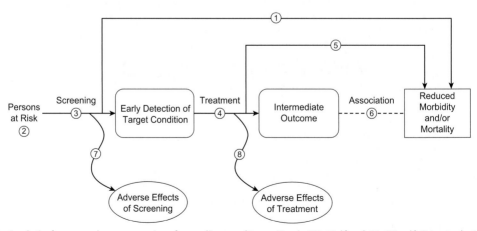

Fig. 1. Analytic framework on screening for a disease. (*From* Harris RP, Helfand M, Woolf SH, et al. Current methods of the US Preventive Services Task Force: a review of the process. Am J Prev Med 2001;20(Suppl 3):21–35; with permission.)

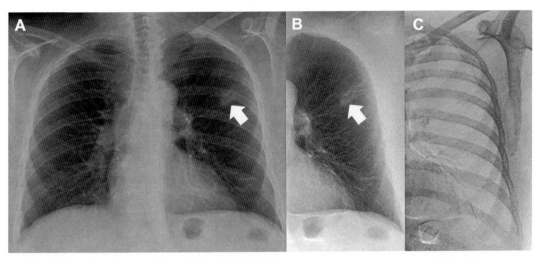

Fig. 2. A 66-year-old woman with significant smoking history underwent dual-energy chest radiography (CXR) for clinically suspected pneumonia. Traditional frontal view (*A*) and dual-energy soft tissue image (*B*) show the lung nodule (*arrows*). Bone image (*C*) shows no calcifications. On surveillance CXR, the lesion became more prominent, which warranted further evaluation with CT (see **Fig. 3**).

have evaluated the effectiveness of chest radiography (CXR) either alone or in conjunction with sputum cytology for lung cancer screening. Most of the case-controlled trials were performed in Japan. Two of the largest trails were performed in the Miyagi prefecture[4] and Okayama prefecture.[5]

The Miyagi prefecture trial[4] evaluated a mass-screening program for lung cancer since 1982 with CXR and sputum for those with 30 pack-years (pack-years = packs of cigarettes smoked per day multiplied by the number of years smoked) or more of smoking history. The study analysis was

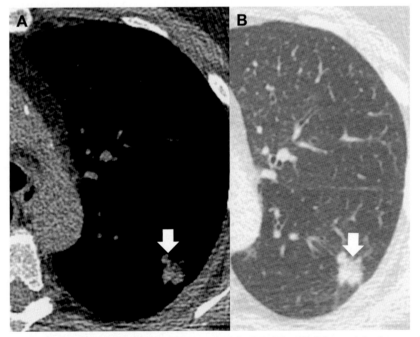

Fig. 3. Low-dose CT axial images confirm the presence of a lobulated 2-cm left lower-lobe lung nodule with no calcifications (*arrow A, B*). Based on the lesion morphology, primary bronchogenic malignancy was suspected. There were no thoracic or upper-abdominal lesions concerning for metastatic disease. This patient later underwent a fluorodeoxyglucose positron emission tomography scan (see **Fig. 4**) for preoperative evaluation.

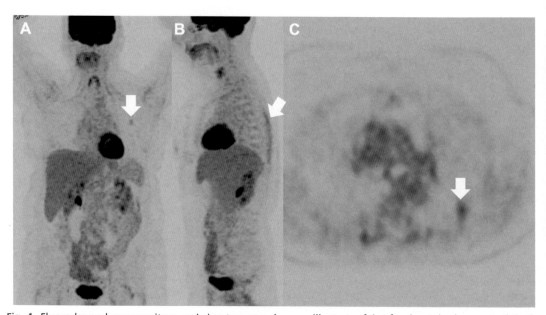

Fig. 4. Fluorodeoxyglucose positron emission tomography scan illustrates faint focal uptake (*arrow A–C*) in the left lower-lobe lesion, and there were no other suspicious avid areas. This patient underwent left lower-lobe surgical resection, and the postoperative diagnosis was stage 1A non–small cell lung carcinoma (T1N0M0).

conducted in the population that was screened in 1989 (n = 284 226). The patients (n = 328) were defined as patients who died of primary lung cancers between the ages of 40 and 79 years. The patients were compared against matched (by gender, year of birth, location, and smoking habits) controls (n = 1886). The smoking-adjusted odds ratio (OR) was 0.54, suggesting that screening was capable of reducing 46% of the risk of death from lung cancer. The Okayama prefecture trial[5] offered screening for the general public who had national health insurance and were living in 34 municipalities of the Okayama prefecture between 1991 and 1996 (n = 247 537). The CXR examinations for all participants and sputum cytology for high-risk participants were offered annually. The patients (n = 412) were participants aged between 40 and 79 years who died of lung cancer during the study period. Randomly selected controls (n = 3490) were matched by age, gender, and living location. Smoking-adjusted OR of death from lung cancer for screened versus unscreened individuals within a year before diagnosis was 0.59, suggesting that screening contributes to reducing lung cancer mortality by 41%. There were also OR differences between men (0.67) and women (0.39). Although support emerged from these case-controlled trials for lung cancer screening with CXR, generally case-control study results are considered inferior to RCT results.

The Mayo Lung Project was an RCT on 10 933 patients conducted from 1971 to 1983 that was designed to determine if frequent CXR with sputum cytology was an effective screening strategy for lung cancer.[6] Male patients (45 years of age or older) who had smoked at least one pack of cigarettes per day in the last year formed the study population. Patients were divided into 2 groups: one receiving CXR and sputum cytology every 4 months and the other annually. Each group was screened for 6 years with subsequent 1- to 5-year follow-ups. A stage shift was demonstrated with more frequent screening, with 91 prevalence cancers found of which 49 (54%) underwent curative resection, a significantly higher proportion than the 15% of lung cancer cases diagnosed clinically at the Mayo Clinic population over the same time frame. The group screened every 4 months had cancers more frequently diagnosed at stage I or II (48% vs 32%), which were more likely to be resectable at the time of diagnosis (46% vs 32%) and had a better 5-year survival (33% vs 15%) than the group screened annually. Ninety-four out of the 206 (46%) lung cancers diagnosed in the group screened more frequently underwent curative resection compared with only 51 out of 160 (32%) cancers in the group screened annually. Despite these differences, the mortality rates in both groups were similar at the 20-year follow-up. The lack of statistical power left open the possibility that a small reduction could have been missed with a larger sample size.

The Memorial Sloan-Kettering lung cancer screening program conducted from 1974 to 1982 compared annual CXR with or without sputum cytology every 4 months in 10 040 men older than 45 years who were current or recent smokers of at least one pack of cigarettes per day.[7] The screening time period varied between 5–8 years. A total of 53 prevalence lung cancers were detected: 23 in the CXR-only group and 30 in the sputum cytology group. A total of 235 incidence lung cancers were detected: 121 in the CXR-only group and 114 in the sputum cytology–screened group. In addition, there were 100 interval lung cancers detected either by symptoms or a non-screening radiograph, 81 of which were stage II to III at diagnosis. Cytology alone only detected 9 out of the 30 prevalence cancers and 18 out of the 114 incidence cancers, most of which were of squamous cell histology. It was thought that the cancers detected by sputum cytology alone were slow growing and would have eventually been identified on a future screening CXR without having an impact on disease-specific mortality. Based on the technology and analysis of sputum at that time, they concluded that sputum cytology did not warrant use in lung cancer screening. Of the prevalence cancers detected, 14 out of 30 (47%) were stage I in the sputum-screened group compared with 8 out of 23 (35%) in the CXR-only group. Of the incidence cancers, 45 out of 114 (39%) were discovered at stage I in the sputum-screened group compared with 50 out of 121 (41%) in the CXR-only group. Although the 5-year survival from lung cancer (35%) in both study groups was better than the general population of clinically diagnosed lung cancers at the time (10%), this study was not designed to demonstrate a reduction in mortality.

The Johns Hopkins Lung Project had a similar design to the Memorial Sloan-Kettering study.[8] It too evaluated whether the addition of sputum cytology to annual CXR reduced lung cancer mortality. A total of 10 387 men who were either current or recent smokers using at least one pack of cigarettes per day were enrolled from 1972 to 1983 and randomly assigned to either sputum cytology every 4 months with annual CXR or annual CXR alone. Each group was screened for 5 to 7 years. A total of 79 prevalence lung cancers were detected (40 in the CXR-only group and 39 in the dual screen group), and 396 incidence lung cancers were detected (202 in the CXR-only group and 194 in the dual screen group). Of the incidence cancers, 194 were interval cancers detected by either symptoms or a non-screening radiograph. Cytology alone detected 11 out of the 39 prevalence cancers and 22 out of the 194 incidence cancers. Nearly all of the cancers detected by cytology alone were of squamous cell histology and thought to be slowly growing tumors. There was no survival benefit with the addition of sputum cytology to annual CXR. Fifty-seven percent of the cancers detected by either screening examination were diagnosed at stage I compared with only 17% of the interval cancers. Although this study demonstrated a survival benefit in both study groups compared with the general population, this study was not designed to demonstrate a reduction in mortality.

Lastly, the RCT conducted in Czechoslovakia from 1976 to 1983 enrolled 6364 men aged 40 to 64 years who had consumed greater than 150 000 cigarettes each.[9] Patients received either CXR and sputum cytology at the initial presentation and then every 6 months for 3 years or underwent baseline CXR and sputum cytology at enrollment and again only once 3 years later. Incidence cancers in the frequently screened group were earlier in stage (53% vs 21%) and associated with improved 5-year survival (23% vs 0%). Additional data were collected on patients in both groups for up to 6 years and were followed with annual CXR. This study also demonstrated no difference in lung cancer mortality between the two groups. As in the Mayo Lung Project, the lack of statistical power left open the possibility that a small reduction in mortality may have been missed because of the sample size.

Although none of these RCTs demonstrated improved mortality from lung cancer screening with CXR or sputum cytology, CXR could not be completely dismissed as a screening tool because these studies were either not designed to evaluate mortality or lacked sufficient statistical power. As a result, the lung component of the Prostate, Lung, Colorectal, and Ovarian Cancer Screening Trial was initiated to assess the effectiveness of CXR as a screening tool for lung cancer and was designed to answer this question with sufficient statistical power, enrolling 154 901 men and women aged 55 to 74 years from 1993 to 2001 at 10 screening centers across the United States.[10] Participants were assigned either to an intervention group screened with CXR at enrollment and then annually for 3 years or the control group that received usual care. The selection of participants was not based on smoking history because the study also included arms evaluating screening tools for other malignancies. Approximately 45% were never smokers, 42% were former smokers, and 10% were current smokers. Approximately 24 000 enrolled patients were considered at high risk for lung cancer using criteria defined by the NLST as individuals aged 55 to 74 years with a 30-or-more pack-year history of smoking who were either current smokers or former smokers who had stopped smoking within the previous 15 years. The overall adherence rate to screening was 84%. The cumulative lung cancer incidence was similar in both groups. Although lung cancers detected in the intervention group were slightly more likely to be stage I (32% vs 27%), only 20% of lung cancers in this group were detected by screening. During the 13-year follow-up period, 1213 lung cancer deaths occurred in the intervention group compared with 1230 in the usual-care group, with resulting mortality rates of 14.0 and 14.2 per 10 000 person-years, respectively. The study concluded that there was no statistically significant reduction in lung cancer mortality using annual CXR, whether using the entire patient cohort or only patients that would have met NLST entry criteria, finally putting to rest the role of CXR in lung cancer screening (**Figs. 5** and **6**).

LUNG CANCER SCREENING WITH CT

The greater sensitivity of CT over CXR to detect small pulmonary nodules renewed interest in the ability of this diagnostic tool to effectively screen for lung cancer. Numerous prospective single-arm cohort trials were performed during the past 2 decades, all demonstrating a stage shift to lower-stage cancers and improved survival and suffering from the bias of having survival as an outcome measure. None are designed to demonstrate a mortality reduction because of the lack of a control arm. A few of these studies are described here, and the relevant details of many of these trials are tabulated in this article (**Tables 1** and **2**).

The first of these trials was performed in Japan.[11,12] The Hitachi Health Care Center began screening 50- to 69-year-old current or former employees and their spouses in 1998, most of whom were current or former smokers with an average age of 57 years.[12] Patients with 1 or more 8- to 10-mm noncalcified pulmonary nodules underwent standard-dose CTs 1, 3, and

6 months later to demonstrate a lack of growth; when growth was demonstrated, sampling of the lesion was recommended. If there was no growth, patients were returned to annual CT screening. Patients with nodules 5- to 7-mm in size continued annual screening CT with no additional intervention. CT examinations were performed at 10-mm slice thickness, which reduces the detectability of smaller lung nodules, particularly those less than 5 mm in size. In a similar program, Hitachi Medical Center began screening patients aged 50 years or older with low-dose CT in 2001[11] (average age 64 years). For patients with 1 or more nodules 5- to 10-mm in size, standard-dose CTs were performed at 1, 3, and 6 months; if there was no growth, they were returned to annual screening. If growth was demonstrated, further evaluation with confirmatory tests was recommended. Nodules greater than 10 mm were sampled at both centers. A total of 25 385 patients underwent baseline screening at both sites, detecting 169 prevalence cancers (mean diameter 18 mm), 154 of which were stage I. A total of 36 529 subsequent annual screening examinations were performed, resulting in the discovery of 41 incidence cancers (mean diameter 14 mm), 37 of which were stage I. All but 7 cancers were treated with surgical resection. Seventy percent of patients were followed for a minimum of 5 years (average 5.7 years), with follow-up continued until February 2011. Of the 210 patients diagnosed with lung cancer, 19 deaths were attributed to that cancer. The estimated 5-year survival was 90% for all patients with lung cancer and 97% for patients with stage IA cancers. There was no significant difference in survival among patients with lung cancer diagnosed at baseline or during subsequent annual CT screening. The study concluded that lung cancers detected by CT had a good prognosis but that the impact of screening for lung cancer on mortality at the community level needed to be determined.

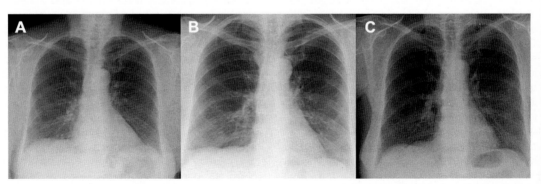

Fig. 5. A 73-year-old NLST participant with screen negative at baseline (*A*), year 1 (*B*), and year 2 (*C*) single-view CXRs. At year 2, this patient also underwent a noncontrast chest CT for chronic nonproductive cough (see **Fig. 6**).

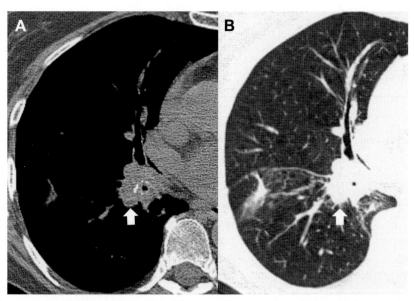

Fig. 6. Soft tissue window (*A*) and lung window (*B*) images illustrate the right lower-lobe speculated lung lesion (*arrows*) suspicious for primary lung malignancy. Pathologic conditions from bronchoscopic tissue sampling confirmed squamous cell carcinoma. Fluorodeoxyglucose positron emission tomography scan also had focal avidity in this lesion, and there were no other suspicious avid areas. This patient refused surgery and underwent definitive external beam radiation therapy.

Early Lung Cancer Action Project Study

The first US single-arm prospective cohort study was the Early Lung Cancer Action Project (ELCAP).[13] This study screened 1000 volunteers aged 60 years or older (54% men, 91% whites, median age 67 years) with a 10–pack-year or more smoking history who underwent both 2-view CXR and low-dose chest CT (140 kVp, 40 mA, 2/1 pitch, 10-mm collimation, 5-mm image reconstruction overlap) at enrollment. A positive CT screen was defined as 1 to 6 noncalcified or indeterminate nodules. Patients with a positive screen 5 to 10 mm in size subsequently underwent a standard-dose CT at 1, 3, 6, 12, and 24 months to confirm lack of growth, returning to annual screening if the nodules resolved; nodules greater than 10 mm underwent tissue sampling, and patients with nodules less than 5 mm returned to annual low-dose screening.

The first publication of baseline incidence screens demonstrated that CT examinations were positive slightly more than 3 times than CXRs were positive (23% vs 7%; 95% confidence interval [CI] 21–26), malignancy was detected 4 times more frequently with CT (2.7% vs 0.7%; CI 1.8–3.8 and 0.3–1.3, respectively), and 6 times more stage I cancers were detected with CT (2.3% vs 0.4%; CI 1.5–3.3 and 0.1–0.9, respectively). Overall, 233 participants had a baseline positive CT of which 27 (12%) were lung cancer: 23 out of 27 were stage 1 (85%) and 20 out of 27 (74%) were not detected by CXR. Of the 23 cancers measuring less than 20 mm, all were detected by CT and only 4 by CXR. The study concluded that screening with low-dose CT resulted in lung cancers diagnosed at an earlier stage and with a higher than the cure rate than symptom-detected lung cancers. Although the data from this study were limited because of the small sample size and lack of a control arm, it was a catalyst for the many more studies that followed (refer to **Tables 1** and **2**).

The ELCAP, later extended as New York-Early Lung Cancer Project, subsequently reporting on 6295 screened patients (51.2% were women, 87.1% were white, median age was 66 years, median smoking history was 40 pack-years) enrolled between 2000 and 2003.[14] The primary differences from the initial report were caused by advances in technology, including the use of multidetector CT scanners resulting in thinner slices (1.25 mm compared with the earlier 10.0 mm) and workstation-based interpretation instead of film based. A total of 5134 and 880 participants received a subsequent 1- and 2-year annual CT screen, respectively. Screening examinations were considered negative, positive (solid/part-solid nodules ≥5 mm or nonsolid nodules ≥8 mm), or semipositive (solid/part-solid ≤5 mm or nonsolid nodules <8 mm). The recommended management also varied from the initial report. Patients with

Table 1
Summary of single-arm prospective screening studies for lung cancer using CT

Principal Author/ Study Name	Time Frame	Interval Between Screens (mo)	Enrollees	Age (y)	mA	kVp	Pitch	Collimation
ELCAP[13]	1993–1998	6–18	1000	≥60	140	40	2.0	10.0
Sobue et al[37]	1993–1998	6	1611	40–79	120	50	2.0	10.0
Kaneko et al[38]	1993–1998	12	1669	≈63	120	50	2.0	10.0
Sone et al[39]	1996–1999	12	5483	≈64	120	50/20	2.0	10.0
Bach et al[17]	1998–2002	12	3246	≈60	NR	NR	NR	NR
Chong et al[40]	1999–2003	6, 12	6406	46–85	120	50	NR	NR
Swensen et al[16]	1999–2003	12	1520	≥50	120	40	1.5	5.0
Gohagan et al[41]	2000	12	1660	55–74	40–120	60	2.0	5.0
Pastorino et al[42]	2001–2002	24	1035	50–84	140	40	2.0	10.0
Novello et al[43]	2001	12	520	≈59	120	33	1.5	8.8
Garg et al[a,44]	2001	3, 6, 12, 24	92	≈66	NR	200	2.0	5.0
Picozzi et al[45]	200–2003	3, 6, 9, 12	60	57–78	120–140	20–43	2.0	10.0
Stephenson et al[46]	NR	N/A	87	47–88	140	40	NR	10.0
Macredmond et al[47]	NR	12	449	50–74	NR	50	2.0	10.0
Bastarrika et al[48]	NR	12	911	≈55	120–140	43/20	1.5	8.0
Diederich et al[49]	NR	12	817	40–78	120	50	NR	5.0
NY-ELCAP[14]	2000–2003	12	6295	≥60	120	40	1.5/2.0	1.25/10.0
I-ELCAP[15]	1993–2005	7–18	31 567	40–85	120	40	1.5	1.25
Nawa et al[a,11]	1998–2006	12	25 385	≈60	120	50	2.0	10.0
Wilson et al[50]	2002–2006	12	3642	50–79	140	40–60	NR	2.5
Fukijawa et al[51]	2001–2007	24	2550	50–87	120	50	NR	10.0
Menezes et al[52]	2003–2007	12	3352	50–80	120	40–60	NR	1.0–1.25
Veronesi et al[53]	2004–2006	12	5201	≥50	140	30	1.75	2.5

Abbreviations: ELCAP, Early Lung Cancer Action Project; I-ELCAP, International-Early Lung Cancer Action Project; NR, Not Reported; NY-ELCAP, New York-Early Lung Cancer Action Project.
    [a] Nawa: CT parameters were those used at Hitachi Health Care Center.

nodules less than 5 mm returned to annual screening, whereas those with nodules 5 to 14 mm underwent either follow-up CT in 3 months or an immediate fluorodeoxyglucose positron emission tomography (FDG-PET) scan, with growth on CT or FDG-PET uptake proceeding with a recommendation for tissue sampling. For nodules 15 mm or larger, immediate sampling, PET scan, or a 1-month follow-up CT after 2 weeks of antibiotics were recommended; nodules with negative PET scan, a negative sampling result, or decreasing size were followed with a 12-month CT scan.

Positive and semipositive test results were found in 906 (14.4%) and 1722 (27.0%) patients, respectively. A total of 502 patients with positive test results (55%) and 1453 (84.4%) patients with semipositive test results underwent additional workup before their next annual screening, including 134

biopsy recommendations, 110 of which were performed, revealing 101 primary lung cancers. In subsequent annual screening CT cycles, positive test results were found in 361 participants (6%) and 151 of them (41.8%) underwent additional workup before their next annual repeat screening. Of the 31 biopsy recommendations, 24 were performed, revealing 22 lung cancers.

Of the prevalence cancers, the average diameter was 14 mm, all but 2 were resectable, and 81 out of 121 cancers were stage I. Of the incidence cancers, the average size was 8 mm and 3 had evidence of lymph node metastasis at diagnosis, all of which were of small cell histology. The 10-year survival was estimated to be 80% regardless of stage and 92% for those diagnosed with stage I disease. The study concluded that screening with low-dose CT detected lung cancer

Table 2
Summary of single-arm prospective screening studies for lung cancer using CT

Principal Author/ Study Name	Baseline Screening Examinations	Incidence Screening Examinations	Positive Studies or Patients with Nodules (Prevalence/Incidence)	Prevalence Cancers	Incidence Cancers	Mean Size (mm)	Stage I (%)
ELCAP[13]	1000	2184	233/30	27	7	14	85
Sobue et al[37]	1611	7891	186/721	8	16	16	88
Kaneko et al[38]	1669	9993	NR	24 (total)	24 (total)	12	78
Sone et al[39]	5483	8303	279/309	23	37	13	100
Bach et al[17]	3246	NR	NR	144 (total)	144 (total)	NR	67
Chong et al[40]	6406	10,932	NR	11	12	NR	NR
Swensen et al[16]	1520	5541	782/336	31	30	16	74
Gohagan et al[41]	1586	1398	325/228	30	8	NR	53
Pastorino et al[42]	1035	996	199/99	11	11	18	55
Novello et al[43]	519	NR	241	5	6	NR	NR
Garg et al[44]	92	N/A	30	2	NR	NR	100
Picozzi et al[45]	60	87	20/13	1	2	NR	NR
Stephenson et al[46]	87	N/A	12	4	N/A	NR	75
Macredmond et al[47]	449	922	105/6	2	3	NR	NR
Bastarrika et al[48]	911	424	440	11	2	NR	100
Diederich et al[49]	817	1735	378/89	11	10	17	70
NY-ELCAP[14]	6295	6014	906/361	101	20	13	88
I-ELCAP[15]	31 567	27 456	27 381/4186	405	74	12	85
Nawa et al[11]	25 385	36 529	NR	169	41	17	91
Wilson et al[50]	3642	3423	1477/256	53	27	NR	58
Fukijawa et al[51]	2550	755	337	15	0	14	100
Menezes et al[52]	3352	3572	600/351	56	6	20	82
Veronesi et al[53]	5201	4821	2754/2198	55	37	15	66

Abbreviations: ELCAP, Early Lung Cancer Action Project; I-ELCAP, International-Early Lung Cancer Action Project; NR, Not Reported; NY-ELCAP, New York-Early Lung Cancer Action Project.

at an early stage when it is more likely to be cured, resulting in improved patient survival.

International-Early Lung Cancer Project

The International-Early Lung Cancer Project was a conducted from 1993 to 2005 at multiple institutions across multiple countries.[15] A total of 31 567 participants aged 40 to 85 years received baseline screening with and subsequent annual screening low-dose CT examinations, with 27 456 annual CT screens performed anywhere from 7 to 18 months following the baseline CT. The study was different from many other prospective single-arm cohort studies in that it included other patients at risk for lung cancer, including exposure to asbestos, beryllium, uranium, radon, and second-hand smoke. The median number of pack-years was 30. A positive CT screen was defined as a solid nodule greater than 5 mm, a nonsolid nodule greater than 8 mm, or an endobronchial nodule. Recommendations for the management of positive studies were similar to the ELCAP study, but the management was left up to each individual and the referring clinicians. There were 4186 positive prevalence screens and 1460 incidence screens. A total of 535 biopsies were performed, resulting in a diagnosis of lung cancer in 479 patients and metastasis or lymphoma in an additional 13. There were 405 prevalence lung cancers detected at baseline, 74 incidence cancers detected on follow-up screening, and 5 interval cancers detected between screenings. Of the 484 cancers, 412 (85%) were stage I; the average diameter was 13 mm for prevalence cancers and 9 mm for incidence cancers. Three hundred two of the patients with clinical stage I disease underwent surgical resection within 1 month of diagnosis, with a 5-year survival rate of 92%. The estimated 10-year survival of all patients with lung cancer was 80% and 88% for those with clinical stage I disease. As of 2006, 75 (16%) patients had died of lung cancer. Lung cancer detection rates were 1.3% for baseline screening and 0.3% on subsequent annual screening. This study again demonstrated that screening with low-dose CT detects lung cancer at an earlier stage when curative surgery can be offered.

Mayo Clinic Trial

In 1999, 1520 men and women with an average age of 59 years and with a smoking history of at least 20 pack-years were enrolled in the Mayo Clinic screening using annual low-dose CT and sputum cytology at baseline and then annually for 4 years.[16] Recommendations for follow-up of nodules were as follows: for nodules smaller than 4 mm, a CT was performed in 6 months; for nodules 4 to 8 mm, a CT was performed at 3 months; and for 8- to 20-mm nodules, a CT was performed as soon as possible and consideration was given to a contrast-enhanced CT or PET scan. For nodules larger than 20 mm, a biopsy was performed. Compliance rates for each subsequent annual screening was 98%, 96%, 95%, and 80%, respectively. A total of 1118 (74%) participants had noncalcified nodules detected at least once during the screening process, of which 61% were smaller than 4 mm, 37% were 4 to 7 mm, 8% were 8 to 20 mm, and less than 1% were larger than 20 mm. A total of 1646 nodules were identified on the baseline CT and 847 new nodules were identified on subsequent annual screens. The rate of false-positive studies was 92% to 96%. Thirteen participants underwent 15 surgeries for benign disease, none of which experienced mortality from surgery. Sixty-eight cancers were detected in 66 participants, including 31 prevalence cancers, 34 incidence cancers, and 3 interval cancers. The average size of both prevalence and incidence cancers together was 14 mm, and the most common histology was adenocarcinoma followed by squamous cell carcinoma. Only 17 incidence cancers were stage I, failing to demonstrate a significant stage shift unlike earlier screening trials. There were 9 deaths from lung cancer (1.6 per 1000 person-years).

Lung cancer mortality rates in men aged older than 50 years were similar in this CT study (2.8) and the Mayo Lung Project (2.0), which evaluated CXR as a lung cancer–screening tool.[6,16] A comparison of stage distribution between the two studies failed to show a significant difference in the rates of non–small cell lung cancer diagnosed at stage I or in the number of cancers diagnosed at an advanced stage. The investigators concluded that, although CT allows for the detection of many cancers at an early stage, this might be attributed to overdiagnosis bias rather than a true stage shift given the high number of adenocarcinomas (74% of prevalence cancers and 37% of incidence cancers), many of which were of bronchioalveolar histology. If a true stage shift had occurred, the number of advanced-stage cancers that were diagnosed would have been expected to decrease. The rates of diagnosis of advanced disease were not significantly different in this study (33%) than the Mayo Lung CXR Project (45%). However, the lack of statistical power in this study prohibited any definitive conclusion from being reached.[6,16]

BACH Study

This study to assess the impact of lung cancer screening on patient outcomes was conducted at 3 centers: Istituto Tumoris in Milan, Italy, the Mayo Clinic, and the Moffitt Cancer Center.[17] Noncalcified nodules were managed using a protocol similar to the Mayo Clinic CT screening study.[16] Lung cancer events were compared with prediction models developed to estimate an individual's risk of being diagnosed with or dying of lung cancer. A total of 3246 current or former smokers with average smoking histories of approximately 40 pack-years and a mean age of 60 years were enrolled. All patients were offered a low-dose CT scan at enrollment and annually for 3 years at the Mayo Clinic and the Istituto Tumoris and for 4 years at the Moffitt Cancer Center. Patients were followed an average of 3.7 years. One hundred forty-four lung cancers were diagnosed at a rate of 13.9 per 1000 person-years, a much higher frequency than the 4 per 1000 person-years predicted without screening. Stage I or II cancers were diagnosed in 96 patients, 12 of which resulted in death during the study. Death from lung cancer diagnosed at any stage occurred in 38 patients (3.5 per 1000 person-years), similar to that demonstrated in studies using CXR as a screening tool. Twenty participants who died of lung cancer during the study were either not diagnosed (6), diagnosed with advanced-stage disease (13), or had small cell lung cancer (7). The investigators concluded that early detection with CT screening did not seem to reduce the rate of lung cancer diagnoses at an advanced stage and it did not seem to reduce the risk of death from lung cancer. They concluded that the increased frequency of lung cancer diagnoses was likely attributed to overdiagnosis and that screening with CT failed to detect early stage cancers that were likely to progress and eventually cause death. The study was limited because of the small number of study participants and a short follow-up period. Lung cancers were confirmed after 649 positive CT scans (3.6%) and 279 positive CXR examinations (5.5%).

NLST

Given the conflicting results of single-arm cohort studies and the inability of that study design to demonstrate a mortality reduction, the US National Cancer Institute funded NLST, a multicenter randomized trial initiated in 2002.[2] The primary endpoint of NLST was lung cancer mortality. The NLST enrolled 53 454 current or former heavy smokers, aged 55 to 74 years, at 33 US medical centers (Refer to **Box 1** for enrollment criteria). Patients were randomized to receive either low-dose chest CT (refer to **Table 3** for scan parameters) or single frontal-view CXR annually for 3

> **Box 1**
> **NLST study enrollment criteria**
>
> *Inclusion*
> - 55 to 74 years of age
> - Current smokers (at least 30 pack-years)
> - Former smokers (at least 30 pack-years, quit within the prior 15 years)
>
> *Exclusion*
> - Prior diagnosis of cancer
> - Chest CT within 18 months before enrollment
> - Hemoptysis
> - Unexplained weight loss of greater than 6.8 kg (15 lb) in the preceding year
>
> *Data from* Aberle DR, Adams AM, Berg CD, et al. Reduced lung-cancer mortality with low-dose computed tomographic screening. N Engl J Med 2011;365(5):395–409.

years. Some centers collected biologic blood, sputum, and urine specimens that were placed in a biorepository for future analysis. All centers collected data for cost-effectiveness, quality of life, and smoking cessation. Low-dose CT scans were all acquired on multidetector scanners of 4 detectors or more, with an average effective dose of approximately 1.5 mSv.[18] Screening compliance was 95% for the CT group and 93% for

Table 3
NLST low-dose CT acquisition parameters

Patient positioning	Supine with arms elevated above head
Inspiration	Suspended maximal
Voltage	120–140 kVp
Tube current—time current (mAs)	40–80 (dependent on participant body habitus)
Pitch	1.25–2.0
Detector collimation	≤2.5 mm
Nominal reconstructed section width	1.0–3.2 mm
Reconstruction interval	1.0–2.5 mm
Reconstruction algorithm	Soft tissue or thin section
Scan time	≤24 s

Data from Aberle DR, Adams AM, Berg CD, et al. Reduced lung-cancer mortality with low-dose computed tomographic screening. N Engl J Med 2011;365(5):395–409.

CXR group. From the time of enrollment, 144 103 person-years (total number of years that each member was present in the study) in the low-dose CT group and 143 368 person-years in the CXR group were accrued.

A positive CT screen was defined as a noncalcified lung nodule at least 4 mm in diameter. Thirty-nine percent of the CT group and 16% of the CXR group had a positive screen at least once over 3 annual screens. Twenty-seven percent of the positive CT screens occurred at baseline CT, 28% at year 1, and 17% at year 2. Nine percent of the positive CXR screens occurred at enrollment, 5% at year 1, and 4% at year 2. Lung cancers were confirmed after 649 positive CT scans (3.6%) and 279 positive CXR examinations (5.5%). Following a positive test, patients underwent further workup based on local practice, with general study recommendations for guidance. The subsequent testing in each is tabulated in **Table 4**.

Among the 649 patients with CT screen–detected cancer, major complications from the diagnostic evaluation occurred in 11.6% (n = 75), intermediate complications in 14.6% (n = 95), and minor complications in 2.2% (n = 14), with 10 deaths occurring within 2 months of the evaluations. Among the 279 patients with CXR screen–detected cancer, major complications from the diagnostic evaluation occurred in 8.6% (n = 24), intermediate complications in 12.5% (n = 35), and minor complications in 2.2% (n = 6), with 3.9% (n = 11) of the deaths occurring within 2 months of the evaluations.

More than one-third of the screen-detected cancers were in the bronchoalveolar cell carcinoma–adenocarcinoma malignancy spectrum. Half of the screen-detected cancers in the CT arm

were stage 1, whereas only less than one-third were stage 1 in the CXR arm. As expected, early stage tumors were detected more often in the CT arm, and late-stage tumors were detected more often in the CXR arm. An inoperability decision based on staging alone (stage 3b or higher) would have rendered approximately one-third of the CT-detected cancers and nearly half of the CXR-detected cancers unresectable (**Tables 5** and **6**).

There were 356 deaths (247 per 100 000 person-years) from lung cancer in the CT group compared with 443 (309 per 100 000 person-years) in the CXR group, a 20% relative reduction in lung cancer–specific mortality in the CT group. In addition, there was a 6.7% reduction in all-cause mortality in the CT group. Several additional analyses are underway, the most significant of which is the cost-effectiveness analysis, a critical element in discussions of public health policy around the use of CT for screening. NLST is the first study to demonstrate a reduction in lung cancer–specific mortality using low-dose CT. It is unlikely that overdiagnosis bias plays a significant role because only 95 of the 646 cancers detected by screening in the CT group and 13 of the 276 cancers detected by screening with CXR were of the slowly growing bronchioalveolar histology, representing 20% of all stage IA cancers in the CT group and 9% of all stage IA cancers in CXR group.

European RCTs

Several studies are underway and have reported some initial results. Individually, none are large

Table 4
NLST: follow-up

Follow-up Methods	CT Arm	CXR Arm
Any diagnostic follow-up N (%)	17 702 (72.1)	4953 (85.0)
Clinical procedure (%)	58.9	56.4
Imaging FU (%)	57.9	78.4
Percutaneous biopsy (%)	1.8	3.5
Bronchoscopy (%)	3.8	4.5
Surgery (%)	4.0	4.8
Other procedures (%)	1.8	2.5

Abbreviation: FU, Follow-up.
   Data from Aberle DR, Adams AM, Berg CD, et al. Reduced lung-cancer mortality with low-dose computed tomographic screening. N Engl J Med 2011;365(5):395–409.

Table 5
Histology of screen-detected cancers in NLST by trial arms

Cancer Types	CT Arm (N = 1060) (%)	CXR Arm (N = 941) (%)
BAC	10.5	3.8
Adenocarcinoma	36.3	35.2
Squamous-cell carcinoma	23.2	22.1
Large-cell carcinoma	3.9	4.6
Non–small cell carcinoma/others	12.5	17.0
Small cell carcinoma	13.1	17.1
Carcinoid	0.6	0.2

Abbreviation: BAC, Bronchoalveolar carcinoma.
   Data from Aberle DR, Adams AM, Berg CD, et al. Reduced lung-cancer mortality with low-dose computed tomographic screening. N Engl J Med 2011;365(5):395–409.

Table 6
Stage distribution of NLST cancers

Cancer Stages	CT Detected (N = 1060)		CXR Detected (N = 941)	
	(No.)	(%)	(No.)	(%)
1a	416	40.0	196	21.1
1b	104	10.0	93	10.0
2a	35	3.4	32	3.4
2b	38	3.7	42	4.5
3a	99	9.5	109	11.7
3b	122	11.7	122	13.1
4	226	21.7	335	36.1

Data from Aberle DR, Adams AM, Berg CD, et al. Reduced lung-cancer mortality with low-dose computed tomographic screening. N Engl J Med 2011;365(5):395–409.

enough to be able to demonstrate a statistically significant reduction in lung cancer mortality. It is hoped that combining these studies may be able to do this. The DANTE trial (Detection and Screening of Early Lung Cancer by Novel Imaging Technology and Molecular Essays) is an RCT performed in Italy.[19] A total of 2472 men aged 60 to 74 years with at least 20 pack-years of smoking history, half of which underwent low-dose CT at enrollment and then annually for 4 years, and a control group that received usual care were enrolled from 2001 to 2006. Depiscan, a pilot trial in France, was initiated in 2002 to assess the feasibility of performing a large-scale national lung cancer screening trial, GranDepiscan.[20] A total of 765 current or recently former smokers aged 50 to 75 years with at least 15 pack-years of smoking history were enrolled, half undergoing low-dose CT and half CXR.

Nederlands-Leuvens Longkanker Screenings Onderzoek (NELSON) is a large Dutch-Belgium randomized lung cancer screening trial launched in 2003.[21,22] Approximately 16 000 participants, nearly all men, aged 50 to 75 years who were current or recently former smokers (quit 10 or < years ago) with at least a 20 pack-year history of smoking at 4 centers. Enrollees underwent either low-dose CT using a 16 detector CT scanner at baseline and at years 1 and 3 or usual care. NELSON is the first trial to use semi-automated volumetric nodule assessment to classifying examinations as positive, negative or indeterminate based on size, nodule characteristics, location and nodule growth (doubling time). Patients with negative test results were rescheduled for a CT scan in year 4. For patients with indeterminate

results, a repeat scan was made 1 year later (year 3) or they required a repeat scan 6 to 8 weeks later. Participants with positive test results were referred to a chest physician for workup and diagnostic assessment. Doubling time considerations in this study were, a positive scan was defined as a doubling time of less than 400 days, a negative screen as a doubling time of more than 600 days, and an indeterminate screen as a doubling time of 400 to 600 days.

The Danish Lung Cancer Screening Trial (DLCST) is an RCT that enrolled patients from 2004 to 2010 comparing low-dose CT with usual care; the 10-year follow-up is still being collected.[23] A total of 4104 patients aged 50 to 70 years who were current or recently former smokers with 20 pack-years of smoking history all received health questionnaires and spirometry annually for 5 years, with the experimental arm also receiving annual low-dose CT scans using a 16-detector CT scanner. The primary study end point being assessed is lung cancer mortality. DLCST is being performed in collaboration with the NELSON trial, with pooling of data from both studies to occur on completion.

ITALUNG is an RCT initiated in 2004 at 3 centers in Italy.[24] The 3206 patients received either annual low-dose CT for 4 years or usual care. The CT scanners that were used were either single detectors or 4-detector CT scanners. A positive test was defined as a noncalcified nodule greater than or equal to 5 mm or a nonsolid nodule greater than or equal to 10 mm. Low-dose CT, FDG-PET, and fine-needle aspiration were used to evaluate positive studies. The Multicentric Italian Lung Detection project[25] is an RCT initiated in 2005 that enrolled 50- to 75-year-old current or recently former smokers with at least a 20 pack-year history of smoking randomized to receive either low-dose CT with a 16-channel CT scanner and primary prevention or only primary prevention. The CT-screened group was further divided into half that received CT annually and the other half every 2 years. Both of these Italian studies use automated volumetric nodule assessment.

The United Kingdom Lung Screen (UKLS) is an RCT that began in 2011 with a pilot, with the expectation of enrolling 28 000 patients to receive either low-dose CT on a 16-detector scanner or usual care.[26] Patients enrolled are 50 to 75 years of age at a high risk for lung cancer. The risk is determined by a model developed by the Liverpool Lung Project, which includes variables, such as age, sex, smoking duration, family history of lung cancer, and occupational exposures. The UKLS study design is unique in that participants will receive only a single screen at baseline and not multiple screens, as uses a risk model to determine risk. The UKLS study design is unique in that participants will receive only a single screen at baseline and not multiple screens, and uses a risk model to determine risk.

OTHER CONSIDERATIONS
Characteristics of Missed Cancers in Low-Dose CT Screening Trials

Lung cancers missed on low-dose screening CT are either the result of a detection error, when the abnormality is not identified, or interpretation error, when the abnormality is identified but misinterpreted. In an analysis of 32 missed lung cancers on CT in a Japanese screening program using CT images with a 10-mm slice thickness, 20 were detection errors and 13 interpretation errors.[27] Interpretation errors were not subtle and exhibited features often associated with benign lesions, nearly all of which were misdiagnosed as tuberculosis or another inflammatory lesion. They often existed on the background of complex lung disease, such as emphysema or fibrosis. Of the detection errors, the average size of the lung cancers was 10 mm, nearly all were ground-glass nodules with or without a solid component, and many were subtle, exhibited an appearance similar to a pulmonary vessel, or were obscured by adjacent hilar structures. Advances in computer-aided diagnosis (CAD) may reduce false negatives. For example, in one study, CAD detected 80% (N = 18) of the lung cancers missed in one low-dose CT screening program.[28]

Evolution of Technology

Since the initial CT screening trials began, there have been significant improvements in CT-scanner technology. Newer CT scanners, including those used in the recently conducted lung cancer screening trials, use thinner slice thickness and reconstruction intervals than in the past, typically 1.0 to 1.5 mm, which increases the detection rate for small lung nodules but also increases the number of images per examination for the radiologist to interpret. The improved spatial resolution and faster acquisition times of modern multidetector CT scanners permit more-robust CAD and volume measurements of pulmonary nodules across these larger datasets. These applications may be useful to improve the detection of nodules and changes in nodule size over time across the diversity of readers, from dedicated thoracic radiologist to general radiologists who interpret fewer thoracic CT examinations. Maximum-intensity projection image reconstructions are increasingly used in the interpretation of thoracic CT

examinations, often routinely reconstructed at the CT scanner or generated on basic radiology workstations or advanced applications workstations and, like CAD, this also increases the detection rate and efficiency for detecting lung nodules.

CAD

Nodule detection on the large CT datasets reconstructed at 1.0- to 1.5-mm slice thickness is challenging not only because of the large number of images that contributes to reader fatigue but also challenges in detecting nodules that are central or perivascular in location. The abilities of CAD and radiologists in detecting pulmonary nodules are complementary, with CAD more adept at detecting centrally located nodules, whereas radiologists have greater sensitivity for detecting peripheral nodules.[29] When used together, the overall sensitivity for the detection nodules that are larger than 4 mm in size may increase to almost 90%.[30] However, the limitations of CAD that currently prevent the widespread application in clinical practice include the false-positive rate of approximately of 3 to 20 per CT scan. This rate is most commonly caused by vessels (54%), pleura (24%), and scar (12%).[29] In addition, there are workflow limitations caused by the lack of seamless integration into routine radiology workstations of CAD software that are slowly being overcome.

Volumetric Nodule Evaluation and Nodule Doubling Time

The determination of lung nodule growth or lack thereof is the mainstay of clinical algorithms for the evaluation of indeterminate lung nodules less than 8 mm in size, which includes most of the lung nodules detected with screening CT. Precise and reproducible measurements are critical to estimate growth rates. A doubling time of 20 to 400 days generally indicates a nodule is malignant, whereas a doubling time of greater than 400 days or smaller than 20 days generally indicates benign behavior.[31]

Most of these nodules are benign. With nodule growth comes an increased likelihood of cancer and more-aggressive interventions that range from PET-CT and percutaneous or bronchoscopic sampling to resection. Measurement of nodule diameter and change in diameter over time has been the standard method for evaluating growth but is well known to be inaccurate and lacks reproducibility within a reader, across readers, and across measurement tools and is more difficult the smaller the nodules are in diameter.[32] Furthermore, asymmetric nodule growth may not be detectable if the largest diameter is used. Computer-assisted characterization tools, specifically nodule segmentation and volume calculation, consider the 3-dimensional nature of nodules for more-precise size estimation and, therefore, improved calculation of nodule doubling time. The reproducibility of semiautomated volume measurements is high (approximately 90%). Volume measurements in spherical, smoothly margined nodules may be highly reproducible.[33] However, repeated measurements of the same intermediate-sized (50–500 mm^3), irregular nodules may vary by approximately 10%, which is a number that is not insignificant given that lung cancers are more likely to exhibit these characteristics.[34]

Radiation Dose and Downstream Testing Following a Positive Screen

The potential benefits of lung cancer screening with low-dose CT need to be considered in conjunction with the potential risks and costs. Every effort must be made to reduce the radiation dose from CT given the large number of people that would be affected if screening is implemented. Reducing radiation can be accomplished by reducing the tube current, increasing pitch, or decreasing tube voltage without compromising the diagnostic utility. The risk of radiation-induced lung cancer needs to be considered even when using low-dose CT. Although the risk of radiation-induced malignancy of solid organs decreases as the age at the time of exposure increases, the risk of radiation-induced lung cancer increases with the age at the time of exposure throughout adulthood. The greatest risk of radiation-induced lung cancer occurs when exposed at 55 years of age. In addition, damage to the lung from radiation and from smoking may act synergistically to produce an elevated risk of radiation-induced lung cancer in the population that would benefit most from screening. The NLST study was able to decrease the average effective dose of a screening examination to 1.5 mSv.

Even further dose reductions may be possible because of the recent improvements in CT scanning technology, such as advanced image reconstruction methodologies.

Overdiagnosis and False-Positive Studies

There is also a risk of morbidity and mortality from interventions that might occur during the evaluation of false-positive studies. The presence of nodules on baseline screening examinations is high and has ranged from 4% to 56%. New nodules detected on interval screening examinations have ranged from 5% to 13%. The frequency of nodules detected by CT may vary by region.

Although the rates of false-positive studies are high, the NLST demonstrated that most nodules can be managed noninvasively, either with follow-up CT or FDG-PET imaging. The NLST also demonstrated that the number of procedures performed on false-positive studies is low and complications from such procedures are exceedingly rare.

Overdiagnosis is inherent in any screening test. It is difficult to assess to what degree this occurs in lung cancer screening. The harmful effects resulting from overdiagnosis include the psychological distress associated with the diagnosis of lung cancer as well as the morbidity and mortality associated with unnecessary medical procedures.

Cost-Effectiveness

Many inherent relationships affect the cost-effectiveness of lung cancer screening with CT. The cost per quality-adjusted life-year (QALY) increases as the rate of overdiagnosis increases and as the prevalence of lung cancer decreases. The cost per QALY is also likely to be highest in the first 2 years of screening, when more nodules are detected that require follow-up studies to document stability. The cost-effective analysis data from the NLST are currently being analyzed and will be useful data to determine whether CT screening could be implemented on a large scale with acceptable costs. The ongoing European RCTs will also be able to provide valuable information as to whether screening with CT can be cost-effective.

WHAT IS NEXT?

Numerous studies have tried to demonstrate the impact of lung cancer screening, first with CXR alone or in combination with sputum analysis and then with CT screening. Although the other methodologies have not, NLST-CT screening has convincingly shown to decrease mortality from lung cancer. The implications of such widespread screening in the United States and worldwide is vast, both in terms of required resources and the potential for improved health outcomes. Before the recommendation can be made to screen for lung cancer with low-dose CT, the results of the NLST should ideally be confirmed by other trials. Given the resources that were dedicated to the NLST, it is unlikely another study of similar magnitude will be possible. Many RCTs are currently being conducted in Europe and might be able to confirm reduced mortality from lung cancer screening. Although none individually will be able to achieve the same statistical power of the NLST, a meta-analysis might be able to provide sufficient evidence to recommend screening for lung cancer with low-dose CT in high-risk individuals.

Many additional questions remain regarding the optimal implementation of a mass-screening program. Will the effective screening for lung cancer and the treatment of curable disease be as successful in the community at large as it was at the centers that participated in the NLST? What population of current or former smokers stands to benefit from screening? Should screening be extended to those with exposure to other known carcinogens? At what age should screening begin and for what duration? What is the most effective screening interval? What criteria should be used to define a positive screen to detect cancers while minimizing the number of false-positive studies? What is the appropriate role of FDG-PET imaging in the workup of a positive screen? Although some of these questions may be answered by the numerous currently ongoing European trials, others may require additional studies designed specifically to answer these questions.

LUNG CANCER SCREENING GUIDELINES

Medical professional societies have been cautious about endorsing screening since the NLST results were reported pending the results of the cost-effectiveness analysis. However, the American Cancer Society and the American College of Radiology have recommended that individuals interested in screening do so in a multidisciplinary program as part of an ongoing research program. In the last few months, the National Comprehensive Cancer Network has published lung cancer screening guidelines using low-dose CT.[35] These guidelines issue a detailed management plan for managing screen results. Similarly, the American Lung Association has also recommended low-dose CT screening for people who meet the NLST study criteria.[36]

SUMMARY

The authors conclude by mentioning that it is important to screen populations who would gain the most benefit from CT lung cancer screening. It is critical to have an organized framework to provide lung cancer screening both to diagnose and subsequently manage the results. A multidisciplinary approach will be the best way to catch this deadly disease at an early stage and to have a significant impact in the health care of patients with lung cancer.

REFERENCES

1. Siegel R, Naishadham D, Jemal A. Cancer statistics, 2012. CA Cancer J Clin 2012;62(1):10–29.

2. Aberle DR, Adams AM, Berg CD, et al. Reduced lung-cancer mortality with low-dose computed tomographic screening. N Engl J Med 2011; 365(5):395–409.

3. Harris RP, Helfand M, Woolf SH, et al. Current methods of the US Preventive Services Task Force: a review of the process. Am J Prev Med 2001; 20(Suppl 3):21–35.

4. Sagawa M, Tsubono Y, Saito Y, et al. A case-control study for evaluating the efficacy of mass screening program for lung cancer in Miyagi Prefecture, Japan. Cancer 2001;92(3):588–94.

5. Nishii K, Ueoka H, Kiura K, et al. A case-control study of lung cancer screening in Okayama Prefecture, Japan. Lung Cancer 2001;34(3):325–32.

6. Fontana RS, Sanderson DR, Taylor WF, et al. Early lung cancer detection: results of the initial (prevalence) radiologic and cytologic screening in the Mayo Clinic study. Am Rev Respir Dis 1984; 130(4):561–5.

7. Melamed MR, Flehinger BJ, Zaman MB, et al. Screening for early lung cancer. Results of the Memorial Sloan-Kettering study in New York. Chest 1984;86(1):44–53.

8. Frost JK, Ball WC Jr, Levin ML, et al. Early lung cancer detection: results of the initial (prevalence) radiologic and cytologic screening in the Johns Hopkins study. Am Rev Respir Dis 1984;130(4):549–54.

9. Kubik A, Polak J. Lung cancer detection. Results of a randomized prospective study in Czechoslovakia. Cancer 1986;57(12):2427–37.

10. Oken MM, Hocking WG, Kvale PA, et al. Screening by chest radiograph and lung cancer mortality: the Prostate, Lung, Colorectal, and Ovarian (PLCO) randomized trial. JAMA 2011;306(17):1865–73.

11. Nawa T, Nakagawa T, Mizoue T, et al. Long-term prognosis of patients with lung cancer detected on low-dose chest computed tomography screening. Lung Cancer 2012;75(2):197–202.

12. Nawa T, Nakagawa T, Kusano S, et al. Lung cancer screening using low-dose spiral CT: results of baseline and 1-year follow-up studies. Chest 2002; 122(1):15–20.

13. Henschke CI, McCauley DI, Yankelevitz DF, et al. Early Lung Cancer Action Project: overall design and findings from baseline screening. Lancet 1999;354(9173):99–105.

14. NY-ELCAP Investigators. CT Screening for lung cancer: diagnoses resulting from the New York Early Lung Cancer Action Project. Radiology 2007;243(1):239–49.

15. Henschke CI, Yankelevitz DF, Libby DM, et al. Survival of patients with stage I lung cancer detected on CT screening. N Engl J Med 2006; 355(17):1763–71.

16. Swensen SJ, Jett JR, Hartman TE, et al. CT screening for lung cancer: five-year prospective experience. Radiology 2005;235(1):259–65.

17. Bach PB, Jett JR, Pastorino U, et al. Computed tomography screening and lung cancer outcomes. JAMA 2007;297(9):953–61.

18. Larke FJ, Kruger RL, Cagnon CH, et al. Estimated radiation dose associated with low-dose chest CT of average-size participants in the National Lung Screening Trial. AJR Am J Roentgenol 2011;197(5): 1165–9.

19. Infante M, Lutman FR, Cavuto S, et al. Lung cancer screening with spiral CT: baseline results of the randomized DANTE trial. Lung Cancer 2008;59(3): 355–63.

20. Blanchon T, Brechot JM, Grenier PA, et al. Baseline results of the Depiscan study: a French randomized pilot trial of lung cancer screening comparing low dose CT scan (LDCT) and chest X-ray (CXR). Lung Cancer 2007;58(1):50–8.

21. Ru Zhao Y, Xie X, de Koning HJ, et al. NELSON lung cancer screening study. Cancer Imaging 2011; 11(Spec No A):S79–84.

22. Xu DM, Gietema H, de Koning H, et al. Nodule management protocol of the NELSON randomised lung cancer screening trial. Lung Cancer 2006; 54(2):177–84.

23. Pedersen JH, Ashraf H, Dirksen A, et al. The Danish randomized lung cancer CT screening trial–overall design and results of the prevalence round. J Thorac Oncol 2009;4(5):608–14.

24. Lopes Pegna A, Picozzi G, Mascalchi M, et al. Design, recruitment and baseline results of the ITA-LUNG trial for lung cancer screening with low-dose CT. Lung Cancer 2009;64(1):34–40.

25. Marchiano A, Calabro E, Civelli E, et al. Pulmonary nodules: volume repeatability at multidetector CT lung cancer screening. Radiology 2009;251(3): 919–25.

26. Baldwin DR, Duffy SW, Wald NJ, et al. UK Lung Screen (UKLS) nodule management protocol: modelling of a single screen randomised controlled trial of low-dose CT screening for lung cancer. Thorax 2011;66(4):308–13.

27. Li F, Sone S, Abe H, et al. Lung cancers missed at low-dose helical CT screening in a general population: comparison of clinical, histopathologic, and imaging findings. Radiology 2002;225(3): 673–83.

28. Armato SG 3rd, Li F, Giger ML, et al. Lung cancer: performance of automated lung nodule detection applied to cancers missed in a CT screening program. Radiology 2002;225(3):685–92.

29. Yuan R, Vos PM, Cooperberg PL. Computer-aided detection in screening CT for pulmonary nodules. AJR Am J Roentgenol 2006;186(5):1280–7.

30. Das M, Muhlenbruch G, Heinen S, et al. Performance evaluation of a computer-aided detection algorithm for solid pulmonary nodules in low-dose and standard-dose MDCT chest examinations and its influence on radiologists. Br J Radiol 2008; 81(971):841–7.

31. Yankelevitz DF, Reeves AP, Kostis WJ, et al. Small pulmonary nodules: volumetrically determined growth rates based on CT evaluation. Radiology 2000;217(1):251–6.

32. Bogot NR, Kazerooni EA, Kelly AM, et al. Interobserver and intraobserver variability in the assessment of pulmonary nodule size on CT using film and computer display methods. Acad Radiol 2005; 12(8):948–56.

33. Wang Y, van Klaveren RJ, van der Zaag-Loonen HJ, et al. Effect of nodule characteristics on variability of semiautomated volume measurements in pulmonary nodules detected in a lung cancer screening program. Radiology 2008;248(2):625–31.

34. Gietema HA, Wang Y, Xu D, et al. Pulmonary nodules detected at lung cancer screening: interobserver variability of semiautomated volume measurements. Radiology 2006;241(1):251–7.

35. NCCN clinical practice guidelines in oncology: lung cancer screening. 2012. Available at: http://www.nccn.org/professionals/physician_gls/pdf/lung_screening.pdf. Accessed June 22, 2012.

36. American Lung Association. Providing guidance on lung cancer screening to patients and physicians. 2012. Available at: http://www.lung.org/lung-disease/lung-cancer/lung-cancer-screening-guidelines/lung-cancer-screening.pdf. Accessed June 22, 2012.

37. Sobue T, Moriyama N, Kaneko M, et al. Screening for lung cancer with low-dose helical computed tomography: anti-lung cancer association project. J Clin Oncol 2002;20(4):911–20.

38. Kaneko M, Kusumoto M, Kobayashi T, et al. Computed tomography screening for lung carcinoma in Japan. Cancer 2000;89(Suppl 11):2485–8.

39. Sone S, Takashima S, Li F, et al. Mass screening for lung cancer with mobile spiral computed tomography scanner. Lancet 1998;351(9111):1242–5.

40. Chong S, Lee KS, Chung MJ, et al. Lung cancer screening with low-dose helical CT in Korea: experiences at the Samsung Medical Center. J Korean Med Sci 2005;20(3):402–8.

41. Gohagan JK, Marcus PM, Fagerstrom RM, et al. Final results of the Lung Screening Study, a randomized feasibility study of spiral CT versus chest X-ray screening for lung cancer. Lung Cancer 2005;47(1):9–15.

42. Pastorino U, Bellomi M, Landoni C, et al. Early lung-cancer detection with spiral CT and positron emission tomography in heavy smokers: 2-year results. Lancet 2003;362(9384):593–7.

43. Novello S, Fava C, Borasio P, et al. Three-year findings of an early lung cancer detection feasibility study with low-dose spiral computed tomography in heavy smokers. Ann Oncol 2005;16(10):1662–6.

44. Garg K, Keith RL, Byers T, et al. Randomized controlled trial with low-dose spiral CT for lung

cancer screening: feasibility study and preliminary results. Radiology 2002;225(2):506–10.

45. Picozzi G, Paci E, Lopez Pegna A, et al. Screening of lung cancer with low dose spiral CT: results of a three year pilot study and design of the randomised controlled trial 'Italung-CT'. Radiol Med 2005;109(1–2):17–26.

46. Stephenson SM, Mech KF, Sardi A. Lung cancer screening with low-dose spiral computed tomography. Am Surg 2005;71(12):1015–7.

47. MacRedmond R, Logan PM, Lee M, et al. Screening for lung cancer using low dose CT scanning. Thorax 2004;59(3):237–41.

48. Bastarrika G, Garcia-Velloso MJ, Lozano MD, et al. Early lung cancer detection using spiral computed tomography and positron emission tomography. Am J Respir Crit Care Med 2005;171(12):1378–83.

49. Diederich S, Wormanns D, Semik M, et al. Screening for early lung cancer with low-dose spiral CT:

prevalence in 817 asymptomatic smokers. Radiology 2002;222(3):773–81.

50. Wilson DO, Weissfeld JL, Fuhrman CR, et al. The Pittsburgh Lung Screening Study (PLuSS): outcomes within 3 years of a first computed tomography scan. Am J Respir Crit Care Med 2008; 178(9):956–61.

51. Fujikawa A, Takiguchi Y, Mizuno S, et al. Lung cancer screening–comparison of computed tomography and X-ray. Lung Cancer 2008;61(2): 195–201.

52. Menezes RJ, Roberts HC, Paul NS, et al. Lung cancer screening using low-dose computed tomography in at-risk individuals: the Toronto experience. Lung Cancer 2010;67(2):177–83.

53. Veronesi G, Bellomi M, Mulshine JL, et al. Lung cancer screening with low-dose computed tomography: a non-invasive diagnostic protocol for baseline lung nodules. Lung Cancer 2008;61(3):340–9.

Evaluation and Management of Indeterminate Pulmonary Nodules

Philip A. Hodnett, MD[a,b,*], Jane P. Ko, MD[a,b]

KEYWORDS

- Solitary pulmonary nodule • Indeterminate • Computed tomography • Nodule characterization
- Lung cancer • Management • Guidelines

KEY POINTS

- Pulmonary nodules are routinely detected on computed tomography of the chest.
- Once a pulmonary nodule is identified, the key question for management of pulmonary nodules is their characterization.
- Management decisions should not be based on nodule size alone. Central, laminar, or dense diffuse patterns of calcification are indicators of benignancy.
- Increasing patient age generally correlates with increasing likelihood of malignancy.

INTRODUCTION

Although several clinical and radiologic features may suggest the diagnosis, many solitary pulmonary nodules remain indeterminate after conventional evaluation. If there are no definite benign morphologic findings, the solitary pulmonary nodule is classified as an indeterminate, possibly malignant lesion. The solitary pulmonary nodule (SPN) remains a frequently encountered finding on multidetector computed tomography (MDCT).[1] Since the first instillation of a clinical CT scanner, repeated advances in CT technology have resulted in the rapid growth in the use of MDCT[2] and, thus, significant increase in the detection of lung nodules.[3]

Lung nodules may be caused by a variety of disorders, including neoplasm, infection, inflammation, and vascular and congenital abnormalities. Although most incidentally discovered pulmonary nodules are benign, 1 in 13 men and 1 in 16 women will be diagnosed with lung cancer, with an estimated 20% to 30% of these patients presenting with an SPN.[4]

The occurrence of malignancy for an SPN, such as in mass screening studies with both plain radiography and CT, low.[5,6] This low and reflects the higher sensitivity of CT for small lung nodules that have a lesser likelihood of malignancy.[7] The high mortality associated with lung cancer emphasizes the need for detection and characterization of SPNs so that benign lesions can be distinguished from their malignant counterparts.

Options for nodule characterization include noninvasive and minimally-invasive techniques. Many nodules remain indeterminate and require surveillance, further imaging evaluation, or tissue sampling for definitive diagnosis. This has practical importance so that patients with a benign SPN are not referred for unnecessary surgical

No grant funding or other support was provided for this work.

[a] Thoracic Imaging Department of Radiology, New York University Langone Medical Center, IRM 236, 560 First Avenue, New York, NY 10016, USA; [b] Division of Thoracic Imaging, Department of Radiology, New York University; School of Medicine, New York University Langone Medical Center, 560 First Avenue, New York, NY 10016, USA

* Corresponding author. Thoracic Imaging, Department of Radiology, New York University Langone Medical Center; New York University School of Medicine, 560 First Avenue, New York, NY 10016.
E-mail address: phodnett33@gmail.com

0033-8389/12/$ – see front matter © 2012 Elsevier Inc. All rights reserved.

resection, while avoiding mischaracterization of a small malignant SPN that may represent resectable (ie, curable) early-stage lung cancer as benign. The aims of this article are to review the role of imaging and to address and evaluate strategies for the evaluation and management of indeterminate pulmonary nodules.

DEFINITION

According to the Nomenclature Committee of the Fleischner Society, a "pulmonary nodule" is defined as a sharply-defined circular opacity that is 2 to 30 mm in diameter.[8] A micronodule is a discrete, small, round, focal opacity; a variety of diameters have been used in the past to define a micronodule. Use of the term is most often limited to a nodule with a diameter of less than 5 mm[9] or less than 3 mm.[10] The term "nodule" is reserved for opacities less than 3 cm in diameter, based on the fact that most solitary lung lesions larger than 3 cm in diameter (termed *masses*) are malignant. First, when considering a radiographically detected SPN, it is important to ascertain if the density in question is truly solitary, lies within the lung, and represents a nodule. Up to 50% of patients with suspected SPNs detected radiographically actually are proved to have multiple nodules on CT evaluation.[11] This is particularly important because multiple lung nodules may represent, for example, either metastatic or granulomatous disease, depending on the clinical scenario.[12] Multiple small incidental nodules in a patient are considered independently when lacking a distinctive relationship to structures within the secondary lobule.[13]

In contrast, multiple nodules distributed within the lungs in a pattern in relation to the secondary pulmonary lobule, such as centrilobular or perilymphatic, are considered to be a single entity, with different diagnostic considerations, of which an in-depth discussion is beyond the scope of this article. Centrilobular nodules are round or ovoid poorly-defined pulmonary opacities approximately 5 to 8 mm in diameter and suggestive of entities such as respiratory bronchiolitis and hypersensitivity pneumonitis. Perilymphatic nodules aligned in regions of the subpleural lung and bronchovascular bundles where lymphatics are prevalent imply diseases such as sarcoidosis, silicosis, and lymphangitic carcinomatosis.

FREQUENCY

The prevalence of noncalcified SPNs is largely based on lung cancer screening studies, with nodules detected in selected individuals reported in 8% to 51% of baseline screenings.[14] The wide variation in the prevalence of SPNs may be partially explained by the use of different imaging methods (chest radiography, CT), varying radiography techniques, varying percentage of smokers and their degree of smoking (former, current, and heavy) included in each study population, and the diverse geographic location of the studies (United States, Japan, Germany, and Italy). Other factors that may affect lung nodule prevalence of lung nodules include the technical quality of the imaging study and interobserver variation related to radiologists' interpretation of the images. However, the true prevalence of pulmonary nodules may be underestimated in these lung cancer screening studies constrained by z-axis spatial resolution; not surprisingly, CT examinations using 10-mm section thickness detect approximately half the number of nodules compared with those using 1.25 to 5 mm.[15] The latest MDCT systems has isotropic spatial resolution with a pixel dimension in 3 planes of 0.5 to 0.7 mm, which result in increased pulmonary nodule detection.[16] Pulmonary nodules tend to be less than 10 mm; up to 96% of noncalcified nodules are <10 mm; of these, 72% are <5 mm.[17]

NODULE DETECTION
Radiography

Although chest radiography remains the most commonly ordered radiologic examination, it has low sensitivity for demonstrating pulmonary nodules and a high false-positive rate.[18] The Early Lung Cancer Action Project (ELCAP)[5] described a detection rate for noncalcified nodules with low-dose CT that was 3 times greater than that with chest radiography. In general radiologic practice, bronchogenic carcinomas have been reported as missed on chest radiography (ie, an undetected lesion is evident retrospectively) in 19% of cases[19]; this rate has varied from 12% to 90%, depending on study design.[20] Potentially resectable non–small-cell lung cancer (NSCLC) lesions not identified on chest radiography are predominantly peripheral (85%) and upper lobe (72%) in location.[21] This is particularly worrisome given that NSCLC tends to progress from early-stage to late-stage disease, especially if several years pass between examinations. The detection of pulmonary nodules on screen-film radiographs is notoriously unreliable, with Muhm and colleagues[22] reporting that 90% of peripheral nodules and 75% of perihilar nodules identified during a lung cancer screening program were visible in retrospect on an earlier radiograph. Missed nodules may reflect an incomplete visual survey by the evaluator[23] or a nodule's low conspicuity when located in the upper lung, centrally,[24] or over other structures such as the clavicle or hilar vessels (**Fig. 1**).

Developments in image acquisition and computer-assisted image analysis techniques for chest radiography have been primarily driven by recognized challenges and limitations of the technique. Dual-energy subtraction (DES) reduces anatomic noise by subtracting bony structures overlying the lungs in a chest radiograph, and advances in flat panel detector technology have enabled improved DES imaging with digital radiography technology.[25] DES technique is based on imaging with differing peak kilovoltage values and aids in more clearly depicting calcification[26] and potentially characterizing pulmonary nodules as benign, as well as having improved sensitivity for noncalcified nodules.[27] Bone-subtraction technology, based on postprocessing techniques that enable removal of the overlying bony structures, has recently been introduced as an alternative to DES. Nodule detection may be improved on chest radiographs with temporal image subtraction, in which the aim is to selectively enhance areas of interval change, accomplished by subtracting a patient's previous chest radiograph from the current one.[28] The quality of the technique is inherently dependent on the success of 2-dimensional registration.[29] Computer-aided detection (CAD) and computer-aided diagnosis (CADx) technology has slowly made its way into the clinical arena. The clinical role of radiography-based CAD and CADx technology is highly debated and continuously evolving.[30] An early CAD program marked approximately 40% of the lung cancers that were missed in a lung cancer screening program, but it made an average of 15 false-positive marks per image.[31] This technology has a complementary role in clinical practice as a second opinion, possibly enhancing accuracy and improving efficiency, although documented limitations of CAD include the false-positive markings.[32,33]

MDCT

MDCT is typically performed for a nodule identified on chest radiography and not determined to be stable through comparison with prior radiographs. CT is considered the current gold standard for the detection of lung nodules.[34] The latest commercially released MDCT systems are increasingly complex, with 128 or more detectors-row configurations and temporal resolutions on the order of 0.3 msec. The greater degree of spatial and contrast resolution provided by MDCT affords improved sensitivity and specificity for pulmonary nodule detection.[35] Since its introduction, MDCT technology continues to advance with an increasing number of detector rows and more rapid scan acquisition times. Given the low attenuation of the lungs, the evaluation of the lungs is tolerant to lower doses than for the soft tissues and mediastinum. Therefore, to minimize patient irradiation, it has been suggested that low-dose CT be performed for the follow-up of lung nodules.[36] Tube current modulation techniques for maintaining a standard image quality throughout a CT examination while adjusting for overall patient size and varying thicknesses of the patient in the x, y, and z planes will also minimize irradiation,

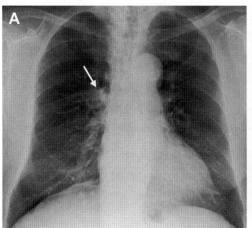
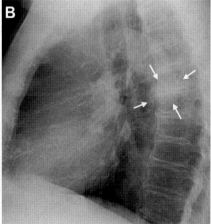

Fig. 1. Perihilar lung cancer. On posteroanterior radiography (*A*), the nodular density (*arrow*) projecting just above the right hilum is difficult to visualize given the location close to the vasculature. The nodule (*arrows*) appears as a vague density that projects over the spine (*B*), another location that hinders identification of lung nodules.

particularly for smaller patients.[37–39] Consistency of CT protocols across varying CT scanner models and manufacturers will also ensure standard degrees of exposure to patients and can be assessed by comparing the volume CT dose index, which is a measure of the radiation output of the CT machine to a scanned volume of a standardized phantom.[40]

Parameters for chest CT are determined to maximize temporal and spatial resolution. In terms of temporal resolution, MDCT chest CT typically entails a rapid gantry rotation time to decrease the duration of the CT examination and minimize the time required for sustained breathholding by the patient. Typically, a 25- to 35-cm field of view (FOV) is used and adjusted according to a patient's size to maximize spatial resolution. Given the use of a standard 512 × 512 imaging matrix, smaller FOVs result in smaller pixel sizes (0.48–0.68 mm for standard FOVs vs 0.20–0.29 mm for targeted FOVs) and thus improve spatial resolution.[41] High-frequency reconstruction algorithms enhance edges and spatial resolution but amplify image noise and therefore are best used for the assessment of the lung parenchyma and bones. Although reconstructions are typically in the order of 3- to 5-mm section thickness for a nontargeted FOV, thin-section CT scans in the order of 2 mm and smaller in thickness through an area of interest greatly improves nodule assessment, decreasing partial volume effect and increasing spatial resolution.[42] A high-frequency algorithm increases spatial resolution and is optimum for evaluation of a nodule's borders, shape, and architecture. Soft-tissue algorithms in distinction facilitate assessment of attenuation by minimizing image noise and potentially high-attenuation pixels that might be interpreted as calcifications. Particularly for nodules with a complex nature, such as ground-glass or mixed solid and ground-glass attenuation nodules, thin-section images on the order of 1 mm may be beneficial for assessing the morphology and change in these features, if follow-up evaluation is performed.[43] The thin-section volume data are beneficial for computer-assisted evaluation methods and provide valuable images for planning transbronchial biopsy.

Pulmonary nodule detection on 5-mm sections is reported to be on the order of 69% for nodules smaller than 6 mm and 95% for nodules measuring 6 mm or larger.[44] Small nodule size was shown to be a major factor contributing to difficulty in the detection of nodules, as well as central or lower lobe location, complex background of other disease, or decreased nodule attenuation (Fig. 2).[45] Ko and colleagues[46] in a study evaluating the effect of image compression on lung nodule detection, confirmed that ground-glass nodules (GGNs) were detected less frequently than solid nodules (65% vs 83%); in addition, decreased sensitivity for central compared with peripheral nodules was revealed (61% vs 80%). Nodules that were not located adjacent to the pleura were similarly not detected as well. Although detection of pulmonary nodules by MDCT is improved with reduced slice thickness,[47] reader fatigue can be created by the 5-fold increased number of images generated.[48] The use of postprocessing techniques such as maximum intensity projection (MIP) methodology has been shown to improve detection rates of pulmonary nodules in comparison with axial images that are not postprocessed. In the MIP algorithm, only the highest-attenuation voxels along lines projected through the selected plane of volume data are selected to create the final image. MIP images with a slab thickness of 8 mm has been reported to be superior in the detection of pulmonary nodules to all other tested techniques.[49]

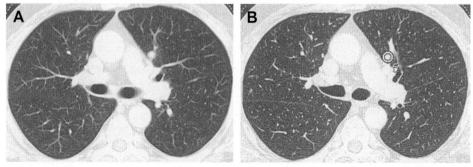

Fig. 2. Nodule detected with use of CAD. On a 5-mm axial CT section (A), a 6-mm nodule, located between the mediastinum is difficult to identify given the close proximity to vasculature. CAD marking (B), displayed as a circle on a 1-mm axial section, indicates the nodule. The CAD candidate marks are typically processed using image data on the order of 1 mm.

CAD

Given the challenges in nodule detection, CAD has been primarily developed as a second reader and has been shown to increase reader detection of nodules (**Fig. 2**). A secondary interpreter role aims at having CAD complement a radiologist's initial evaluation of a CT examination for nodules. CAD nodule candidate marks are viewed after an initial radiologist read and accepted or rejected. CAD has been shown in multiple studies to increase radiologist sensitivity in the detection of pulmonary nodules, although often with a concomitant increase in the number of false-positive results.[50,51] The number of false-positive marks presented to the reader by CAD has decreased as the quality of MDCT data for analysis by such systems has improved, in addition to further development of computer algorithms. A study comparing the performance of radiologists and CAD for pulmonary nodule detection on thin-section thoracic CT scans demonstrated a substantially higher detection of nodules (76%) compared with double reading (50%).[52] Important in this study is the reported low rate of false-positives (3%), typically related to branching points of vessels, artifact, or central vessels. It is interesting that the experience level of the radiologist may influence the benefit of CAD. Awai and colleagues[53] reported that radiology residents showed significant improvement for nodule detection but there was no significant improvement for board-certified radiologists.

However, most of the development of CAD for nodule detection has focused primarily on solid nodules only. GGNs remain one of the major difficulties encountered by nodule detection software development.[54,55] In the literature, lung CAD techniques can be divided into 2 groups: intensity-based and model-based methods. Intensity-based detection methods use the assumption that lung nodules have relatively higher intensity than those of the lung parenchyma. CAD techniques for identifying GGNs are therefore hindered by the reduced nodule contrast and lower attenuation.[56] Future direction may involve shape (model)-based techniques to improved performance.[57]

NODULE SIZE AND CAUSE

The smaller the nodule, the more likely it is to be benign, with 80% of benign nodules measuring less than 2 cm in diameter.[58–60] The prevalence of malignancy in nodules that measure less than 5 mm is exceedingly low (range, 0%–1%), with the exception of one small retrospective study[61] that reported both of 2 nodules smaller than 5 mm in diameter as malignant.[15] However, small size alone does not exclude lung cancer. In a study by Ginsberg and colleagues[62] of resected nodules on video-assisted thoracoscopy, 15% of malignant nodules are less than 1 cm in diameter and approximately 42% are less than 2 cm in diameter. In this investigation, a resected SPN was more likely to be malignant if the patient had a known cancer. Thus, the clinical context of the patient in whom a nodule is reported is important, particularly malignancy. The current knowledge relating to the significance of small pulmonary nodules largely reflects data from lung cancer screening trials in patients with significant smoking histories.[17,63,64] In the Fleischner Society statement,[36] even in high-risk patients, the likelihood that nodules measuring less than 5 mm represented lethal cancers is described to be less than 1%.

The differential diagnosis for a solitary pulmonary nodule includes benign and malignant causes (**Table 1**). More specifically, inflammation (infectious and noninfectious), neoplasia (both benign and malignant), and developmental (vascular and hamartomatous) causes are considerations. Most benign pulmonary nodules represent granulomas (80%), hamartomas (10%), and intrapulmonary lymph nodes.[65]

NODULE MORPHOLOGY, LOCATION, AND SHAPE

Evaluation of specific morphologic features of a solitary pulmonary nodule with MDCT imaging techniques can help differentiate benign from

Table 1 Causes of solitary pulmonary nodules	
Neoplastic malignant	Primary lung malignancies (non–small cell, small cell, carcinoid, lymphoma); solitary metastasis
Benign	Hamartoma; arteriovenous malformation; hematoma; pulmonary venous varix
Infectious	Granuloma; round pneumonia; abscess; septic embolus
Noninfectious	Amyloidoma; intrapulmonary lymph nodule; rheumatoid (necrobiotic) nodule; Wegener granulomatosis; focal scarring; infarct; sarcoid
Congenital	Sequestration; bronchogenic cyst; bronchial atresia with mucoid impaction

malignant nodules. Several morphologic features may help in determining the risk of malignancy in a nodule. In small nodules, location, shape, and grouping may be used to predict benignity. Most malignant solitary pulmonary nodules occur in the upper lobes,[66] whereas benign nodules are equally distributed throughout both upper and lower lobes. Frequently, bilateral, apical segmental, subpleural nodules are identified with somewhat irregular margins, likely reflecting post-inflammatory fibrosis.[36] Perifissural nodules have a low likelihood of malignancy if in a patient without a history of preexisting malignancy. These nodules may represent lymphoid tissue and intraparenchymal lymph nodes, which are increasingly recognized as a benign cause of a solitary pulmonary nodule identified.[67] CT signs suggestive of intraparenchymal lymph nodes (**Fig. 3**) include a subpleural location[68] within 15 mm of a pleural surface and a coffee-bean shape with a fine, linear opacity connecting them to a pleural surface.[69] Published data from the Nederlands-Leuvens Longkanker Screenings ONderzoek (NELSON) screening trial[70] indicated no cancers originating from smoothly marginated nodules or nodules attached to fissures, pleura, or adjacent vessels with many intrapulmonary lymph nodes meeting these criteria. In a screening population, Ahn and colleagues[43] demonstrated that none of the 159 perifissural nodules developed into lung cancer, thus suggesting a low-malignancy potential.

Shape has also been investigated as a predictor. Polygonal shape (concave surfaces on all sides and straight border at points of pleural contact) is highly specific for benign disease.[3] Nodules with this appearance tended to be focal condensations or nodules of fibrosis. The ratio of the maximum transverse dimension to the maximum perpendicular length (3-dimensional ratio) of a nodule was found to be significantly larger in benign nodules than in malignant nodules. Round nodules are therefore more likely to be malignant than are tubular or flat-shaped nodules, which may represent intrapulmonary lymph nodes, granulomas, or

nodular fibrosis. When combining 3 nodule features, Takashima and colleagues[60] reported that a predominantly solid attenuation and subpleural location or polygonal shape or 3-dimensional ratio was associated with the highest sensitivity (63% and 60%) for 2 reviewers.

NODULE CONTOUR

Nodule margins and contours can be classified as smooth, lobulated, irregular, or spiculated. Lobulation (**Fig. 4**) is attributed to differing growth rates within both primary and secondary malignancies, whereas spiculated margins are usually thought to be reflective of malignant infiltration along the interstitium.[71] Lobular nodules have a higher likelihood for malignancy.[72] There is, however, significant overlap regarding nodule margins and lobulation, with up to 25% of benign nodules having lobular morphology (**Fig. 5**). Pulmonary nodules in biopsy-proved lung cancer and nodule metastases may also manifest smooth, well-defined margins; Siegelman and colleagues[73] reported 21% of nodules with a well-defined and smooth border as malignant. Smooth borders and the presence of a pleural tail are seen in a range of benign and malignant entities and are therefore of little practical assistance.[74] Although spiculation has a high predictive value for malignancy[75] (90%), infection and inflammation nodule causes can have a similar appearance. Concave margins had 100% specificity for benignity and 43% to 48% sensitivity, respectively.[60]

CAVITATION

Cavitation can occur in both benign and malignant nodules secondary to infectious and other

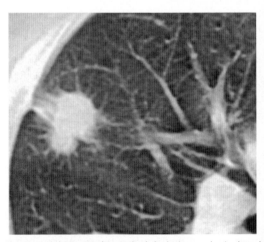

Fig. 4. Axial CT scan shows the lobulation and spiculated margin features of an adenocarcinoma. A pleural tail extends to the pleural surface, in addition to the irregular spiculations on the lateral aspect of the nodule.

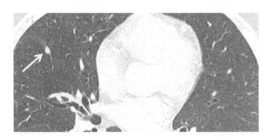

Fig. 3. Perifissural nodule (*arrow*) with a coffee bean shape. Lesions in this region are frequently related to intraparenchymal lymph nodes.

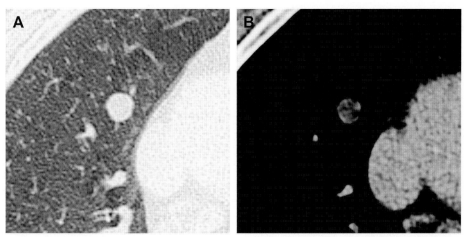

Fig. 5. Lobulated hamartoma. Axial lung window 1.0-mm image reconstructed using a high-frequency reconstruction filter (*A*) demonstrates a slightly lobulated nodule border. The nodule on thin-section low-frequency reconstruction axial 1.0-mm section (*B*) shows low-attenuation areas consistent with macroscopic fat. No calcification is identified in this lesion.

inflammatory conditions as well as in primary and metastatic tumors. Cavitation in primary lung malignancies is more commonly associated with squamous cell histology.[76] Malignant nodules typically have thick, irregular inner cavity walls, whereas benign cavitary nodules generally have smooth, thin walls, although considerable overlap limits discrimination (**Fig. 6**). Cavity wall thickness cannot reliably differentiate benign from malignant nodules; of cavitary nodules with a wall thickness between 5 and 15 mm, 51% were found to be benign and 49% were malignant.[77] Nodules with a wall thickness greater than 15 mm are more likely to be malignant, whereas those with a wall thickness of 4 mm or less are usually benign. Irregularity of the inner cavity wall is identified more frequently in malignant as opposed to benign cavitary nodules.[78] Notching of the outer wall, similarly, is more common in malignant cavitary nodules.

Irregularity of the outer cavitary wall is identified, similarly, in both benign and malignant lesions in one investigation.[78]

AIR BRONCHOGRAMS, AIR BRONCHIOLOGRAMS, OR "BUBBLY" LUCENCIES

A study comparing the internal features of indeterminate pulmonary GGNs on CT with their characteristics suggestive of malignancy evaluated the presence of cavitation, air bronchograms, and pseudocavitation (**Fig. 7**). Pseudocavitation, or spherical areas of air attenuation, may be present in cases of bronchioalveolar cell (BAC) carcinoma,[79] representing lucencies that mimic cavitation caused by distended alveoli and bronchi spared from involvement of tumor cells surrounding yet not obliterating these structures (lepidic growth). The presence of air bronchograms or cystic or "bubbly" lucencies within an SPN is highly suggestive of pulmonary carcinoma including BAC and mucinous adenocarcinoma, although lymphoma and occasional benign lesions, such as organizing pneumonia and mass-like sarcoidosis, can have air bronchograms.

NODULE ATTENUATION AND SUBSOLID NODULES

Patterns of calcification may be helpful in discriminating benign from malignant pulmonary nodules. When CT section thickness is 5 mm, partial volume effect may render detection of calcification within nodules difficult. CT, particularly thin-section CT, allows objective, qualitative assessment of

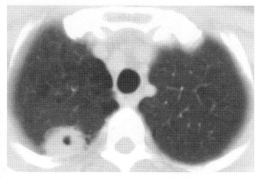

Fig. 6. Wegener granulomatosis. Shown is a benign cavitary right upper lobe nodule with a smooth, thin inner cavity wall.

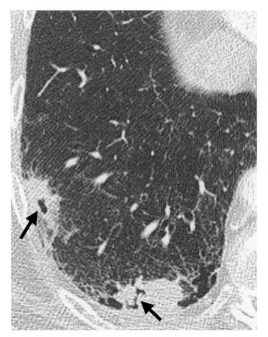

Fig. 7. Air bronchograms and pseudocavitation in known mucinous adenocarcinoma of the lung. Lucencies are present in 2 lower lobe soft tissue large nodules with irregular margins.

calcification.[65] There are 4 benign patterns of calcification: central, diffuse solid, laminated, and "popcorn like." These patterns, not frequently detected, are specific for benign disease, with central, concentric or lamellated (**Fig. 8**), or completely homogeneous calcification typically reflecting

granulomatous response to prior infection.[80] Dense, uniform calcification is a strong indicator of benign disease and present in 14% of subcentimeter nodules detected at baseline in one lung cancer screening study.[81] Popcorn calcification is typical of hamartomas and is caused by chondroid calcification.[82] Another classic feature of hamartomas is the presence of fat with internal density ranging between −40 and −120 Hounsfield units (HU) (**Figs. 5** and **8**), allowing this diagnosis to be made with confidence in a smooth nodule measuring less than 2.5 cm in diameter. Hamartomas, however, are relatively rare, and at least a third of hamartomas contain neither fat nor calcium. Stippled, amorphous, or eccentric calcifications (**Fig. 9**) are indeterminate patterns in an SPN and may be seen in malignancy.[83] Patients with a documented history of osteosarcoma or chondrosarcoma may present with lung metastases demonstrating "benign" patterns of calcification.[84] Intratumoral calcifications may be seen in lung cancer; however, these tend to occur in larger, more centrally located lesions.[85] Last, although fat content typically suggests a hamartoma, other causes of nodular densities with fat include liposarcoma and focal lipoid pneumonia.

Pulmonary subsolid nodules are defined as "rounded" areas of homogeneous or heterogeneous "increased" ground-glass attenuation in CT scans, which are lower in density with regard to surrounding soft tissue structures such as vessels.[86] Subsolid nodules can be classified further as either part-solid (**Fig. 10**), when areas of parenchymal architecture are obscured completely within the nodule, or nonsolid, when the nodule is pure ground-glass attenuation and harbors no areas of soft tissue density.[87] In the Early Lung Cancer Action Program study,[86] pure GGNs had an 18% incidence of malignancy, with partly

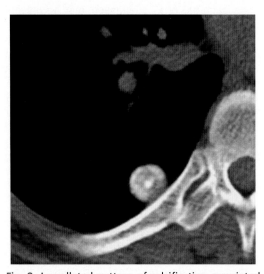

Fig. 8. Lamellated pattern of calcification associated with granulomatous disease. The "target" pattern of calcification is manifested by central calcification with concentric rings and a peripheral rim of calcification.

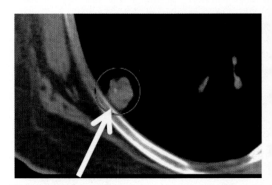

Fig. 9. Eccentric calcification. Lobulated nodule with low attenuation areas correlate with macroscopic fat indicating a hamartoma. A small eccentric solitary calcification is also present, which is an indeterminate pattern that is nonspecific.

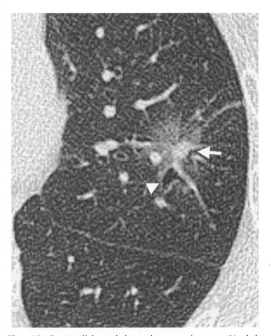

Fig. 10. Part-solid nodule: adenocarcinoma. Nodule with ground-glass attenuation has an eccentric solid component (*white arrow*) in the lesion. There is a dilated airway (*arrowhead*) in the periphery of this nodule. This lesion proved to be a lung cancer on resection and was mutation positive for epidermal growth factor receptor, correlating with responsiveness to tyrosine kinase inhibitor therapy for lung cancer.

solid nodules having the highest incidence of malignancy (63%). Solid nodules, on the other hand, had an incidence rate of 7%.[86] The persistent presence of a solitary GGN usually supports the diagnosis of BAC or mixed adenocarcinoma with BAC, atypical adenomatous hyperplasia (AAH) (which is now believed to be a precursor to adenocarcinoma), and, less frequently, inflammatory causes such as organizing pneumonia and focal interstitial fibrosis.[88] Pulmonary lymphoproliferative disorder is another, although less common cause, of a GGN. When multiple GGNs are present, multiple synchronous adenocarcinomas are a consideration including other causes such as eosinophilic lung disease.[89]

Adenocarcinoma is composed of a spectrum of entities with varying malignant behavior ranging from preneoplasia of AAH to BAC to invasive adenocarcinoma. The development of collapse fibrosis and ultimately invasion is a result of the continuum of pathologic changes that leads to stepwise progression for some but not all adenocarcinomas.[90] Recently, the pathologic classification of adenocarcinoma has changed, developed by the International Association for the Study of Lung Cancer.[91] The changes include an end to the use of the term "BAC," to be replaced by "adenocarcinoma in situ," representing tumors with lepidic growth without invasive features.[92] Minimally invasive carcinoma refers to any lesion 3 cm or smaller in which there is 5 mm or less of invasive areas, not necessarily in one location.

When CT imaging is compared to pathology, investigation has demonstrated that subsolid nodules containing some solid components correlate with lesions demonstrating collapse fibrosis, active fibroblast proliferation, and invasive features seen with higher grades of adenocarcinoma.[90,93] Lesions greater than 1 cm are more likely to represent adenocarcinoma than AAH. Nodular sphericity and internal air bronchograms have been described as findings on thin-section helical CT that can differentiate between BAC and AAH,[79] although there is overlap in their imaging appearance. A large number of studies have compared CT to the previous Noguchi and World Health Organization pathologic classification systems. Thus, with the new International Association for the Study of Lung Cancer classification, it is unclear in terms of the correlation of CT with the newer classification.

In terms of differentiating benign from malignant subsolid nodules, Li and colleagues[94] reported that the margin characteristics and the sizes of GGNs were not useful in differentiating between benign and malignant lesions. Round shape was found more frequently in pure ground-glass malignant lesions rather than in benign lesions. Mixed GGNs with central solid attenuation and peripheral ground-glass regions were associated more often with malignant entities. In their evaluation of persistent nodules,[88] Kim and colleagues also did not find any significant differences in morphologic features among benign and malignant causes of persistent GGNs. However, Lee and colleagues[95] identified a size greater than 8 mm and a lobulated border for pure GGNs as being predictive of malignancy.

CT HALO SIGN

The halo sign is identified as an ill-defined rim of ground-glass attenuation surrounding a pulmonary nodule.[96] The finding is nonspecific and may represent BAC, hemorrhage, or inflammation, initially described in the setting of invasive fungal *Aspergillus* infection (**Fig. 11**). Inflammatory and infectious causes, particularly organizing pneumonia, can sometimes demonstrate a reverse-halo sign, where a central focal area of ground-glass attenuation is surrounded by a peripheral rim of consolidation.[97]

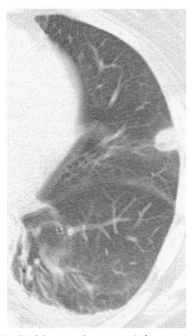

Fig. 11. Evolving pulmonary infarct. A well-circumscribed nodular peripheral density abutting the lingular visceral pleura lacked air bronchograms on axial CT section. Three weeks earlier, the finding had ground-glass opacity in the periphery with poorly-defined margins and a broad base of contact with the pleura.

NODULE GROWTH

An important and cost-effective step in the evaluation of a solitary pulmonary nodule is determining whether growth has occurred by comparing its size on a current image with that on prior images. Assessment is performed visually and can be quantified. Doubling time, representing the time required for a nodule to double in volume, for most malignant nodules is between 30 and 400 days.[98] Nodules that double more rapidly than 30 days are typically benign and related to infection, although lymphoma and metastases may on occasion demonstrate rapid growth. Doubling times greater than 400 days have been associated with benign entities such as hamartomas (**Fig. 12**). Interestingly, however, Hasegawa and colleagues[99] conducted a growth rate analysis of small lung cancers detected during a 3-year mass screening program. They classified nodules as ground-glass opacity, as ground-glass opacity with a solid component, or as solid. Mean volume doubling times were 813, 457, and 149 days, respectively, for these 3 types, all of which were significantly different (**Fig. 13**). Thus, GGNs that are lung cancer can exhibit very long doubling times (**Fig. 14**). Persistent GGNs that represent lung cancer may also progress by increasing density with or without concomitant size increase. GGNs have been infrequently described as decreasing in size, reflecting

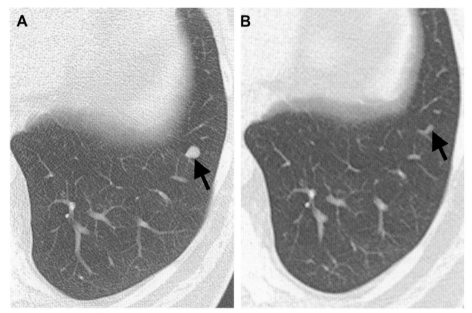

Fig. 12. Increasing small peripheral carcinoid. The well-circumscribed, smoothly marginated nodule in the left lower lobe on axial CT scan (*A*) grew from a small nodule (*arrow*) as shown in an axial image from a study obtained 5.5 years earlier (*B*).

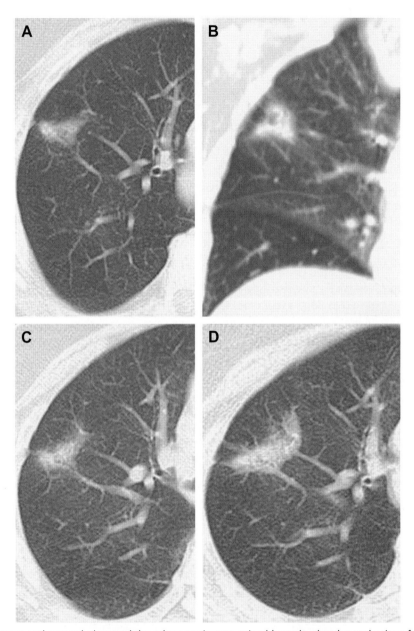

Fig. 13. Air space and ground-glass nodule: adenocarcinoma, mixed bronchoalveolar and acinar features. Axial (*A*) chest CT scan demonstrates a lesion showing branching on the axial projection, whereas the coronal view (*B*) demonstrates the rounded nature, thus supporting the utility of including multiple planes in the evaluation. Axial CT sections for studies at 11 months (*C*) and 22 months (*D*) later showed an increase in the lesion in terms of size and density. Malignancy was proven by resection and pathologic examination.

increasing fibrosis. Thus, continued interval chest CT follow-up is warranted in this setting.[100]

Additionally, it can be difficult to reliably detect growth in small nodules of less than 1 cm.[101] Traditionally, pulmonary nodule measurement has involved 2-dimensional caliper measurement of the largest nodule diameter, its perpendicular breadth, and the average of the largest lengths. Significant intrareader and interreader variability has been reported using 2-dimensional measurements and electronic caliper placement, particularly in lesions with spiculated margins.[102,103] For example, a 5-mm nodule can double in volume during a 6-month period (malignant growth rate), but its diameter will increase by only 1.25 to 6.25 mm. For a nodule to double in volume, the change in nodule diameter is approximately 26%.[104]

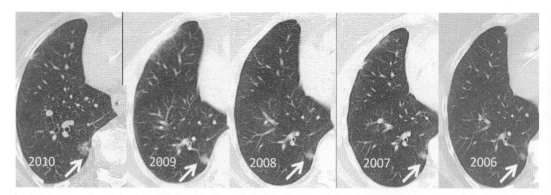

Fig. 14. Increased nodule size and density. A small nodule increased slowly over time in terms of size and density. Note the change in the border morphology in addition to one with a more lobulated appearance. Adenocarcinoma with lepidic components can increase in density without a large appreciable change in overall size.

VOLUMETRIC ANALYSIS

To overcome these limitations, volume measurement has been suggested as a more reproducible and reliable means for assessing growth. Although manual volumetry is time consuming, automated techniques are increasingly available. Variability in volumetric analysis may particularly affect measurement of perivascular, speculated, and pleura-based nodules[105] and also may vary depending on whether intravenous contrast is administered.[106] Volumetric techniques, however, are also susceptible to error. Variability of lung nodule software in patients scanned 3 times in the same session has been reported to have an interscan volumetric variation of ±20%.[107] Applications of volumetric 3-dimensional measurement tools include characterization of lung nodules in addition to measurement of known malignancy/whether expressed in the longest dimension or in volume. Increasing use of volumetric software will be facilitated by integration with clinical workflow via picture archiving and communication systems.

NODULE ENHANCEMENT

Contrast-enhanced CT can be used to further non-invasively assess lung nodules. This has been investigated as a method to differentiate benign and malignant nodules, with the degree of enhancement directly related to the likelihood of malignancy and the vascularity of the nodule.[108] Enhancement of a nodule of less than 15 HU after contrast material administration is strongly predictive of a benign lesion, whereas enhancement of more than 20 HU typically indicates malignancy (sensitivity, 98%; specificity, 73%; accuracy, 85%).[109] Regions of interest placed to measure attenuation measurements should comprise approximately 70% of the nodule diameter with measurement performed on mediastinal window settings to reduce partial volume averaging. This technique is performed so that contiguous thin sections are reviewed. Application of this technique should not be performed on lesions with calcium, areas of fluid attenuation representing obvious necrosis on precontrast CT scans, or ground-glass opacity.

Dual-energy CT allows material differentiation of iodine and thus simultaneously provides a virtual non–contrast-enhanced (VNC) and an iodine-enhanced image from a single image acquisition after the administration of iodine contrast material (**Fig. 15**).[110] Technology for dual-energy CT imaging includes dual- and single-source systems. This technique may eliminate the need to acquire non-enhanced CT before scanning with intravenous contrast, thus reducing patient's radiation exposure.[111] Chae and colleagues[111] investigated the accuracy of both VNC and iodine-enhanced images for the evaluation of pulmonary nodule. In their study, the VNC image demonstrated 85% of the calcifications in nodules that were visible on a true non–contrast-enhanced CT. Diagnostic quality for VNC images was the same as for true noncontrast imaging in 77.6% or inferior yet diagnostic in 16.3%, respectively. HU differences between VNC and true non–contrast-enhanced evaluation was 4.3 on average with a 95% confidence interval of −14.6 to 23.3 HU. In terms of iodine-enhanced images in comparison to traditional nodule enhancement, the average difference was −0.5 HU (95% confidence interval of −17.6 to 16.5 HU). Sensitivity for malignancy using iodine-enhanced images using 20 HU as a cutoff was 92%, whereas specificity was 70%.

PET CT EVALUATION

Positron emission tomography (PET) provides in vivo functional mapping of 2-deoxy-2[^{18}F]

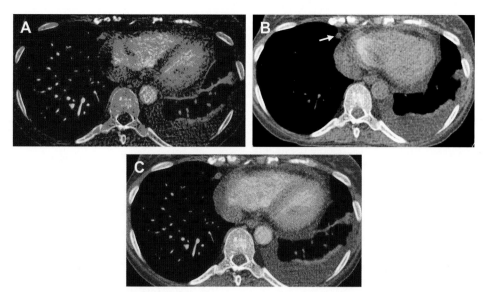

Fig. 15. Nodular metastasis with enhancement. Dual-energy CT imaging performed with intravenous contrast with subsequent material decomposition reveals iodine distributed in a small nodule on iodine-enhanced image (*A*). Nodule is shown in the VNC image in the right middle lobe (*B*). The VNC image is generated during the same process as the iodine-enhanced image. An overlay of the iodine-enhanced and VNC (*C*) images can be performed for better correlation of iodine and anatomic information.

fluoro-D-glucose (FDG) uptake, which is elevated in neoplastic lesions (**Fig. 16**).[112,113] The value of PET CT in the diagnosis of pulmonary nodules is well documented with meta-analysis–reported sensitivity of 90% and specificity of 83% for diagnosing malignancy.[114] The high specificity of FDG PET for the diagnosis of benign lesions has important clinical utility. Lesions with low FDG uptake may be considered benign; however; these lesions should be followed radiologically because of false-

negative results.[115] Certain histologic types such as low-grade adenocarcinoma, BAC,[116] and carcinoid tumors may give rise to false-negative FDG evaluations. In addition, the diagnostic performance of PET decreases considerably for lesions of less than 6 mm. False-positive results may also be seen with infectious or inflammatory processes and granulomatous disorders such as granulomatosis with polyangiitis (Wegener granulomatosis) or sarcoidosis. In some circumstances,

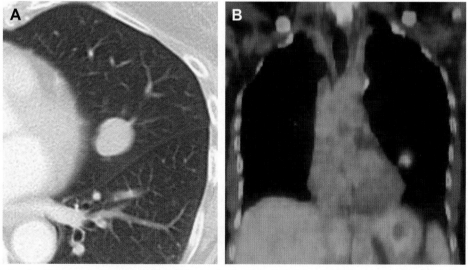

Fig. 16. Carcinoid tumor with FDG PET uptake. A well-circumscribed, smoothly marginated mildly lobulated nodule in the lingula (*A*) had increased FDG uptake on fused PET CT image (*B*). Carcinoid lesions may not have abnormal uptake.

FDG PET can be used to direct tissue biopsy and to identify which lesions or portions of lesions are metabolically active and most likely to yield a definitive tissue result.[117]

NODULE BIOPSY

In pursuing a tissue diagnosis of a suspected lung cancer, there is a range of procedures from which to choose. Transthoracic needle aspiration and biopsy, bronchoscopy, video-assisted thoracoscopic surgery, or thoracotomy may be performed. The method of diagnosis depends on the type of lung cancer, the size and location of the primary tumor, the presence of metastasis, and the overall clinical status of the patient. Studies have shown that the diagnostic sensitivity of bronchoscopy for peripheral lung cancer is 78% but only 34% for lesions with a diameter of less than 2 cm.[118] The decision of whether to pursue a diagnostic bronchoscopy for a lesion that is suspicious for lung cancer largely depends on the location of the lesion in terms of whether it is central or peripheral.[119,120]

For peripheral lung lesions, the sensitivity of transthoracic needle aspiration biopsy (TNAB) is higher than that of bronchoscopy. Percutaneous fine-needle biopsy is accurate for diagnosing malignancy, with reported sensitivities varying from 70% to 100%[121–123] Nodules that are ideal for percutaneous sampling are accessible without crossing major vascular structures and fissures.[124] In patients who have lung cancer, TNAB sampling has approximately a 90% chance of providing confirmation of the diagnosis with a low false-positive rate rendering a positive finding for cancer reliable. The confirmation of a benign diagnosis is more problematic when performing needle aspiration alone. Acquiring a biopsy sample at time of TNAB after the acquisition aspiration increases the diagnostic yield for benign diagnosis from 12% to 75%.[125]

TNAB is generally regarded as a safe procedure with limited morbidity and extremely rare mortality.[126] Complications, most notably pneumothorax, occur in approximately 5% to 30% of patients.[127–129] A recent study confirms previous reports that older age and the presence of chronic obstructive pulmonary disease increase complication rates,[130] with more than 6% of CT-guided biopsies that result in pneumothorax requiring a chest tube, a clinically important complication.

Thoracotomy remains the most invasive but effective means to obtain a histologic diagnosis. The operative mortality of thoracotomy is 3% to 7% for malignant nodules and less than 1% for benign nodules.[131,132] Decreased perioperative mortality and hospital stays have been achieved with the development of video-assisted thoracoscopy.[61]

PULMONARY NODULE MANAGEMENT STRATEGIES
Pretest Probability of Malignancy

The approach to managing pulmonary nodules is multidisciplinary, with input from pulmonologists, surgeons, and radiologists. The evaluation of a pulmonary nodule has been summarized by the American College of Chest Physicians Clinical Practice Guidelines.[14] Specific clinical features determined to be significant predictors of malignancy are older age, smoking history, and personal history of cancer greater than 5 or more years prior to nodule detection.

The clinical probability of malignancy in patients with SPNs assists in directing appropriate management strategies. Current quantitative models for the risk of malignancy incorporate the patient's personal risk factors for lung cancer as well as characteristics of the lung lesion itself. Bayesian theory and neural network–based methods using factors such as smoking history and age have been studied.[59,133,134] A multiple logistic regression model[135] identified 4 independent risk factors for predicting malignancy: positive smoking history, older patient age, larger nodule diameter, and time since smoking cessation. The respective odds ratios for these factors were 7.9, 2.2 (for each decade of life), 1.1 (for each mm), and 0.6 (for each decade since stopping smoking).[135]

Decision-analysis models have suggested that most effective management strategies for solitary pulmonary nodules depend on the probability of an SPN being malignant. The most pertinent strategy in terms of cost-effectiveness was simple surveillance for nodules with a low probability of malignancy (<5%), immediate surgical resection for those with a high probability of malignancy (≥60%), and biopsy or noninvasive imaging evaluation with FDG PET or nodule enhancement CT for those with a probability of malignancy between 5% and 60%.[136]

Fleischner Society Guidelines

On the basis of collective evidence that suggests that a substantial number of solitary pulmonary nodules are benign,[13,137] the Fleischner Society issued a set of guidelines in 2005 for the management of indeterminate nodules incidentally detected during CT examinations performed for clinical purposes other than lung cancer screening.[36] Their development was in response to a perceived need for guidance in the management and follow-up of small nodules that are frequently detected with MDCT technology. Of note, the Fleischner guidelines do not apply to patients with a history of malignancy, those younger than 35 years unless there is a known primary cancer, and those with a fever, in whom the nodules may have an infectious cause. For pulmonary nodule a follow-up noncontrast, thin-collimation, low-dose CT scan is recommended by the Fleischner Society. Risk factors are considered in these guidelines and include smoking, family history of lung cancer, and environmental exposures.

Given that 99% of all nodules that measure 4 mm or less are benign and that these small opacities are seen very frequently on thin-section CT examinations, systematic CT reassessment is no longer recommended for those with low risk. A single CT examination can be performed at 12 months in high-risk individuals. For nodules measuring between 4 and 8 mm, surveillance is the most appropriate strategy, with 2-year stability considered an indicator of benignity. The timing of these examinations varies according to the nodule size (4–6 or 6–8 mm) and type of patient whether low or high risk for having malignancy. Different management options apply to nodules greater than 8 mm, including study of enhancement on CT, PET CT, percutaneous needle biopsy, or video-assisted thoracoscopic resection. In high-risk patients, the optimal strategy probably remains that of biopsy or nodule resection.

GGN Management

Proposed interim management guidelines for ground-glass and subsolid pulmonary nodules have been proposed by Godoy and Naidich.[89] It is currently debated whether pure GGNs that are less than 5 mm necessarily require follow-up CT studies given their association with AAH; for those larger than 5 mm, follow-up is requisite pending better definition of their true nature.

Nodules with pure ground-glass attenuation that are larger than 5 mm represent AAH or BAC and initially assessed, such as at 3 months with subsequent annual evaluation, to identify any invasive adenocarcinomas presenting as a pure GGN. The duration of surveillance at this point has not been established but probably is longer than that for solid counterparts given the slow growth rates associated with pure GGNs. It should be noted that 20% to 25% will prove to be benign at resection; surgery should be considered especially if the nodule is enlarging or if there is an increase in attenuation or development of a solid component. Persistent lesions with mixed solid component and ground-glass attenuation should also be presumed malignant, and further evaluation with FDG PET and surgical resection should be considered, particularly for those with solid components comprising more than half of the nodule. TNAB can also be considered in accessible lesions. High-resolution thin-section evaluation of ground-glass–containing lesions will assist in characterizing the degree of soft tissue and interval change in solid and ground-glass components.

Adherence to Guidelines

A recent study[138] assessing adherence to Fleischner Society guidelines for management of small lung nodules reported that surveyed radiologists, when given potential nodule management scenarios, made management selections that were consistent with the Fleischner guidelines in 34.7% to 60.8% of responses. A significantly higher rate of concordance occurred in those who were aware of the Fleischner guidelines (77.8%), had written policies based on them, were working in a teaching practice setting, practiced in a group with at least one member having fellowship training in thoracic radiology, and had fewer than 5 years of experience practicing radiology. Even though the respondents reported high awareness and use of the Fleischner guidelines, conformance varied. There are many reasons offered for this apparent inconsistent approach.[139] The American College of Chest Physicians systematic review of evidence-based clinical guidelines regarding the management of pulmonary nodules concludes that assessment of risk factors, including risks/benefits of biopsy, surgery, and further observation, is critical, and patient preference plays a role.[14] Additionally, there is interreader variability in 2-dimensional measurements involving electronic caliper placement when measuring noncalcified pulmonary nodules.[140] Similarly, CT measurement of a nodule has limitations with a well-described "zone of transition" of the distance between nonaerated solid tumor and surrounding nonneoplastic pulmonary parenchyma.[141] The authors stress that this consideration is especially a limitation for radiologic assessment of subcentimeter subsolid nodules.

SUMMARY

With the use of MDCT as a diagnostic modality, the incidental detection of solitary subcentimeter pulmonary nodules has increased substantially. If there are no definite benign morphologic findings, the solitary pulmonary nodule must be classified as an indeterminate, possibly malignant lesion.

Many solitary pulmonary nodules have similar features, and malignant nodules may be inaccurately classified as benign after radiologic assessment of size, margins, contour, and internal characteristics. Patients with an indeterminate pulmonary nodule should be evaluated with knowledge of expert consensus-based recommendations for performing follow-up CT scans and tissue sampling. Clinical management of these incidental nodules relies not only on imaging characteristics but also on patient risk factors for malignancy, the weighing of the risks and benefits of further investigation, and consideration of patient preference.

REFERENCES

1. Brandman S, Ko JP. Pulmonary nodule detection, characterization, and management with multidetector computed tomography. J Thorac Imaging 2011;26(2):90–105.

2. Huppmann MV, Johnson WB, Javitt MC. Radiation risks from exposure to chest computed tomography. Semin Ultrasound CT MR 2010;31(1):14–28.

3. Edey AJ, Hansell DM. Incidentally detected small pulmonary nodules on CT. Clin Radiol 2009;64(9):872–84.

4. Truong MT, Sabloff BS, Ko JP. Multidetector CT of solitary pulmonary nodules. Thorac Surg Clin 2010;20(1):9–23.

5. Henschke CI, McCauley DI, Yankelevitz DF, et al. Early lung cancer action project: a summary of the findings on baseline screening. Oncologist 2001;6(2):147–52.

6. Good CA, Wilson TW. The solitary circumscribed pulmonary nodule; study of seven hundred five cases encountered roentgenologically in a period of three and one-half years. JAMA 1958;166(3):210–5.

7. Midthun DE. Solitary pulmonary nodule: time to think small. Curr Opin Pulm Med 2000;6(4):364–70.

8. Hansell DM, Bankier AA, MacMahon H, et al. Fleischner Society: glossary of terms for thoracic imaging. Radiology 2008;246(3):697–722.

9. Remy-Jardin M, Remy J, Wallaert B, et al. Subacute and chronic bird breeder hypersensitivity pneumonitis: sequential evaluation with CT and correlation with lung function tests and bronchoalveolar lavage. Radiology 1993;189(1):111–8.

10. Brauner MW, Lenoir S, Grenier P, et al. Pulmonary sarcoidosis: CT assessment of lesion reversibility. Radiology 1992;182(2):349–54.

11. Costello P, Anderson W, Blume D. Pulmonary nodule: evaluation with spiral volumetric CT. Radiology 1991;179(3):875–6.

12. Hanamiya M, Aoki T, Yamashita Y, et al. Frequency and significance of pulmonary nodules on thin-section CT in patients with extrapulmonary malignant neoplasms. Eur J Radiol 2012;81(1):152–7.

13. Henschke CI, McCauley DI, Yankelevitz DF, et al. Early Lung Cancer Action Project: overall design and findings from baseline screening. Lancet 1999;354(9173):99–105.

14. Gould MK, Fletcher J, Iannettoni MD, et al. Evaluation of patients with pulmonary nodules: when is it lung cancer? ACCP evidence-based clinical practice guidelines (2nd edition). Chest 2007;132(Suppl 3):108S–30S.

15. Wahidi MM, Govert JA, Goudar RK, et al. Evidence for the treatment of patients with pulmonary nodules: when is it lung cancer? ACCP evidence-based clinical practice guidelines (2nd edition). Chest 2007;132(Suppl 3):94S–107S.

16. Boone JM. Multidetector CT: opportunities, challenges, and concerns associated with scanners with 64 or more detector rows. Radiology 2006;241(2):334–7.

17. Swensen SJ, Jett JR, Sloan JA, et al. Screening for lung cancer with low-dose spiral computed tomography. Am J Respir Crit Care Med 2002;165(4):508–13.

18. Austin JH, Romney BM, Goldsmith LS. Missed bronchogenic carcinoma: radiographic findings in 27 patients with a potentially resectable lesion evident in retrospect. Radiology 1992;182(1):115–22.

19. Quekel LG, Kessels AG, Goei R, et al. Miss rate of lung cancer on the chest radiograph in clinical practice. Chest 1999;115(3):720–4.

20. Turkington PM, Kennan N, Greenstone MA. Misinterpretation of the chest x ray as a factor in the delayed diagnosis of lung cancer. Postgrad Med J 2002;78(917):158–60.

21. Shah PK, Austin JH, White CS, et al. Missed non-small cell lung cancer: radiographic findings of potentially resectable lesions evident only in retrospect. Radiology 2003;226(1):235–41.

22. Muhm JR, Miller WE, Fontana RS, et al. Lung cancer detected during a screening program using four-month chest radiographs. Radiology 1983;148(3):609–15.

23. Samuel S, Kundel HL, Nodine CF, et al. Mechanism of satisfaction of search: eye position recordings in the reading of chest radiographs. Radiology 1995;194(3):895–902.

24. Kundel HL, Nodine CF, Toto L. Searching for lung nodules. The guidance of visual scanning. Invest Radiol 1991;26(9):777–81.

25. Tagashira H, Arakawa K, Yoshimoto M, et al. Detectability of lung nodules using flat panel detector with dual energy subtraction by two shot method: evaluation by ROC method. Eur J Radiol 2007;64(2):279–84.

26. Fischbach F, Freund T, Rottgen R, et al. Dual-energy chest radiography with a flat-panel digital

detector: revealing calcified chest abnormalities. AJR Am J Roentgenol 2003;181(6):1519–24.

27. Balkman JD, Mehandru S, DuPont E, et al. Dual energy subtraction digital radiography improves performance of a next generation computer-aided detection program. J Thorac Imaging 2010;25(1):41–7.

28. Kano A, Doi K, MacMahon H, et al. Digital image subtraction of temporally sequential chest images for detection of interval change. Med Phys 1994;21(3):453–61.

29. Ishida T, Ashizawa K, Engelmann R, et al. Application of temporal subtraction for detection of interval changes on chest radiographs: improvement of subtraction images using automated initial image matching. J Digit Imaging 1999;12(2):77–86.

30. McAdams HP, Samei E, Dobbins J 3rd, et al. Recent advances in chest radiography. Radiology 2006;241(3):663–83.

31. Matsumoto T, Yoshimura H, Giger ML, et al. Potential usefulness of computerized nodule detection in screening programs for lung cancer. Invest Radiol 1992;27(6):471–5.

32. MacMahon H, Engelmann R, Behlen FM, et al. Computer-aided diagnosis of pulmonary nodules: results of a large-scale observer test. Radiology 1999;213(3):723–6.

33. Johkoh T, Kozuka T, Tomiyama N, et al. Temporal subtraction for detection of solitary pulmonary nodules on chest radiographs: evaluation of a commercially available computer-aided diagnosis system. Radiology 2002;223(3):806–11.

34. Sieren JC, Ohno Y, Koyama H, et al. Recent technological and application developments in computed tomography and magnetic resonance imaging for improved pulmonary nodule detection and lung cancer staging. J Magn Reson Imaging 2010;32(6):1353–69.

35. Fischbach F, Knollmann F, Griesshaber V, et al. Detection of pulmonary nodules by multislice computed tomography: improved detection rate with reduced slice thickness. Eur Radiol 2003;13(10):2378–83.

36. MacMahon H, Austin JH, Gamsu G, et al. Guidelines for management of small pulmonary nodules detected on CT scans: a statement from the Fleischner Society. Radiology 2005;237(2):395–400.

37. Angel E, Yaghmai N, Jude CM, et al. Monte Carlo simulations to assess the effects of tube current modulation on breast dose for multidetector CT. Phys Med Biol 2009;54(3):497–512.

38. Angel E, Yaghmai N, Jude CM, et al. Dose to radiosensitive organs during routine chest CT: effects of tube current modulation. AJR Am J Roentgenol 2009;193(5):1340–5.

39. McCollough CH, Bruesewitz MR, Kofler JM Jr. CT dose reduction and dose management tools: overview of available options. Radiographics 2006;26(2):503–12.

40. McCollough CH, Primak AN, Braun N, et al. Strategies for reducing radiation dose in CT. Radiol Clin North Am 2009;47(1):27–40.

41. Moses DA, Ko JP. Multidetector CT of the solitary pulmonary nodule. Semin Roentgenol 2005;40(2):109–25.

42. Swensen SJ, Morin RL, Aughenbaugh GL, et al. CT reconstruction algorithm selection in the evaluation of solitary pulmonary nodules. J Comput Assist Tomogr 1995;19(6):932–5.

43. Ahn MI, Gleeson TG, Chan IH, et al. Perifissural nodules seen at CT screening for lung cancer. Radiology 2010;254(3):949–56.

44. Diederich S, Semik M, Lentschig MG, et al. Helical CT of pulmonary nodules in patients with extrathoracic malignancy: CT-surgical correlation. AJR Am J Roentgenol 1999;172(2):353–60.

45. Gurney JW. Missed lung cancer at CT: imaging findings in nine patients. Radiology 1996;199(1):117–22.

46. Ko JP, Rusinek H, Naidich DP, et al. Wavelet compression of low-dose chest CT data: effect on lung nodule detection. Radiology 2003;228(1):70–5.

47. Park EA, Goo JM, Lee JW, et al. Efficacy of computer-aided detection system and thin-slab maximum intensity projection technique in the detection of pulmonary nodules in patients with resected metastases. Invest Radiol 2009;44(2):105–13.

48. Rubin GD. Data explosion: the challenge of multidetector-row CT. Eur J Radiol 2000;36(2):74–80.

49. Kawel N, Seifert B, Luetolf M, et al. Effect of slab thickness on the CT detection of pulmonary nodules: use of sliding thin-slab maximum intensity projection and volume rendering. AJR Am J Roentgenol 2009;192(5):1324–9.

50. Hirose T, Nitta N, Shiraishi J, et al. Evaluation of computer-aided diagnosis (CAD) software for the detection of lung nodules on multidetector row computed tomography (MDCT): JAFROC study for the improvement in radiologists' diagnostic accuracy. Acad Radiol 2008;15(12):1505–12.

51. White CS, Pugatch R, Koonce T, et al. Lung nodule CAD software as a second reader: a multicenter study. Acad Radiol 2008;15(3):326–33.

52. Rubin GD, Lyo JK, Paik DS, et al. Pulmonary nodules on multi-detector row CT scans: performance comparison of radiologists and computer-aided detection. Radiology 2005;234(1):274–83.

53. Awai K, Murao K, Ozawa A, et al. Pulmonary nodules: estimation of malignancy at thin-section helical CT-effect of computer-aided diagnosis on performance of radiologists. Radiology 2006;239(1):276–84.

54. Kim KG, Goo JM, Kim JH, et al. Computer-aided diagnosis of localized ground-glass opacity in the lung at CT: initial experience. Radiology 2005; 237(2):657–61.

55. Jacobs C, Sanchez CI, Saur SC, et al. Computer-aided detection of ground glass nodules in thoracic CT images using shape, intensity and context features. Med Image Comput Comput Assist Interv 2011;14(Pt 3):207–14.

56. Okada T, Iwano S, Ishigaki T, et al. Computer-aided diagnosis of lung cancer: definition and detection of ground-glass opacity type of nodules by high-resolution computed tomography. Jpn J Radiol 2009;27(2):91–9.

57. Ye X, Lin X, Beddoe G, et al. Efficient computer-aided detection of ground-glass opacity nodules in thoracic CT images. Conf Proc IEEE Eng Med Biol Soc 2007;2007:4449–52.

58. Zwirewich CV, Vedal S, Miller RR, et al. Solitary pulmonary nodule: high-resolution CT and radiologic-pathologic correlation. Radiology 1991; 179(2):469–76.

59. Gurney JW, Swensen SJ. Solitary pulmonary nodules: determining the likelihood of malignancy with neural network analysis. Radiology 1995; 196(3):823–9.

60. Takashima S, Sone S, Li F, et al. Small solitary pulmonary nodules (< or =1 cm) detected at population-based CT screening for lung cancer: reliable high-resolution CT features of benign lesions. AJR Am J Roentgenol 2003;180(4): 955–64.

61. Suzuki K, Nagai K, Yoshida J, et al. Video-assisted thoracoscopic surgery for small indeterminate pulmonary nodules: indications for preoperative marking. Chest 1999;115(2):563–8.

62. Ginsberg MS, Griff SK, Go BD, et al. Pulmonary nodules resected at video-assisted thoracoscopic surgery: etiology in 426 patients. Radiology 1999; 213(1):277–82.

63. Gohagan J, Marcus P, Fagerstrom R, et al. Baseline findings of a randomized feasibility trial of lung cancer screening with spiral CT scan vs chest radiograph: the Lung Screening Study of the National Cancer Institute. Chest 2004;126(1):114–21.

64. Church TR. Chest radiography as the comparison for spiral CT in the National Lung Screening Trial. Acad Radiol 2003;10(6):713–5.

65. Zerhouni EA, Spivey JF, Morgan RH, et al. Factors influencing quantitative CT measurements of solitary pulmonary nodules. J Comput Assist Tomogr 1982;6(6):1075–87.

66. Swensen SJ, Silverstein MD, Ilstrup DM, et al. The probability of malignancy in solitary pulmonary nodules. Application to small radiologically indeterminate nodules. Arch Intern Med 1997; 157(8):849–55.

67. Bankoff MS, McEniff NJ, Bhadelia RA, et al. Prevalence of pathologically proven intrapulmonary lymph nodes and their appearance on CT. AJR Am J Roentgenol 1996;167(3):629–30.

68. Sykes AM, Swensen SJ, Tazelaar HD, et al. Computed tomography of benign intrapulmonary lymph nodes: retrospective comparison with sarcoma metastases. Mayo Clin Proc 2002;77(4): 329–33.

69. Hyodo T, Kanazawa S, Dendo S, et al. Intrapulmonary lymph nodes: thin-section CT findings, pathological findings, and CT differential diagnosis from pulmonary metastatic nodules. Acta Med Okayama 2004;58(5):235–40.

70. Xu DM, van der Zaag-Loonen HJ, Oudkerk M, et al. Smooth or attached solid indeterminate nodules detected at baseline CT screening in the NELSON study: cancer risk during 1 year of follow-up. Radiology 2009;250(1):264–72.

71. Heitzman ER, Markarian B, Raasch BN, et al. Pathways of tumor spread through the lung: radiologic correlations with anatomy and pathology. Radiology 1982;144(1):3–14.

72. Xu DM, van Klaveren RJ, de Bock GH, et al. Limited value of shape, margin and CT density in the discrimination between benign and malignant screen detected solid pulmonary nodules of the NELSON trial. Eur J Radiol 2008;68(2):347–52.

73. Siegelman SS, Zerhouni EA, Leo FP, et al. CT of the solitary pulmonary nodule. AJR Am J Roentgenol 1980;135(1):1–13.

74. Girvin F, Ko JP. Pulmonary nodules: detection, assessment, and CAD. AJR Am J Roentgenol 2008;191(4):1057–69.

75. Winer-Muram HT. The solitary pulmonary nodule. Radiology 2006;239(1):34–49.

76. Onn A, Choe DH, Herbst RS, et al. Tumor cavitation in stage I non-small cell lung cancer: epidermal growth factor receptor expression and prediction of poor outcome. Radiology 2005; 237(1):342–7.

77. Woodring JH, Fried AM. Significance of wall thickness in solitary cavities of the lung: a follow-up study. AJR Am J Roentgenol 1983;140(3):473–4.

78. Honda O, Tsubamoto M, Inoue A, et al. Pulmonary cavitary nodules on computed tomography: differentiation of malignancy and benignancy. J Comput Assist Tomogr 2007;31(6):943–9.

79. Oda S, Awai K, Liu D, et al. Ground-glass opacities on thin-section helical CT: differentiation between bronchioloalveolar carcinoma and atypical adenomatous hyperplasia. AJR Am J Roentgenol 2008; 190(5):1363–8.

80. Erasmus JJ, Connolly JE, McAdams HP, et al. Solitary pulmonary nodules: part I. Morphologic evaluation for differentiation of benign and malignant lesions. Radiographics 2000;20(1):43–58.

81. Diederich S, Wormanns D, Semik M, et al. Screening for early lung cancer with low-dose spiral CT: prevalence in 817 asymptomatic smokers. Radiology 2002;222(3):773–81.

82. Hamper UM, Khouri NF, Stitik FP, et al. Pulmonary hamartoma: diagnosis by transthoracic needle-aspiration biopsy. Radiology 1985;155(1):15–8.

83. Mahoney MC, Shipley RT, Corcoran HL, et al. CT demonstration of calcification in carcinoma of the lung. AJR Am J Roentgenol 1990;154(2):255–8.

84. Seo JB, Im JG, Goo JM, et al. Atypical pulmonary metastases: spectrum of radiologic findings. Radiographics 2001;21(2):403–17.

85. Grewal RG, Austin JH. CT demonstration of calcification in carcinoma of the lung. J Comput Assist Tomogr 1994;18(6):867–71.

86. Henschke CI, Yankelevitz DF, Mirtcheva R, et al. CT screening for lung cancer: frequency and significance of part-solid and nonsolid nodules. AJR Am J Roentgenol 2002;178(5):1053–7.

87. Ko JP. Lung nodule detection and characterization with multi-slice CT. J Thorac Imaging 2005;20(3): 196–209.

88. Kim HY, Shim YM, Lee KS, et al. Persistent pulmonary nodular ground-glass opacity at thin-section CT: histopathologic comparisons. Radiology 2007; 245(1):267–75.

89. Godoy MC, Naidich DP. Subsolid pulmonary nodules and the spectrum of peripheral adenocarcinomas of the lung: recommended interim guidelines for assessment and management. Radiology 2009;253(3):606–22.

90. Noguchi M, Shimosato Y. The development and progression of adenocarcinoma of the lung. Cancer Treat Res 1995;72:131–42.

91. Travis WD, Brambilla E, Noguchi M, et al. International Association for the Study of Lung Cancer/ American Thoracic Society/European Respiratory Society international multidisciplinary classification of lung adenocarcinoma. J Thorac Oncol 2011; 6(2):244–85.

92. Travis WD, Brambilla E, Noguchi M, et al. International Association for the Study of Lung Cancer/ American Thoracic Society/European Respiratory Society: international multidisciplinary classification of lung adenocarcinoma: executive summary. Proc Am Thorac Soc 2011;8(5):381–5.

93. Aoki T, Nakata H, Watanabe H, et al. Evolution of peripheral lung adenocarcinomas: CT findings correlated with histology and tumor doubling time. AJR Am J Roentgenol 2000;174(3):763–8.

94. Li F, Sone S, Abe H, et al. Malignant versus benign nodules at CT screening for lung cancer: comparison of thin-section CT findings. Radiology 2004; 233(3):793–8.

95. Lee HJ, Goo JM, Lee CH, et al. Predictive CT findings of malignancy in ground-glass nodules on thin-section chest CT: the effects on radiologist performance. Eur Radiol 2009;19(3):552–60.

96. Georgiadou SP, Sipsas NV, Marom EM, et al. The diagnostic value of halo and reversed halo signs for invasive mold infections in compromised hosts. Clin Infect Dis 2011;52(9):1144–55.

97. Kim SJ, Lee KS, Ryu YH, et al. Reversed halo sign on high-resolution CT of cryptogenic organizing pneumonia: diagnostic implications. AJR Am J Roentgenol 2003;180(5):1251–4.

98. Lillington GA, Caskey CI. Evaluation and management of solitary and multiple pulmonary nodules. Clin Chest Med 1993;14(1):111–9.

99. Hasegawa M, Sone S, Takashima S, et al. Growth rate of small lung cancers detected on mass CT screening. Br J Radiol 2000;73(876):1252–9.

100. Kakinuma R, Ohmatsu H, Kaneko M, et al. Progression of focal pure ground-glass opacity detected by low-dose helical computed tomography screening for lung cancer. J Comput Assist Tomogr 2004; 28(1):17–23.

101. Yankelevitz DF, Henschke CI. Does 2-year stability imply that pulmonary nodules are benign? AJR Am J Roentgenol 1997;168(2):325–8.

102. Zhao B, Yankelevitz D, Reeves A, et al. Two-dimensional multi-criterion segmentation of pulmonary nodules on helical CT images. Med Phys 1999; 26(6):889–95.

103. Yankelevitz DF, Gupta R, Zhao B, et al. Small pulmonary nodules: evaluation with repeat CT–preliminary experience. Radiology 1999;212(2): 561–6.

104. Erasmus JJ, McAdams HP, Connolly JE. Solitary pulmonary nodules: part II. Evaluation of the indeterminate nodule. Radiographics 2000;20(1): 59–66.

105. Wang Y, de Bock GH, van Klaveren RJ, et al. Volumetric measurement of pulmonary nodules at low-dose chest CT: effect of reconstruction setting on measurement variability. Eur Radiol 2010;20(5): 1180–7.

106. Rampinelli C, De Fiori E, Raimondi S, et al. In vivo repeatability of automated volume calculations of small pulmonary nodules with CT. AJR Am J Roentgenol 2009;192(6):1657–61.

107. Goodman LR, Gulsun M, Washington L, et al. Inherent variability of CT lung nodule measurements in vivo using semiautomated volumetric measurements. AJR Am J Roentgenol 2006;186(4): 989–94.

108. Swensen SJ. Functional CT: lung nodule evaluation. Radiographics 2000;20(4):1178–81.

109. Swensen SJ. Lung nodules: enchantment with enhancement. J Thorac Imaging 1995;10(2):89–90.

110. Johnson TR, Krauss B, Sedlmair M, et al. Material differentiation by dual energy CT: initial experience. Eur Radiol 2007;17(6):1510–7.

111. Chae EJ, Song JW, Seo JB, et al. Clinical utility of dual-energy CT in the evaluation of solitary pulmonary nodules: initial experience. Radiology 2008; 249(2):671–81.

112. Lowe VJ, Fletcher JW, Gobar L, et al. Prospective investigation of positron emission tomography in lung nodules. J Clin Oncol 1998;16(3):1075–84.

113. Patz EF Jr, Lowe VJ, Hoffman JM, et al. Focal pulmonary abnormalities: evaluation with F-18 fluorodeoxyglucose PET scanning. Radiology 1993; 188(2):487–90.

114. Rohren EM, Turkington TG, Coleman RE. Clinical applications of PET in oncology. Radiology 2004; 231(2):305–32.

115. Erasmus JJ, McAdams HP, Patz EF Jr, et al. Evaluation of primary pulmonary carcinoid tumors using FDG PET. AJR Am J Roentgenol 1998;170(5): 1369–73.

116. Higashi K, Ueda Y, Seki H, et al. Fluorine-18-FDG PET imaging is negative in bronchioloalveolar lung carcinoma. J Nucl Med 1998;39(6):1016–20.

117. Hain SF, Curran KM, Beggs AD, et al. FDG-PET as a "metabolic biopsy" tool in thoracic lesions with indeterminate biopsy. Eur J Nucl Med 2001;28(9): 1336–40.

118. Rivera MP, Mehta AC. Initial diagnosis of lung cancer: ACCP evidence-based clinical practice guidelines (2nd edition). Chest 2007;132(Suppl 3): 131S–48S.

119. Saita S, Tanzillo A, Riscica C, et al. Bronchial brushing and biopsy: a comparative evaluation in diagnosing visible bronchial lesions. Eur J Cardiothorac Surg 1990;4(5):270–2.

120. Cox ID, Bagg LR, Russell NJ, et al. Relationship of radiologic position to the diagnostic yield of fiberoptic bronchoscopy in bronchial carcinoma. Chest 1984;85(4):519–22.

121. Flower CD, Verney GI. Percutaneous needle biopsy of thoracic lesions—an evaluation of 300 biopsies. Clin Radiol 1979;30(2):215–8.

122. Klein JS, Zarka MA. Transthoracic needle biopsy. Radiol Clin North Am 2000;38(2):235–66, vii.

123. Klein JS, Salomon G, Stewart EA. Transthoracic needle biopsy with a coaxially placed 20-gauge automated cutting needle: results in 122 patients. Radiology 1996;198(3):715–20.

124. Moore EH. Technical aspects of needle aspiration lung biopsy: a personal perspective. Radiology 1998;208(2):303–18.

125. Boiselle PM, Shepard JA, Mark EJ, et al. Routine addition of an automated biopsy device to fine-needle aspiration of the lung: a prospective assessment. AJR Am J Roentgenol 1997;169(3):661–6.

126. Geraghty PR, Kee ST, McFarlane G, et al. CT-guided transthoracic needle aspiration biopsy of pulmonary nodules: needle size and pneumothorax rate. Radiology 2003;229(2):475–81.

127. Miller JA, Pramanik BK, Lavenhar MA. Predicting the rates of success and complications of computed tomography-guided percutaneous core-needle biopsies of the thorax from the findings of the pre-procedure chest computed tomography scan. J Thorac Imaging 1998;13(1):7–13.

128. Westcott JL, Rao N, Colley DP. Transthoracic needle biopsy of small pulmonary nodules. Radiology 1997;202(1):97–103.

129. Westcott JL. Percutaneous transthoracic needle biopsy. Radiology 1988;169(3):593–601.

130. Wiener RS, Schwartz LM, Woloshin S, et al. Population-based risk for complications after transthoracic needle lung biopsy of a pulmonary nodule: an analysis of discharge records. Ann Intern Med 2011;155(3):137–44.

131. Daly BD, Faling LJ, Diehl JT, et al. Computed tomography-guided minithoracotomy for the resection of small peripheral pulmonary nodules. Ann Thorac Surg 1991;51(3):465–9.

132. Krasna MJ, Deshmukh S, McLaughlin JS. Complications of thoracoscopy. Ann Thorac Surg 1996; 61(4):1066–9.

133. Gurney JW. Determining the likelihood of malignancy in solitary pulmonary nodules with Bayesian analysis. Part I. Theory. Radiology 1993;186(2): 405–13.

134. Gurney JW, Lyddon DM, McKay JA. Determining the likelihood of malignancy in solitary pulmonary nodules with Bayesian analysis. Part II. Application. Radiology 1993;186(2):415–22.

135. Gould MK, Ananth L, Barnett PG. A clinical model to estimate the pretest probability of lung cancer in patients with solitary pulmonary nodules. Chest 2007;131(2):383–8.

136. Cummings SR, Lillington GA, Richard RJ. Estimating the probability of malignancy in solitary pulmonary nodules. A Bayesian approach. Am Rev Respir Dis 1986;134(3):449–52.

137. Swensen SJ. CT screening for lung cancer. AJR Am J Roentgenol 2002;179(4):833–6.

138. Eisenberg RL, Bankier AA, Boiselle PM. Compliance with Fleischner Society guidelines for management of small lung nodules: a survey of 834 radiologists. Radiology 2010;255(1):218–24.

139. MacMahon H. Compliance with Fleischner Society guidelines for management of lung nodules: lessons and opportunities. Radiology 2010; 255(1):14–5.

140. Revel MP, Bissery A, Bienvenu M, et al. Are two-dimensional CT measurements of small noncalcified pulmonary nodules reliable? Radiology 2004; 231(2):453–8.

141. Zhang L, Yankelevitz DF, Henschke CI, et al. Zone of transition: a potential source of error in tumor volume estimation. Radiology 2010;256(2): 633–9.

The 7th Edition of the TNM Staging System for Lung Cancer
What the Radiologist Needs to Know

Constantine A. Raptis, MD*, Sanjeev Bhalla, MD

KEYWORDS

- Lung cancer • Staging • Non–small cell lung cancer • Small cell lung cancer
- International Association for the Study of Lung Cancer • TNM staging

KEY POINTS

- The 7th Edition of the TNM staging for lung cancer represents a thorough revision and reassessment of the previous versions.
- The T descriptor includes new size groupings and the reclassification of ipsilateral lobe nodules to T3 and ipsilateral lung, different lobe nodules to T4.
- The N descriptor is unchanged, but a new consensus nodal map has been created.
- The M descriptor is subdivided into M1a for disease in the lungs and pleura, and M1b for disease outside the lungs and pleura.

INTRODUCTION

Although the incidence of lung cancer in the United States has been declining, it is expected to account for 226,160 new cases (14% of all new cancer diagnoses) in the United States in 2012. Despite improved surgical, chemotherapy, and radiation treatment options, survival rates remain low, with 5-year combined survival rates for all stages at 16%. With such a high incidence and poor outcomes, it is not surprising that lung cancer remains the leading cause of cancer-related death in the United States, accounting for 28% of all cases.[1]

Radiologists play an important role in the assessment of this large number of patients with lung cancer. The initial diagnosis of lung cancer is often made on a chest radiograph or computed tomography (CT) examination. Patients undergo key portions of their clinical staging with CT, magnetic resonance (MR) imaging, and positron emission tomography (PET)/CT examinations.

Follow-up after therapy hinges on analysis of serial imaging examinations. Given the important role imaging plays in the care of patients with lung cancer, it is incumbent on the radiologist to have a firm understanding of the TNM (tumor-node-metastasis) staging system used to describe the distribution of disease in lung cancer. The purpose of this article is to review the 7th Edition of the TNM staging system for lung cancer. The steps leading to its creation, important changes from the 6th Edition, and the implications of the descriptors on the final stage groupings are discussed.

THE 7TH EDITION OF THE TNM STAGING SYSTEM FOR LUNG CANCER: HOW DID WE GET HERE?

Before delving into the specifics of the 7th Edition of the TNM staging system for lung cancer, it is important to consider the steps that led to its creation, as this edition represents a thorough revision and reassessment of the previous staging system.

The authors have nothing to disclose.
Cardiothoracic Imaging Section, Mallinckrodt Institute of Radiology at Washington University-St Louis, 510 South Kingshighway Boulevard, Box 8131, St Louis, MO 63110, USA
* Corresponding author.
E-mail address: raptisc@mir.wustl.edu

Radiol Clin N Am 50 (2012) 915–933
http://dx.doi.org/10.1016/j.rcl.2012.06.001
0033-8389/12/$ – see front matter © 2012 Elsevier Inc. All rights reserved.

The first modern TNM staging system for lung cancer was included in the second edition of the *TNM Classification of Malignant Tumors,* published in 1974 by the Union Internationale Contre le Cancer (UICC), and was derived from a staging system proposed by the American Joint Committee on Cancer Task Force on Lung Cancer. This original TNM staging system for lung cancer was based on 2155 cases from the database of Dr Clifton Mountain, the Head of Thoracic Surgery at the M.D. Anderson Cancer Center in Houston.[2–4] Subsequent revisions for the TNM staging system for lung cancer continued to be based on Mountain's database, which had grown to 5319 cases in 1997 at the time of the fifth revision.[5]

Although Mountain's database represented an impressive archive of lung-cancer cases, its use as the basis for the TNM staging system for lung cancer had several flaws. First, it was essentially a single-center database (968 of the 5319 cases were sent to M.D. Anderson for confirmation of stage and histology). In addition, although 5319 cases is a large total number, the individual subgroups were small. This database was also heavily weighted toward patients treated with surgery for lung cancer. While surgery has remained an important treatment option for patients with lung cancer, such options have expanded over the past 30 years to include refined chemotherapy and radiation techniques. The staging of lung cancer has also evolved, and now includes the widespread use of CT and other imaging modalities including MR and PET. Moreover, the previous TNM staging revisions for lung cancer had little internal and no external validation.

In 1996, at a workshop in London sponsored by the International Association for the Study of Lung Cancer (IASLC), the decision was made to pursue the development of an international database of lung-cancer cases that could serve as the basis for future revisions of the TNM staging of lung cancer. Over the next decade, the development of the database represented an international effort that was executed in cooperation with the Cancer Research and Biostatistics (CRAB) center in Seattle, Washington. By the time of the London committee meeting in 2005, 100,869 cases had been submitted to the CRAB database from 45 sources in 20 countries. A total of 81,495 of these cases had the staging and survival information allowing for inclusion in the analysis for the revision of the 7th Edition of the TNM staging for lung cancer. The cases were from the time frame of 1990 to 2000 and included 68,463 non–small cell lung cancer (NSCLC) cases and 13,032 small cell lung cancer (SCLC) cases. The patients included were treated with the full range of possibilities, including 41% with surgery only, 23% with chemotherapy only, 11% with radiation only, and the remainder with a combined approach.[6]

Subcommittees were formed to assess the TNM staging system, including a group focusing on the extent of the tumor (T descriptor), a group for analysis of nodal spread (N descriptor), and a group for analysis of the extent of distant disease (M descriptor). A group was also formed to address the relevance of the current TNM staging system in lung cancer. Additional subcommittees were formed to assess the importance of additional tumor nodules, review the nodal chart, and address other prognostic factors outside of the TNM descriptors. A group was also formed to review and advise on methodology and validation. Using the new larger data set, the subcommittees assigned to revising the staging system determined survival statistics based on the descriptors as well the final groupings. These survival statistics were adjusted for cell type, sex, age, and region of origin. The main determinant in determining outcome was overall survival. In addition, the staging system remained based on the anatomic extent of the tumor. Other factors, such as clinical symptoms and the molecular biology of the tumor, were not assessed. Ultimately, all data were internally validated. External validation was also achieved via tests against the National Cancer Institute's Surveillance, Epidemiology, and End Results (SEER) database. The subcommittees then presented their results and recommendations in a series of articles published in the *Journal of Thoracic Oncology* from 2007 to 2009.[7–15] In 2009, these recommendations were incorporated into the 7th Edition of the TNM staging system for lung cancer (hereafter the 7th Edition), published by the International Union Against Lung Cancer and the American Joint Committee on Cancer.[16]

Based on the effort put forth by the IASLC in its accumulation and review of the newly expanded CRAB database, the new 7th Edition represents a significant step forward in the ability to characterize the extent of disease in patients with lung cancer. While staging systems have many important purposes, including the ability to better define prognosis, assist in the evaluation of treatment planning, and assess the results of treatment, the most relevant purpose of a staging system is its ability to define a common nomenclature that will facilitate the exchange of information between physicians. Although the determination of T, N, and M descriptors as well as overall stage may not be explicitly given in radiology reports, it is the responsibility of the radiologist to understand they key determinants in the staging system and assess for their presence or absence on imaging examinations. Reports based on the current TNM staging of lung cancer ensure that the radiologist remains a central part of the multidisciplinary team. The remainder of this article is dedicated to the specifics of the new staging system, with some emphasis on the changes from previous versions.

T DESCRIPTORS

Assignment of the T descriptor for NSCLC is based on the size of the primary tumor, the extent of invasion of local structures, and the presence and location of additional ipsilateral tumor nodules. In the IASLC assessment of the T descriptor, 18,198 patients met criteria for inclusion by having no distant metastatic disease and complete clinical or pathologic staging. All recommendations were validated internally using a comparison of database subtype and geographic region, as well as externally via comparison with the SEER database.[10]

Tumor Size

For assignment of the T descriptor, tumor size refers to the long-axis diameter of the primary tumor. Size criteria were analyzed in detail by the IASLC T-descriptor subcommittee, in part because a large number of patients had the pathologic staging required to assess tumor size. In the previous edition of the TNM staging for lung cancer, a size cutoff of 3 cm was used to separate T1 from T2 lesions. In the analysis of the new database, survival differences were found to be optimized at additional size thresholds of 2, 3, 5, and 7 cm.

These 4 size thresholds were incorporated into the T descriptor via an analysis of survival data in N0M0 patients who had pathologic staging after complete surgical resection with no residual disease. In patients with primary tumors 2 cm or smaller, 5-year survival was 77% and the mean survival time was not reached. Patients with primary tumors larger than 2 cm but limited to 3 cm in size had a 71% 5-year survival and mean survival time of 113 months. This difference led to the separation of the T1 size descriptor into T1a for primary tumors up to 2 cm and T1b for tumors from 2 cm up to 3 cm in size.

The T2 descriptor was separated in a similar fashion, as N0M0 patients who had complete surgical resection with no residual disease of primary tumors larger than 3 cm up to 5 cm had a 5-year survival of 58% and mean survival time of 81 months, whereas patients with primary tumors larger than 5 cm up to 7 cm had a 5-year survival of 49% and mean survival time of 56 months. These data allowed for stratification of

the T2 descriptor into T2a (>3 cm, ≤5 cm) and T2b (>5 cm, ≤7 cm). In the previous staging system, patients with tumors larger than 7 cm would have remained T2 based on size criteria, but in the IASLC analysis, N0M0 patients who underwent resection with no residual disease and had tumors larger than 7 cm demonstrated a 5-year survival of 35% and mean survival time of 29 months. When using data from clinically staged patients, however, patients who were N0M0 and had primary tumors larger than 7 cm had a 5-year survival of 26% and mean survival time of 17 months, which was similar to that of other clinically staged T3 patients, who had a 5-year survival of 29% with mean survival time of 19 months. Given that the survival data for patients with primary tumors larger than 7 cm was similar to that of other clinically staged T3 patients, primary tumors larger than 7 cm were shifted from T2 to T3. A summary of the changes enacted for size criteria in the 7th Edition is presented in **Table 1**.[10] A key implication for the radiologist is that radiology reports must include the longest dimension of the primary tumor so that the size component of T-staging is performed by the reader.

Local Invasion

The T descriptor in the TNM staging system for lung cancer also assesses local invasion of the primary tumor. In the IASLC analysis of the new database, insufficient data were present for revisions of the local invasion criteria to take place. Reasons cited for this included insufficient patient numbers, inconsistent clinical and pathologic results, and lack of validation.[10] Although no changes were made to the local invasion criteria, they remain an important component of the TNM staging of lung cancer, and are reviewed here.

Chest-wall invasion remains a T3 descriptor in the 7th Edition as do parietal pleura invasion, mediastinal pleural invasion, and parietal pericardium invasion. Visceral pleural invasion (VPI) is also an important component of assigning the T descriptor for lung cancer, and its T descriptor was increased from T1 to T2 in the 6th Edition, even for primary lesions smaller than 3 cm.[17] This descriptor can be relevant regarding whether or not patients with tumors of less than 3 cm in size receive adjuvant chemotherapy following resection.[18] Unfortunately, although VPI plays an important role in the assessment of small tumors, there was a lack of a consistent definition for VPI in the 6th Edition. The IASLC T-descriptor subcommittee could not undertake an analysis of the new database for VPI given that the necessary pathologic information was not submitted. Instead, the IASLC

Table 1
Tumor (T) descriptors of the 7th Edition of the TNM staging system for lung cancer

		T Descriptor
Primary lesion size	≤2 cm	T1a (T1)
	>2 cm, ≤3 cm	T1b (T1)
	>3 cm, ≤5 cm	T2a (T2)
	>5 cm, ≤7 cm	T2b (T2)
	>7 cm	T3 (↑T2)
Local invasion	Visceral pleura	T2a,b (T2)
	Parietal pleura	T3
	Mediastinal pleura	T3
	Parietal pericardium	T3
	Chest wall	T3
	Superior sulcus	T3
	Diaphragm	T3
	Rib	T3
	Phrenic nerve	T3
	Mediastinum	T4
	Heart or great vessels	T4
	Trachea	T4
	Esophagus	T4
	Vertebral body	T4
	Recurrent laryngeal nerve	T4
Airway and atelectasis	Mainstem bronchus >2 cm from carina	T2a,b (T2)
	Mainstem bronchus ≤2 cm from carina	T3
	Carinal invasion	T4
	Atelectasis of less than whole lung	T2a,b (T2)
	Atelectasis of entire lung	T3
Nodules	Same lobe as primary tumor	T3 (↓T4)
	Ipsilateral lung, different lobe	T4 (↓M1)

Changes from the 6th Edition staging system have been placed in parentheses, with the up and down arrows used to indicate whether the specific finding has been upstaged or downstaged.

put forth an article addressing the criteria for VPI based on an analysis of the data available in the literature. The recommendation put forth in the article was for a modified Hammar Classification to be used to assess for VPI, which was defined as invasion beyond the elastic layer, up to and including the visceral pleural surface. Emphasis was placed on the use of elastic stains to better delineate VPI when its presence was in question.[19] The investigators also addressed whether primary tumors with invasion into an adjacent lobe should be classified as T2 or T3, but were unable to find consensus in the literature and thus recommended that tumors with invasion across a fissure into an ipsilateral lobe should remain T2.[19]

Assessment of pleural and chest-wall invasion is not reliable on CT examinations. Whereas frank soft-tissue extension into the chest wall or bone destruction are reliable findings for chest-wall involvement, less flagrant findings, such as contact with the pleura over 3 cm and pleural thickening, are sensitive, but not specific, for pleural involvement. In fact, focal chest-wall pain has long been known to be more specific than CT findings for chest wall and parietal pleural involvement.[20] Newer techniques, which are not widely used, do hold some promise in the assessment of chest-wall invasion in lung cancers. These methods include directed ultrasonography of the lesions as well as the use of dynamic cine MR imaging in the assessment of adherence to the pleural surface.[21–23] Radiologists need to be aware of the limitations of imaging examinations in the assessment of pleural and chest-wall involvement, but should be alert for findings that suggest possible chest-wall or pleural invasion, so that further evaluation can be directed toward these lesions if necessary (**Fig. 1**).

Diaphragm invasion is a T3 descriptor. Mediastinal, heart, great vessel, tracheal, and esophageal invasion are all T4 descriptors. Whereas rib involvement is a T3 descriptor, vertebral body invasion remains a T4 descriptor. Phrenic nerve invasion is a T3 descriptor, whereas recurrent laryngeal nerve invasion remains a T4 descriptor (**Fig. 2**). Superior sulcus tumors are classified according to the structures that are involved. Although a superior sulcus

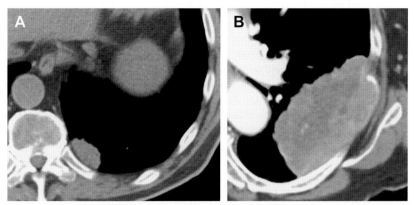

Fig. 1. In (*A*) a 2.8 × 1.7-cm right lower lobe lung cancer is seen abutting the pleural surface over a relatively long length. Although no direct pleural invasion was seen on this examination, this patient was found to have visceral pleural invasion at resection, which results in a T descriptor of T2a. In (*B*) a larger 5 × 9-cm mass is seen in the left lung, with clear invasion of the chest wall and ribs. This mass is a T3 lesion by both size and local invasion criteria.

tumor is T3 at baseline, involvement of a vertebral body or the spinal canal, subclavian vessel involvement, or superior brachial plexus (above C8) involvement upgrade this tumor to the T4 designation.[16,24]

The impact of central airway invasion on the T descriptor remains unchanged in the 7th Edition.

Lesions extending into the mainstem bronchus greater than 2 cm from the carina remain T2 lesions, but are now subdivided as T2a and T2b based on the revised size criteria. Lesions extending into the mainstem bronchus that are 2 cm or more from the carina are T3 lesions, whereas

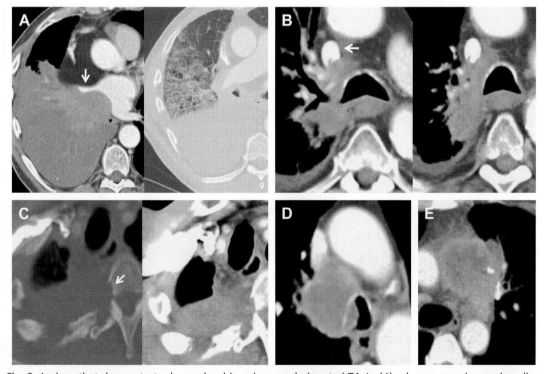

Fig. 2. Lesions that demonstrate deeper local invasion are designated T4. In (*A*) a lung cancer is seen invading into the left atrium and right superior pulmonary vein (*arrow*). Note the resultant venous congestion in the right upper lobe. In (*B*) a lung cancer is seen invading the mediastinum and directly invading the superior vena cava (*arrow*). In (*C*) a right apical lung cancer is seen invading not only ribs but also a thoracic vertebral body (*arrow*). In (*D*) this lung cancer invades not only the mediastinum but also directly invades the trachea. Finally, the patient in (*E*) presented with hoarseness, as a result of recurrent laryngeal nerve involvement by this lung cancer. All of these lesions are designated T4 because of their extensive local invasion.

those that extend to and involve the carina are T4 lesions. Resultant atelectasis is also part of the TNM staging for lung cancer, with lesions causing atelectasis of less than the entire lung classified as T2a or T2b based on size criteria, whereas those that result in atelectasis of the entire lung are T3 (**Fig. 3**).[16] Radiologists can play an important role in the assessment of bronchial involvement and atelectasis, as these findings are discernible on cross-sectional imaging examinations.

Additional Ipsilateral Pulmonary Nodules

The presence of additional tumor nodules was also reviewed in the IASLC subcommittee analysis of the CRAB database. Using the 6th Edition staging system criteria for additional pulmonary nodules, in which a nodule in the same lobe as the primary tumor was T4 and a nodule in the ipsilateral lung but in a different lobe was M1, some important distinctions were determined. First, patients with another nodule in the same lobe who underwent pathologic staging and who were any N and M0 were found to have a 5-year survival of 28% with a mean survival time of 21 months, which was found to be similar to patients who were pathologically designated as T3 for other reasons (5-year survival 31%, mean survival time 24 months). In addition, the patients with nodules in the same lobe as the primary tumor were found to have a statistically significantly improved outcome from patients who were pathologically designated as T4 by other factors (5-year survival 22%, mean survival time 15 months). These findings led to the reclassification of nodules in the same lobe as the primary tumor as T3 in the 7th Edition. In addition, it should be noted that the previously used term "satellite nodules" has been abandoned in favor of "additional tumor nodules."[10] This revision will prevent ambiguity between the typically described satellite nodules seen with benign granulomatous lesions and additional tumor nodules identified in lung cancers.

A similar analysis was performed for nodules in the ipsilateral lung but involving a different lobe from the primary tumor. Using the 6th Edition staging system, these nodules were classified as M1 disease. In the IASLC analysis, patients pathologically staged as M1 owing to ipsilateral nodules in a different lobe who were any N and M0 were found to have a 5-year survival of 22% with a mean survival time of 18 months. This outcome was similar to that of patients pathologically designated as T4 for other reasons, who had a 5-year survival of 22% and mean survival time of 15 months. These findings resulted in the classification of ipsilateral tumor nodules in a different lobe of the primary tumor as T4 in the 7th Edition.[10,16]

Radiologists play an important role in the identification of additional ipsilateral tumor nodules via preoperative imaging studies (**Fig. 4**). Potential additional ipsilateral tumor nodules identified by the radiologist will have a differential diagnosis including metastatic disease from the primary tumor, benign abnormalities, or a synchronous primary tumor. If multiple tumor nodules are found, they can be considered synchronous primaries in the event they are of different histologic cell types. If the nodules are of the same cell type, they can still be considered synchronous primaries if they are pathologically determined to be different subtypes of the same histologic cell type and have no evidence of mediastinal or common nodal drainage metastases. In the settings where synchronous primary tumors are present, the highest T descriptor of the nodules in question is used, with

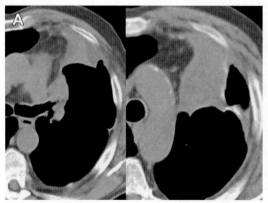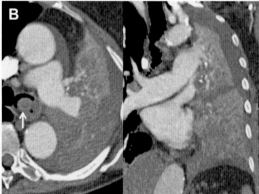

Fig. 3. In (*A*) a 3.1 × 3.6-cm lung cancer obstructing the left upper lobe bronchus leads to atelectasis of the left upper lobe extending to the hilum, but not involving the whole left lung. By both size and invasion criteria, this is a T2a lesion. In (*B*) an endobronchial lesion (*arrow*) results in atelectasis of the entire left lung and is located within 2 cm of the carina, but does not invade it; this is a T3 lesion.

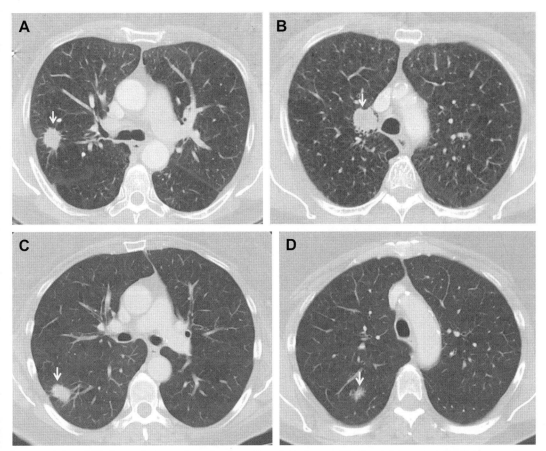

Fig. 4. In (*A*) and (*B*) the patient was found to have 2 nodules (*arrows*) in the right upper lobe. Both were found to represent squamous cell cancer at biopsy, and could not be differentiated as separate primary tumors. Patients with additional tumor nodules in the same lobe are designated T3 in the 7th Edition, decreased from the prior staging system whereby these nodules were deemed T4 disease. In (*C*) and (*D*) a different patient had a primary tumor in the right lower lobe (*C*) and an additional tumor nodule in the right upper lobe (*D*), both found to represent adenocarcinoma on resection. Pathologic analysis could not demonstrate that these lesions were separate primaries and thus, the right upper lobe nodule was considered to represent an additional tumor nodule in the ipsilateral lung but in a different lobe as the primary tumor, making the patient T4.

the number of nodules in parentheses.[24,25] Frequently, the presence of synchronous primary tumors will downstage the T descriptor. For example, a patient with two 2.5-cm tumor nodules without invasion in different lobes of the same lung will be T4 if they are not separate primaries, but only T1b(2) if they are separate primaries.

N DESCRIPTORS

In previous versions of the TNM staging for lung cancer, nodal disease has been characterized as N0 (no nodes involved), N1 (peribronchial, interlobar, or perihilar nodes involved), N2 (ipsilateral mediastinal nodes), or N3 (contralateral mediastinal, hilar, or supraclavicular nodes involved).[17] The IASLC subcommittee on N descriptors set out to review this scheme for the assessment of

nodal disease in NSCLC. From the total CRAB database of 67,725 patients with NSCLC, 38,265 without clinical metastatic disease had available clinical N staging (cN) while 28,371 patients without clinical metastatic disease had pathologic N staging (pN). In the analysis of patients who had clinical N staging, a distinct and statistically significant difference in survival was found in moving between the degree of nodal disease, as patients with cN0, cN1, cN2, and cN3 disease had decreasing 5-year survival rates of 42%, 29%, 16%, and 7%, respectively. Similar findings were identified in the assessment of the patients who were pathologically staged.[12]

One issue that complicated the analysis were discrepancies in the reported data on which lymph node map was used to stage the patients. Over the past 40 years, 2 lymph node maps have evolved

Table 2
Borders of the lymph node stations of the new IASLC consensus nodal map

		Upper Border	Lower Border	Additional Information
Supraclavicular zone	Station #1: Low cervical, supraclavicular, and sternal notch nodes	Lower margin of cricoid cartilage	Clavicles bilaterally and the upper border of the manubrium in the midline	The midline trachea is the divider between 1R and 1L
Upper zone	Station #2: Upper paratracheal nodes	For 2R and 2L: Apex of right/left lung and pleural space extending to the upper border of the manubrium in the midline	For 2R: Intersection of caudal margin of the innominate vein with the trachea For 2L: Superior border of the aortic arch	The divider between 2R and 2L is the left lateral border of the trachea
	Station #3: Prevascular and retrotracheal nodes	For 3a (prevascular) and 3p (retrotracheal): Apex of the chest	For 3a and 3p: The carina	For 3a: Anterior border is the posterior aspect of the sternum and posterior borders are the superior vena cava on the right, the left carotid artery on the left
	Station #4: Lower paratracheal nodes	For 4R: Intersection of the caudal margin or the innominate vein with the trachea For 4L: Upper margin of the aortic arch	For 4R: Lower border of the azygous vein For 4L: Upper rim of the left main pulmonary artery	The divider between 4R and 4L is the left lateral border of the trachea; 4L nodes use the ligamentum arteriosum as their left lateral border
AP zone	Station #5: Subaortic nodes (aortopulmonary window) Station #6: Para-aortic nodes (ascending aorta or phrenic)	Lower border of the aortic arch Line tangential to the upper border of the aortic arch	Upper rim of the left main pulmonary artery Lower border of the aortic arch	Nodes are lateral to the ligamentum arteriosum Nodes are anterior and lateral to the ascending aorta and aortic arch
Subcarinal zone	Station #7: Subcarinal nodes	The carina	The upper border of the lower lobe bronchus on the left, lower border of the bronchus intermedius on the right	Lateral borders defined by the right mainstem bronchus and bronchus intermedius on the right and left mainstem bronchus on the left

Zone	Station			Description
Lower zone	Station #8: Paraesophageal nodes (below carina)	Upper border of the lower lobe bronchus on the left, lower border of the bronchus intermedius on the right	Diaphragm	Nodes lying adjacent to the wall of the esophagus but excluding subcarinal nodes
	Station #9: Pulmonary ligament nodes	Inferior pulmonary vein	Diaphragm	Nodes lying within the pulmonary ligament
Hilar/interlobar zone	Station #10: Hilar nodes	Lower rim of the azygous vein on the right, upper rim of the pulmonary artery on the left	Interlobar region	Nodes immediately adjacent to the mainstem bronchus and hilar vessels including the proximal portions of the pulmonary veins and main pulmonary artery
	Station #11: Interlobar nodes			Between the origins of the lobar bronchi with 2 locations on the right (between RUL and bronchus intermedius as well as between the RML and RLL bronchi) and one on the left (between the LUL and LLL bronchi)
Peripheral zone	Station #12: Lobar nodes			Adjacent to the lobar bronchi
	Station #13: Segmental nodes			Adjacent to the segmental bronchi
	Station #14: Subsegmental nodes			Adjacent to the subsegmental bronchi

The new IASLC consensus nodal map also includes zones for grouping of the nodal stations.
Abbreviations: LLL, left lower lobe; LUL, left upper lobe; RLL, right lower lobe; RML, right middle lobe; RUL, right upper lobe.

for staging lung cancer, the Naruke map and the Mountain-Dressler map.[26,27] While these maps are similar in that they use 14 lymph node stations for lung cancer, with the double-digit stations corresponding to peripheral (N1) stations and single-digit stations corresponding to central (N2) disease, there are some differences. The most important difference arises in the handling of the subcarinal nodal station. In the Mountain-Dressler map, all nodes below the carina extending along the bronchi that are still within the mediastinal pleura and not extending to the lower lobe bronchi and arteries are termed level-7 subcarinal nodes, which categorized them as N2. In the Naruke map, the level 10 nodes, which are peripheral N1 designation nodes, include nodes around the right and left main bronchi. This overlap represents a potential problem in staging between N1 and N2, significant not only for the purposes of the review of the CRAB database but also for the staging of patients. Furthermore, because of difficulties in precisely defining anatomic borders and the language used to describe these borders, consistent labeling of lymph node stations can be difficult. In a study examining the Naruke map, two surgeons present during pulmonary resections showed only a 68.5% concordance rate in the assignment of lymph nodes, with 34.1% of the patients having N1 lymph nodes by one surgeon deemed N2 lymph nodes by the other surgeon.[28]

These irreconcilable differences between the two nodal maps and their impact on the CRAB database and N-descriptor evaluation led to the formation of a smaller group charged with developing a new, more precise consensus nodal map. A radiologist was used in collaboration with the members of the IASLC subcommittee to ensure that the revised nodal map's anatomic boundaries could be discernible on CT examinations used for clinical staging. The result of this group's work was a new nodal map with anatomically distinct and concise definitions. One important change in the new consensus map is the designation of the new level-1 supraclavicular and sternal notch nodes as a separate station from the intrathoracic nodes. Another change particularly relevant for radiologists is moving the division of the right and left level-2 and level-4 nodes from the midline to the left lateral border of the trachea. A lymph node anterior to the trachea would, using the new nodal station definitions, be considered right paratracheal.

In addition to the reconciliation of more precise anatomic borders, the group also proposed the use of grouping the lymph node levels into "zones," which were used by the IASLC N-descriptor group in an attempt to reconcile the differences between the data provided by the Naruke and Mountain-Dressler maps in the CRAB database. The zone concept was proposed for use in future survival analyses, but is not yet recommended for incorporation into standard nomenclature. One potential advantage of using lymph node zones instead of stations includes making it easier to indicate the location of lymph nodes than the previous stations model, particularly in the setting of anatomic boundaries that are difficult to determine on cross-sectional imaging. In addition, large nodal masses that span the relatively smaller nodal stations are also easier to describe using the nodal zones. The new consensus IASLC nodal map definitions including the nodal zones are described in **Table 2**.[11,12,29] The CT locations of the nodal stations are presented in **Fig. 5**.

The N-descriptor subcommittee also attempted to evaluate any influences on survival based on the presence of "skip metastases" (N2 nodal involvement without N1 disease) and the number of involved stations. To include sufficient amounts of patients for the analysis, the nodal stations were grouped into the new nodal zone concept as described above. This work yielded a few interesting results. In the setting of skip metastases, aortopulmonary zone disease without N1 disease was associated with improved outcomes in left upper lobe tumors. However, there was no improved outcome determined for patients with N2 involvement via right paratracheal nodes in the setting of right upper-lobe tumors. As for the potential impact of the number of nodal zones involved, a trend was found. Single-zone N1 disease had a 5-year survival of 48%, multiple-zone N1 disease had a 5-year survival of 35%, single-zone N2 disease had a 5-year survival of 34%, and multiple-zone N2 disease had a 5-year survival of 20%. There was no statistically significant difference in survival between multiple-zone N1 and single-zone N2 disease, thus setting up 3 distinct groups of patients: those with single-zone N1, those with multiple-zone N1 or single-zone N2, and those with multiple-zone N2 disease. Based on these results, the subcommittee explored whether there should be subdivision of the N descriptors, but in analysis with each T-stage category, the subgroups were too small to validate the results. Consequently, no changes were recommended to the N descriptors in the 7th Edition (**Table 3**).[12] Of note, a separate recent single-institution study validated the concept of subdividing the N descriptors by finding a stepwise decrease in survival in similarly amalgamated subdivided N descriptors.[29] It is possible that with

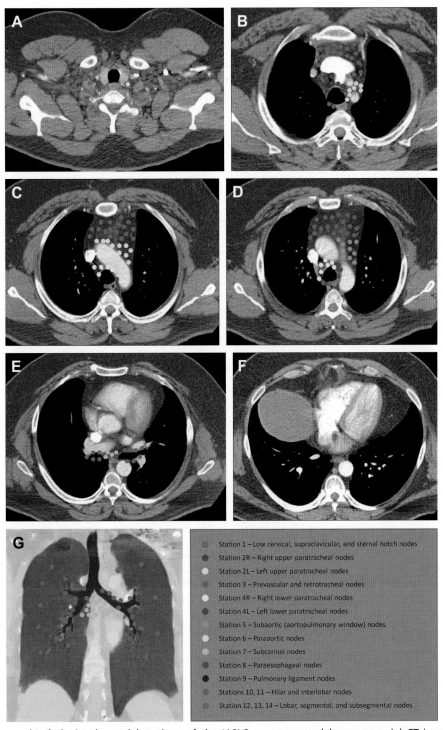

Fig. 5. Images (*A–F*) depict the nodal stations of the IASLC consensus nodal map on axial CT images, while a coronal minimum-intensity projection of a CT image (*G*) is used to depict the locations of the peripheral nodal stations.

larger numbers of patients and more consistent re-porting of lymph node staging, subdivision of the N descriptors will be possible in future revisions of the TNM staging.

In terms of identifying concerning nodes on preoperative imaging, on CT examinations a 10-mm short-axis diameter is typically considered the upper limit of the normal size for lymph

Table 3
Node (N) descriptors of the 7th Edition TNM staging system for lung cancer

N Descriptor	Involved Nodes
N0	No regional lymph node metastasis
N1	Metastasis in ipsilateral intrapulmonary, peribronchial, and hilar nodes (including by direct extension)
N2	Metastasis in ipsilateral mediastinal and/or subcarinal nodes
N3	Metastasis in contralateral mediastinal, contralateral hilar, ipsilateral or contralateral scalene, or ipsilateral or contralateral supraclavicular nodes

nodes.[30] Improvements in sensitivity, specificity, and accuracy in the assessment of mediastinal nodes for metastatic disease were found by Ikezoe and colleagues[31] when using an upper-limit short-axis diameter of 13 mm for subcarinal, precarinal, and tracheobronchial region nodes while using 10 mm for the remaining nodes. Although not widely available during the time during which the CRAB database was collected, PET and PET/CT have also become important imaging modalities for lung cancer, and have also been shown to demonstrate improved accuracy over CT alone in the assessment of nodal disease in patients with lung cancer.[32,33] Ultimately, it should be noted that the value of imaging assessment of nodal disease in patients with lung cancer remains controversial among thoracic surgeons.[34] Even in the modern era, many prefer to stage nodal disease surgically. Nevertheless, familiarity with the new IASLC nodal map and the locations of N1, N2, and N3 nodes assists radiologists in developing an efficient and meaningful search pattern when interpreting and creating reports for examinations of patients with lung cancer.

M DESCRIPTORS

In the 6th Edition of TNM staging for lung cancer, patients with nodules in a different lobe of the ipsilateral lung of the primary tumor, contralateral tumor nodules, and/or distant metastases were classified as having M1 disease.[17] The section on the T descriptors has already addressed the change of nodules in a different lobe of the ipsilateral lung of the primary tumor to T4 in the 7th Edition from M1 in the previous version. The M-descriptor subcommittee also examined the effects of pleural dissemination of tumor (previously T4 in the 6th Edition), contralateral nodules (previously M1), and distant metastases (previously M1) on overall survival. In this analysis, 6596 NSCLC cases with pathologic and/or clinical staging were used. Of these cases, 1106 were patients who were T4 (by the 7th Edition criteria),

any N, M0, 771 cases had pleural dissemination, 369 had contralateral lung nodules, and 4350 had distant metastases. As in the evaluation of the T and N descriptors, the results were internally and externally validated.[9]

In the analysis of the effect of malignant pleural dissemination (effusion or nodules, not by direct extension), a statistically significant survival difference was determined between patients with pleural dissemination (median survival 8 months) and the T4, any N, M0 group, who had a median survival of 13 months. This finding led to the recommendation that pleural dissemination be reclassified as an M descriptor in the 7th Edition.[9] It should also be noted that in the final version of the 7th Edition put forth by the UICC, disseminated pericardial disease was also reclassified as an M descriptor, although it is not explicitly mentioned in the M-descriptor subcommittee's publication.[16]

For the assessment of additional tumor nodules in the contralateral lung, a statistically significant difference in survival was found between the contralateral nodule group median survival of 10 months and the T4, any N, M0 group median survival of 13 months. This finding confirmed the designation of contralateral tumor nodules as an M descriptor. There was a statistically significant improvement in survival in the contralateral nodule group versus the pleural dissemination group ($P = .0235$), and both groups demonstrated a statistically significant improvement in survival versus the 6-month median survival demonstrated by the distant metastases group. Consequently, the decision was made to stratify the M descriptor by designating metastases within the lungs and pleura as M1a and metastases outside the lungs and pleura as M1b (**Table 4**).[9]

Assessment for distant metastatic disease on imaging studies used for staging is a critical phase of treatment planning, as the presence of distant metastatic disease most often precludes patients from surgical resection. In noting suspicious lesions in distant organs, the appropriate biopsies can be performed to appropriately designate

Table 4
Metastasis (M) descriptors of the 7th Edition TNM staging system for lung cancer

M Descriptor	
M1a (M1)	Additional tumor nodules in contralateral lung
M1a (↑T4)	Pleural or pericardial dissemination
M1b (M1)	Distant metastases

Changes from the 6th Edition staging system have been placed in parentheses, with the up and down arrows used to indicate whether the specific finding has been upstaged or downstaged.

patients as M1b. Likewise, a careful description of the location of possible additional tumor nodules is important, as their location in the ipsilateral or contralateral lung affects possible M1a designation in the 7th Edition (Fig. 6). Finally, suspicious findings on CT or PET/CT for malignant pleural or pericardial dissemination including pleural thickening or enhancement, discrete pleural nodules, or increased fluorodeoxyglucose activity in the pleura should warrant further investigation with thoracentesis or thoracoscopic biopsy for patients in whom the presence of a disseminated pleural or pericardial disease is a key factor in M1a designation (Fig. 7).

OTHER TUMORS
Small Cell Lung Cancer

SCLC, which comprises 13% to 20% of all lung cancers, is notable for its rapid growth rate and early dissemination of disease, with the majority of patients presenting with evidence of hematogenous or nodal dissemination. Although the incidence of SCLC has been declining, outcomes remain poor despite initial sensitivity to radiation and chemotherapy.[35,36] The 6th Edition did use

the same TNM staging for SCLC as was used for NSCLC, but the staging system had not been extensively tested given the lack of large cohorts of SCLC with surgical staging.[17] Furthermore, in clinical practice the TNM staging has typically not been used. Rather, SCLC patients have been divided into groups of limited disease (LD) and extensive disease (ED). In an IASLC consensus report from 1989, LD was classified as tumors limited to one hemithorax with regional lymph node metastases including hilar, ipsilateral, and contralateral mediastinal nodes, and ipsilateral and contralateral supraclavicular nodes. Patients with malignant effusions were also considered to have LD. Patients with disease that extended beyond these boundaries were considered to have ED.[37] The LD and ED descriptors also convey some meaning in treatment planning, as patients with LD typically receive chemotherapy and radiation whereas patients with ED receive chemotherapy alone.

The IASLC subcommittee for SCLC was able to perform a more thorough examination of the use of the TNM staging system for SCLC via use of the CRAB database, which contained 12,620 cases of small cell histology, with 8088 having TNM staging. Most patients were staged clinically, as patients with SCLC rarely undergo surgery given the frequent presentation of relatively advanced disease. In the IASLC SCLC subcommittee survival analysis, trends were found with increasing T and N descriptors (using the 6th Edition versions) as well as with increasing stage grouping, although there was some overlap between the groups. Based on these findings, the IASLC subcommittee recommended that TNM staging be incorporated into clinical trials for SCLC stages I to III.[13] One interesting finding from the IASLC analysis was that when using the LD and ED model, patients with LD and disseminated pleural disease were found to have a survival that was intermediate between patients with LD and no pleural disease and those with ED.[13] Although this may seem to represent

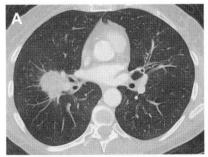
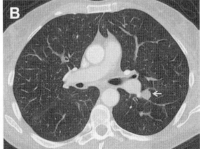

Fig. 6. In (A) the patient has a spiculated right upper lobe lesion, which was found to represent a squamous cell carcinoma. In addition, a metastasis was found in the superior segment of the left lower lobe in (B) (arrow). Metastases to the contralateral lung are deemed M1a disease in the 7th Edition.

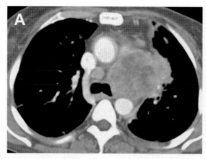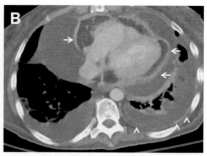

Fig. 7. This patient with adenocarcinoma and extensive mediastinal metastasis (*A*) also had a pericardial effusion with extensive pericardial thickening and enhancement in (*B*) (*arrows*), as well as bilateral pleural effusions with pleural thickening and enhancement (*arrowheads*). These findings were confirmed to represent malignant pleural and pericardial effusions. Disseminated pleural and pericardial disease is now classified as M1a in the 7th Edition, whereas in the 6th Edition pleural and pericardial dissemination was classified as T4 disease.

a limitation of using the 7th Edition for SCLC patients, a separate study investigating the use of the TNM staging system in a retrospective review of 10,660 cases of SCLC from the California Cancer Registry confirmed stratification of survival when using the 7th Edition, and did not find the presence of disseminated pleural disease to represent an intermediate outcome; rather, this study demonstrated patients with disseminated pleural disease to have outcomes similar to those of other patients with M1a disease.[38]

Ultimately, in the final published version of the 7th Edition, the staging system for NSCLC was again recommended for use with SCLC.[16] Certainly further analysis and possible revisions of the SCLC TNM staging system are necessary, and may be possible by adding SCLC patients with improved nodal staging and pleural effusion analysis. Consequently, although the relevance of using the TNM staging for SCLC in clinical practice is not certain at present, inclusion of the staging system in future clinical trials may allow investigators to better assess the benefits of the size of radiation fields, whether prophylactic radiation to noninvolved nodal sites is necessary, and the effects of surgical treatment on lower-stage disease.[13] For radiologists, use of the TNM staging system in SCLC cases requires little change from the norm, with careful assessment of primary tumor (when identifiable) size and local invasion, nodal disease, and metastatic disease required.

Bronchopulmonary Carcinoid Tumors

Bronchopulmonary carcinoid tumors are malignant neuroendocrine tumors that make up 1% to 2% of all pulmonary neoplasms. For neuroendocrine tumors of the lung, there is a classification spectrum ranging from low-grade typical carcinoids and intermediate atypical carcinoids to higher-grade large cell and small cell carcinomas. The distinctions between these neuroendocrine tumors are based on pathologic criteria, including morphology, number of mitoses, necrosis, and histologic grade.[39] Despite the fact that the 6th Edition did not include carcinoids, the TNM system has typically been used to stage patients with carcinoid tumors. The CRAB database included 392 patients with pathologic TNM data for pulmonary carcinoid tumors, and the IASLC performed an analysis of these patients to determine whether the TNM staging system for lung cancer is applicable to carcinoid tumors. External validation was performed via additional comparison with an analysis of 1619 carcinoid cases in the SEER database.[14]

The IASLC analysis of the CRAB and SEER databases determined worsening survival with increasing T, N, and M descriptors as well as with increasing overall stage. Based on these findings, it was recommended that the 7th Edition be applied to carcinoids.[14] There were several limitations in this analysis, including the relatively small number of patients, difficulty in using overall survival as the primary outcome given relatively favorable outcomes in these patients, and the inability to distinguish typical and atypical carcinoids (which have different prognoses) in the database. In addition, patients with multiple nodules were found to have excellent survival, likely because many of these patients had the preinvasive lesion of diffuse idiopathic pulmonary neuroendocrine cell hyperplasia (DIPNECH) and not true metastases (**Fig. 8**).[14] For radiologists this is of particular importance, as recognizing the findings of multiple small (<5 mm) nodules and mosaic attenuation in the setting of a carcinoid tumor should prompt consideration of the diagnosis of DIPNECH on imaging studies.[40,41] Suggesting the diagnosis of DIPNECH on imaging studies

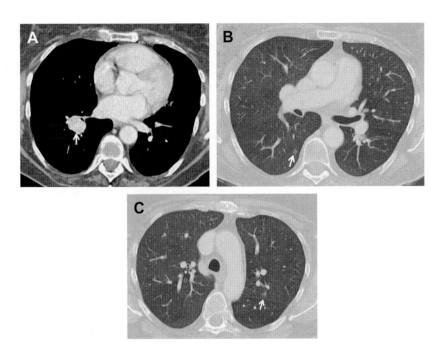

Fig. 8. Contrast-enhanced CT in (*A*) demonstrates a well-circumscribed enhancing nodule in the right lower lobe (*arrow*), which was concerning for a carcinoid tumor. In addition, multiple small (<6 mm) ground-glass nodules (*arrows* in *B* and *C*) were seen on a background of mosaic attenuation. This constellation of findings was consistent with a primary carcinoid tumor and multiple carcinoid tumorlets in the setting of diffuse idiopathic pulmonary neuroendocrine cell hyperplasia (DIPNECH), which was confirmed on resection of the lesion in the right lower lobe. Recognizing these findings is essential so as to not confuse the foci of hyperplasia seen in DIPNECH with metastases from the primary lesion.

can prevent the overstaging of patients with carcinoid tumors when the 7th Edition is used.

STAGE GROUPINGS

The IASLC also performed an analysis of the stage groupings using the 67,725 NSCLC cases from the CRAB database. This analysis used the new 7th Edition TNM descriptors, including the subdivided T descriptors and reclassifications of additional tumor nodules that were previously described. Given the additional number of revised descriptors, the stage groupings have become more complex, with the overall stage grouping scheme depicted in **Table 5**. Additional changes that resulted from the survival analysis included shifting T2b N0 M0 cases from IB to IIA, T2a N1 M0 cases from IIB to IIA, and T4 N0 and N1 M0 cases from IIIB to IIIA. Again, this work was internally and externally validated, and represents a large step forward in the TNM staging for lung cancer.[7]

Although the changes in the stage groupings have little importance for radiologists, there are important implications for clinicians and patients (**Fig. 9**). One important benefit is that the new stage

groupings are better correlated with survival and can be used to better assess patient prognosis. In addition, the new stage groupings hold the potential to alter management strategies. Particularly important groups of patients that may be affected by the new grouping scheme are those with additional tumor nodules in the same lobe as the primary tumor and those with additional tumor nodules in the same lung, but a different lobe. Previously these were T4 and M1 descriptors, but have since been revised to T3 and T4 descriptors, respectively. Consequently, patients with additional tumor nodules in the same lobe that had N1 or N2 disease were previously IIIB and are now IIIA. Likewise, patients with additional tumor nodules in a different lobe of the ipsilateral lung and N0 or N1 disease have been reclassified from IIIB to IIIA. A similar shift into IIIA from higher stages is also seen in patients with T4 disease, based on invasion with concomitant N0 or N1 disease. While it is still important to recognize that management decisions should be based on prospective clinical trials and not the staging system, given that patients with IIIA disease may be surgical candidates while those with IIIB disease are

Table 5
Overall stage groupings with respect to the T, N, and M descriptors in the 7th Edition of the TNM staging of lung cancer

6th Edition T/M Descriptor	7th Edition T/M Descriptor	N0	N1	N2	N3
T1 ($\leq$2 cm)	T1a	IA	IIA	IIIA	IIIB
T1 (>2–3 cm)	T1b	IA	IIA	IIIA	IIIB
T2 ($\leq$5 cm)	T2a	IB	IIA ($\downarrow$IIB)	IIIA	IIIB
T2 (>5–$\leq$7 cm)	T2b	IIA ($\downarrow$IB)	IIB	IIIA	IIIB
T2 (>7 cm)	T3	IIB ($\uparrow$IB)	IIIA ($\uparrow$IIB)	IIIA	IIIB
T3 (invasion)	T3	IIB	IIIA	IIIA	IIIB
T4 (same lobe nodules)	T3	IIB ($\downarrow$IIIB)	IIIA ($\downarrow$IIIB)	IIIA ($\downarrow$IIIB)	IIIB
T4 (extension)	T4	IIIA ($\downarrow$IIIB)	IIIA ($\downarrow$IIIB)	IIIB	IIIB
M1 (ipsilateral lobe nodule)	T4	IIIA ($\downarrow$IV)	IIIA ($\downarrow$IV)	IIIB ($\downarrow$IV)	IIIB ($\downarrow$IV)
T4 (pleural dissemination)	M1a	IV ($\uparrow$IIIB)	IV ($\uparrow$IIIB)	IV ($\uparrow$IIIB)	IV ($\uparrow$IIIB)
M1 (contralateral lung nodule)	M1a	IV	IV	IV	IV
M1 (distant metastasis)	M1b	IV	IV	IV	IV

Changes from the 6th Edition stage groupings are identified in parentheses, with up or down arrows used to indicate whether the group has been upstaged or downstaged. Patients in groups IIIA and below (who may be surgical candidates) are shown in boldface type, unlike those in groups IIIB and above (typically inoperable).

typically deemed inoperable, these changes in the stage groupings have the potential to result in surgical management being used in larger numbers of patients.

LIMITATIONS AND FUTURE DIRECTIONS

The 7th Edition represents a huge leap forward from previous TNM staging systems for lung cancer. It is the first staging system for lung cancer based on a large international database, and is backed by internal and external validation. Despite its many improvements, the new staging system and the project that led to its creation have several important limitations. First, the IASLC analysis was performed in a retrospective fashion. Even more importantly, patient data collected in the database was, in most cases, not designed to be used in a study investigating the TNM staging of lung cancer. Consequently, some data were incomplete for the purposes of TNM staging assessment. For example, many of the specific details of tumor extension were not included, thus precluding detailed analysis of the invasion criteria used in the T descriptor. Other factors, such as lymphangitic spread of tumor, were not included to any extent. In addition, detailed nodal spread was not always reliably recorded, and the database also suffered

from reporting differences based on whether the Mountain-Dressler or the Naruke map was used.

Metastatic disease was assessed, but specific sites were not reliably reported, thus precluding a detailed assessment of the importance of the number of distant metastases as well as the importance of specific sites. Aside from the TNM descriptors, information on histologic type and grade, key factors in other staging systems, were not readily available. Finally, the development of PET and PET/CT over the past two decades has changed the clinical staging of lung cancer, but data from these modalities was not included in the retrospective database.[42]

In an effort to address these limitations, the IASLC has begun the prospective component of its assessment of the lung cancer staging system. In this investigation, the data are being gathered for the purposes of analyzing the TNM staging of lung cancer, and the aforementioned limitations are being addressed. In addition to more detailed assessment of the TNM staging system with prospective data, the prospective arm also aims to assess the importance of new factors such as histologic type and grade, lymphangitic carcinomatosis, and the prognostic impact of PET data, including the maximum standardized uptake value. The recommendations from the prospective project are scheduled to be published in the

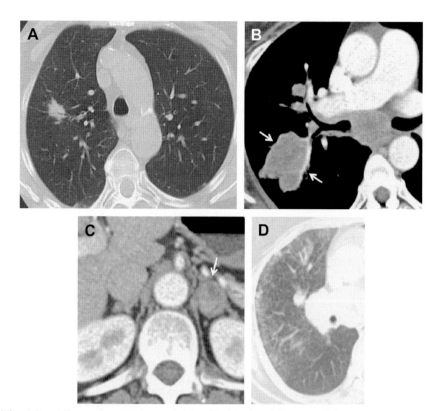

Fig. 9. In (A) a 1.8 × 1.3-cm adenocarcinoma is identified in the right upper lobe, surrounded entirely by lung parenchyma. This mass is a T1a lesion. In the absence of nodal or distant metastases, this patient has an overall stage group of IA with 93% 1-year and 66% 5-year survival based on the TNM staging alone.[15] In (B) a different patient with a right lower lobe adenocarcinoma (*arrow*) and subcarinal nodal metastasis has a left adrenal metastasis in (C) (*arrow*). The presence of distant metastases makes this an M1b lesion. All M1b lesions, regardless of tumor and nodal descriptors, are overall stage group IV. This patient also has nodular septal-line thickening in the right middle and lower lobes, seen in (D), which was worrisome for lymphangitic spread of tumor. Lymphangitic carcinomatosis is not included in the 7th Edition but is to be investigated in the prospective project currently being performed by the IASLC in preparation for the 8th Edition.

Journal of Thoracic Oncology in 2014 for inclusion in the 8th Edition of the TNM classification of malignant tumors in 2016.[42]

interpretation of imaging studies and communication of relevant information in radiology reports.

SUMMARY

The revised 7th Edition of the TNM staging system for lung cancer, based on a large international database, is a significant advance in the staging of lung cancer. The new system is based on improved and more detailed survival analysis, and is backed by internal and external validation. Several changes to the staging system have resulted and are detailed in this article. Given their role in the assessment of patients with lung cancer via the interpretation of imaging studies for initial staging and follow-up, radiologists need to be aware of these changes and have a firm grasp of the overall staging system, thus facilitating better

REFERENCES

1. American Cancer Society. Cancer facts and figures 2012. Atlanta (GA): American Cancer Society; 2012.
2. Watanabe Y. TNM classification for lung cancer. Ann Thorac Cardiovasc Surg 2003;9(6):343–50.
3. UICC. TNM classification of malignant tumors. Geneva (Switzerland): UICC; 1973.
4. Mountain CF, Carr DT, Anderson WA. A system for the clinical staging of lung cancer. Am J Roentgenol Radium Ther Nucl Med 1974;120:130–8.
5. Mountain CF. Revisions in the international system for staging lung cancer. Chest 1997;111:1710–7.
6. Goldstraw P, Crowley JJ. The International Association for the Study of Lung Cancer International

Staging Project on Lung Cancer. J Thorac Oncol 2006;1(4):281–6.

7. Goldstraw P, Crowley JJ, Chansky K, et al. The IASLC Lung Cancer Staging Project: proposals for the revision of the TNM stage groupings in the forthcoming (seventh) edition of the TNM classification of malignant tumours. J Thorac Oncol 2007;2(8): 706–14.

8. Groome PA, Bolejack V, Crowley JJ, et al. The IASLC Lung Cancer Staging Project: validation of the proposals for the revision of the T, N, and M descriptors and consequent stage groupings in the forthcoming (seventh) edition of the TNM classification of malignant tumours. J Thorac Oncol 2007;2(8): 694–705.

9. Postmus PE, Brambilla E, Chansky K, et al. The IASLC Lung Cancer Staging Project: proposals for the revision of the M descriptors in the forthcoming (seventh) edition of the TNM classification of lung cancer. J Thorac Oncol 2007;2(8): 686–93.

10. Rami-Porta R, Ball D, Crowley J, et al. The IASLC Lung Cancer Staging Project T descriptors in the forthcoming (seventh) edition of the TNM classification for lung cancer. J Thorac Oncol 2007; 2(7):593–602.

11. Rusch VW, Asamura H, Watanabe H, et al. The IASLC lung cancer staging project: a proposal for a new international lymph node map in the forthcoming seventh edition of the TNM classification for lung cancer. J Thorac Oncol 2009;4(5): 569–77.

12. Rusch VW, Crowley JJ, Giroux DJ, et al. The IASLC Lung Cancer Staging Project: proposals for the revision of the N descriptors in the forthcoming seventh edition of the TNM classification for lung cancer. J Thorac Oncol 2007;2(7):603–12.

13. Shepherd FA, Crowley JJ, Van Houtee P, et al. The IASLC lung cancer staging project: proposals regarding the clinical staging of small cell lung cancer in the forthcoming (seventh) edition of the tumor, node, and metastasis classification for lung cancer. J Thorac Oncol 2007;2(12):1067–77.

14. Travis WD, Giroux DJ, Chansky K, et al. The IASLC Lung Cancer Staging Project: proposals for the inclusion of broncho-pulmonary carcinoid tumors in the forthcoming (seventh) edition of the TNM classification for lung cancer. J Thorac Oncol 2008;3(11): 1213–23.

15. Chansky K, Sculier JP, Crowley JJ, et al. The International Association for the Study of Lung Cancer Staging Project: prognostic factors and pathologic TNM stage in surgically managed non-small cell lung cancer. J Thorac Oncol 2009; 4(7):792–801.

16. UICC. TNM classification of malignant tumors. 7th edition. New York: Wiley Blackwell; 2009.

17. UICC. TNM classification of malignant tumours. 6th edition. New York: Wiley-Liss; 2002.

18. Tsuboi M, Ohira T, Saji H, et al. The present status of postoperative adjuvant chemotherapy for completely resected non-small cell lung cancer. Ann Thorac Cardiovasc Surg 2007;13:73–7.

19. Travis WD, Brambilla E, Rami-Porta R, et al. Visceral pleural invasion: pathologic criteria and use of elastic stains. J Thorac Oncol 2008;3(12): 1384–90.

20. Glazer HS, Duncan-Meyer J, Aronberg DJ, et al. Pleural and chest wall invasion in bronchogenic carcinoma: CT evaluation. Radiology 1985;157: 191–4.

21. Bandi V, Lunn W, Ernst A, et al. Ultrasound vs. CT in detecting chest wall invasion by tumor: a prospective study. Chest 2008;133:881–6.

22. Akata S, Kajiwara N, Park J, et al. Evaluation of chest wall invasion by lung cancer using respiratory dynamic MRI. J Med Imaging Radiat Oncol 2008; 52:36–9.

23. Kajiwara N, Akata S, Uchida O, et al. Cine MRI enables better therapeutic planning than CT in cases of possible lung cancer chest wall invasion. Lung Cancer 2009;69:203–8.

24. Greaves SM, Brown K, Garon EB, et al. The new staging system for lung cancer: imaging and clinical implications. J Thorac Imaging 2011;26:119–31.

25. Edge SB, Byrd DR, Compton CC, et al. AJCC cancer staging manual. 7th edition. New York: Springer; 2010.

26. Mountain DF, Dressler CM. Regional lymph node classification for lung cancer staging. Chest 1997; 111:1718–23.

27. The Japan Lung Cancer Society. Classification of lung cancer. Tokyo: Kanehara and Co; 2000.

28. Watanabe Y, Ladas G, Goldstraw P. Inter-observer variability in systematic nodal dissection: comparison of European and Japanese nodal designation. Ann Thorac Surg 2002;73:245–9.

29. Lee JG, Lee CY, Bae MK, et al. Validity of International Association for the Study of Lung Cancer proposals for the revision of N descriptors in lung cancer. J Thorac Oncol 2008;3(12):1421–6.

30. Glazer GM, Gross BH, Quint LE, et al. Normal mediastinal lymph nodes: number and size according to American Thoracic Society mapping. AJR Am J Roentgenol 1985;144:261–5.

31. Ikezoe J, Kadowaki K, Morimoto S, et al. Mediastinal lymph node metastases from nonsmall cell bronchogenic carcinoma: reevaluation with CT. J Comput Assist Tomogr 1990;14:340–4.

32. Antoch G, Stattaus J, Nemat AT, et al. Non-small cell lung cancer: dual-modality PET/CT in preoperative staging. Radiology 2003;229:526–33.

33. Dwamema BA, Sonnad SS, Angobaldo JO, et al. Metastases from non-small cell lung cancer: mediastinal

staging in the 1990s—meta-analytic comparison of PET and CT. Radiology 1999;213:530–6.

34. Munden RF, Swisher SS, Stevens CW, et al. Imaging of the patient with non-small cell lung cancer. Radiology 2005;237:803–18.

35. Govindan R, Page N, Morgensztern D, et al. Changing epidemiology of small-cell lung cancer in the United States over the last 30 years: analysis of the surveillance, epidemiologic, and end results database. J Clin Oncol 2008;24:4539–44.

36. Devesa SS, Bray F, Vizcaino AP, et al. International lung cancer trends by histologic type: male:female differences diminishing and adenocarcinoma rates rising. Int J Cancer 2005;117:294–9.

37. Stahel R, Ginsberg R, Havemann K, et al. Staging and prognostic factors in small cell lung cancer: a consensus report. Lung Cancer 1989;5: 119–26.

38. Ou SI, Zell JA. The applicability of the proposed IASLC staging revisions to small cell lung cancer (SCLC) with comparison to the current UICC 6th TNM Edition. J Thorac Oncol 2009;4(3):300–10.

39. Hage R, de la Riviere AB, Seldenrijk CA, et al. Update in pulmonary carcinoid tumors: a review article. Ann Surg Oncol 2003;10(6):697–704.

40. Davies SJ, Gosney JR, Hansell DM, et al. Diffuse idiopathic pulmonary neuroendocrine cell hyperplasia: an under-recognised spectrum of disease. Thorax 2007;62:248–52.

41. Gorshtein A, Gross DJ, Barak D, et al. Diffuse idiopathic pulmonary neuroendocrine cell hyperplasia and the associated lung neuroendocrine tumors. Cancer 2012;118:612–9.

42. Giroux DJ, Rami-Porta R, Chansky K, et al. The IASLC Lung Cancer Staging Project: data elements for the prospective project. J Thorac Oncol 2009;4(6):679–83.

Optimal Imaging Protocols for Lung Cancer Staging
CT, PET, MR Imaging, and the Role of Imaging

Narinder S. Paul, MD[a], Sebastian Ley, MD[a], Ur Metser, MD[b]

KEYWORDS

- Lung cancer staging • Computed tomography • Magnetic resonance imaging
- Hybrid positron emission tomography • Staging algorithm

KEY POINTS

- The majority of patients who present with a diagnosis of lung cancer have advanced disease, and are adequately staged with computed tomography of the thorax and upper abdomen.
- Hybrid positron emission tomography scanning is used in all patients with lung cancer who are considered for curative treatment, to exclude occult disease.
- Magnetic resonance imaging is generally directed toward answering a specific concern, for example, to exclude cerebral metastases.
- Although a comprehensive lung cancer staging algorithm includes access to noninvasive imaging and interventional techniques for tissue sampling, staging algorithms are individualized to the particular circumstances of each patient.

The optimal imaging technique for lung cancer staging requires accurate detection and characterization of the primary lung nodule (≤29 mm) or mass (≥30 mm), and precise assessment of local and distant tumor spread. Chest radiography is the most commonly performed imaging technique for the detection of lung disease. The technique is widely available, easy to perform, of low risk, and relatively inexpensive. However, chest radiography has limitations for accurate detection of early lung cancer because of the superimposition of anatomic structures in the thorax and limited sensitivity in disease detection outside of the thorax.[1] The main imaging modality for the staging of lung cancer is computed tomography (CT), supplemented by positron emission tomography (PET), usually as a hybrid technique in conjunction with CT (PET/CT). Magnetic resonance (MR) imaging is a useful diagnostic tool for specific indications and has the advantage of not using ionizing radiation. This article discusses the optimal imaging protocols for lung cancer staging using CT, PET (PET/CT), and MR imaging, and the role of imaging in patient management.

TECHNICAL CONSIDERATIONS

Sequential advances in CT technology with decrease in gantry rotation to 280 milliseconds and increase in detector coverage up to 160 mm have led to a decrease in scan times and motion artifacts, while reduction in the size of individual detector elements, down to 0.5 mm in diameter, have improved spatial resolution and confidence in delineation of anatomic features.[2] Introduction of respiratory and cardiac gating has reduced image blurring and thereby improved the diagnostic capabilities of CT. The widespread availability of CT and

[a] Division of Cardiothoracic Radiology, University Health Network, Mount Sinai and Women's College Hospital, University of Toronto, Ontario, Canada; [b] Division of Abdominal Radiology, University Health Network, Mount Sinai and Women's College Hospital, University of Toronto, Ontario, Canada
E-mail address: Narinder.Paul@uhn.ca

Radiol Clin N Am 50 (2012) 935–949
http://dx.doi.org/10.1016/j.rcl.2012.06.007
0033-8389/12/$ – see front matter Crown Copyright © 2012 Published by Elsevier Inc. All rights reserved.

the ability to perform a whole-body CT scan in a few seconds mean that CT has a high level of physician preference and patient acceptability. However, incremental use of CT has raised concerns regarding the dramatic increase in population exposure to ionizing radiation.[3] Developments in iterative reconstruction techniques for CT images promise significant reductions in radiation dose, and will help to alleviate these concerns.[4]

Most clinical examinations that use PET are performed on dedicated in-line PET/CT scanners. Hybrid PET/CT scanners offer 2 main advantages over conventional PET scanners. First, attenuation and scatter correction with CT is rapid. This method obviates a prolonged transmission scan, significantly shortening overall study time and improving patient throughput. Second, the spatial resolution of PET is generally inadequate for accurate anatomic localization of pathology. Hybrid imaging with a high-resolution anatomic imaging modality such as CT improves localization and lesion characterization. The advantage of in-line imaging over retrospective software-based coregistration is that the patient undergoing combined PET/CT is not moved physically between the 2 parts of the examination, and there is less frequent misregistration of functional and anatomic data.[5]

MR imaging of lung parenchyma is challenging, owing to respiratory and cardiac motion. There have been significant improvements in staging of bronchogenic carcinoma using MR imaging since the initial study in 1985,[6] with the use of respiratory and cardiac gating/triggering and introduction of new sequences (eg, diffusion-weighted [DW] imaging). These developments have had a substantial impact on image quality and clinical application of MR imaging in staging lung cancer. Although MR imaging is not currently recommended for routine staging of small cell lung cancer (SCLC) or non–small cell lung cancer (NSCLC), it is used to clarify specific areas of concern highlighted on CT, because of the strength of MR imaging in the combined morphologic and functional characterization of hilar or pulmonary lesions. With the introduction of moving table technology, whole-body MR imaging examinations become feasible and can be performed in a routine clinical setting. The recent introduction of MR imaging/PET technology presents exciting research possibilities, but it is too early to understand how this will influence clinical applications.

PATIENT PREPARATION

Many institutions routinely use intravascular iodinated contrast media (CM) for the staging of lung cancer if there is venous access and no contraindications, because of either documented allergic reaction to intravascular iodine or poor renal function (glomerular filtration rate of $\leq$50 mL/s/kg in diabetic patients and $\leq$30 mL/s/kg in nondiabetic patients). Patz and colleagues[7] compared nonenhanced and contrast-enhanced helical acquisitions of the thorax and upper abdomen in 96 patients with a pathologic diagnosis of lung cancer, and concluded that although routine use of intravenous iodinated contrast agent changed the radiologic stage in 4% of patients, it did not significantly affect patient management in their cohort. Subsequent to this study, changes in nodule characterization with dynamic contrast-enhanced CT[8] and more aggressive approaches to patient management with advances in surgery, minimally invasive therapy, and noninvasive treatment have necessitated a higher level of anatomic discrimination and use of CM. An 18-gauge cannula is placed preferably in the left antecubital vein, to reduce streak artifact in the superior vena cava, and 80 to 100 mL of nonionic iso-osmolar or low-osmolar CM containing 320 to 370 mg/mL of iodine is injected at 3 to 5 mL/s using a dual-syringe power injector, followed by a 40-mL saline flush. If abdominal CT is performed, the patient is asked to fast for 4 hours before the examination and 300 to 500 mL of dilute barium suspension is given 30 to 45 minutes before CT to opacify the upper small bowel.

The preparation is similar for PET/CT, as the patient is requested to fast for at least 4 to 6 hours before examination and refrain from any sugar or dextrose-containing fluids (oral or intravenous). The patient is also asked to refrain from strenuous physical activity for 24 to 48 hours before the examination to reduce physiologic uptake of ^{18}F-fluorodeoxyglucose (^{18}F-FDG) in muscle.[9] After arrival in the PET/CT department, the patient's height and weight are recorded and a weight-based dose of ^{18}F-FDG is prepared (for oncology scans, a dose of 0.22 mCi/kg is usual). The patient is interviewed for a history of diabetes mellitus, relevant other current and past medical history, current medications, dates of previous chemotherapy or radiation therapy, the type and date of a lung biopsy or thoracic surgery, and for the presence or absence of recent infection or trauma.[10] All of these parameters may facilitate accurate interpretation of PET findings. The serum glucose is determined to exclude hyperglycemia. At the author's institution a serum glucose level of 9.7 mmol/L (175 mg/dL) is used as a maximum cutoff for performing the procedure. ^{18}F-FDG is injected intravenously and the patient is kept in a quiet room for 1 hour (uptake time) to reduce uptake of

^{18}F-FDG in the neck muscles and larynx. Some institutions administer dilute oral contrast before PET/CT to opacify the upper gastrointestinal tract, but this is not routinely performed for lung tumors at the author's institution.

Patients referred for MR imaging require extensive screening for contraindications to the procedure including claustrophobia, implantation of ferrous material, or devices sensitive to a magnetic field. If gadolinium-based CM is going to be used, the renal function is assessed as for CT.

SCAN PROTOCOLS AND DATA ACQUISITION

Patients who attend for a CT scan are examined supine with arms extended to minimize beam-hardening artifact over the region of the chest. Scout projections are obtained both to delineate the scan range and to prime the tube current modulation software, which ensures optimization of radiation exposure to image noise and provides reductions in the patient's radiation dose.[11] The patient is asked to suspend respiration during inspiration for a few seconds, and image acquisition commences during helical acquisition from the sternal notch to the iliac crest after CM injection; the aim is to image the thorax during opacification of the mediastinal vasculature (20–30 seconds), and the liver is imaged during the portal venous phase (70 seconds). Isotropic images are routinely obtained with modern CT units containing at least 32 detector rows[2] and facilitate review of multiple planar reconstructions (MPR) for assessment of fissural, mediastinal, and chest-wall invasion, and sliding maximum-intensity projections (MIP) for detection of lung nodules.[12] Tube-exposure parameters vary with patient body habitus, but typically a tube potential of 120 to 140 kV and a tube time-current product of 75 to 175 mA will be used. A tube potential of 100 kV can be used in slimmer patients to minimize patient irradiation.[13]

The PET/CT patient is positioned as for CT. A scout topogram is initially performed during continuous table motion, generating an anatomic overview image similar to a conventional radiograph at the locked projection. Topography is performed to define and match the extent of axial examination of CT and PET. The scan range varies, but conventionally is acquired from the skull base to the upper thighs. Although ^{18}F-FDG PET is significantly less sensitive than MR for assessment of brain metastases, these can be identified with PET, and at many institutions the entire brain is covered at PET/CT staging of lung cancer if no recent brain MR image or contrast-enhanced brain CT is available (**Fig. 1**).

Subsequently CT is acquired through the scan range. As patients usually have a PET/CT after a contrast-enhanced staging CT of the thorax and abdomen, only a low-dose non–contrast-enhanced CT is acquired at the time of PET/CT. Scan parameters vary between scanners and institutions; however, typically a tube potential of 120 to 140 kVp and tube current of 60 to 105 mA is used. At PET/CT, CT is usually acquired during quiet respiration for optimal coregistration with PET data, which are acquired over many breathing cycles.[14]

After the CT data are acquired, the patient is repositioned to the PET field of view in the rear of the fused gantry, where the emission scan is obtained. Usually the scan is acquired in the caudocranial direction starting at the upper thighs to limit artifacts from ^{18}F-FDG within the urinary bladder. Normally, between 5 and 7 bed positions are sufficient for the whole-body scan. Depending on the particular scanner and mode of acquisition, each bed position is acquired over 2 to 5 minutes.[15]

Chest MR imaging protocols are fairly simple and do not require electrocardiogram (ECG) gating; however, respiratory-gated techniques are helpful (**Table 1**).[16,17] Scan sequences should be acquired in 2 orientations to visualize lung nodules, and the protocol can be completed in approximately 15 minutes (**Fig. 2**). Additional MR imaging sequences such as DW imaging and first-pass perfusion can be useful in nodule characterization. Dynamic CINE MR images are useful to demonstrate relative motion between tumor and adjacent structures (**Table 2**),[18] to evaluate local invasion. A complete MR imaging protocol requires approximately 60 minutes of examination time.

TUMOR (T) STAGING: ASSESSMENT OF PRIMARY LUNG TUMOR

CT is the gold standard for detection of lung nodules[19] but has limited specificity for small nodules (<10 mm); therefore, consensus guidelines have been developed to facilitate management of indeterminate lung nodules.[20] The T staging for a primary lung cancer requires accurate demarcation of the tumor margin, and thin-slice high-resolution CT is essential for this purpose in small symmetrical[21] and irregular nodules.[22] Petrou and colleagues[23] studied 75 solid lung nodules 3 to 20 mm in diameter imaged with CT, using images reconstructed with 3 different slice thicknesses/reconstruction intervals: 1.25 mm/0.625 mm, 2.5 mm/2 mm, and 5 mm/2.5 mm. The thinner image reconstructions were superior at edge detection and volumetric

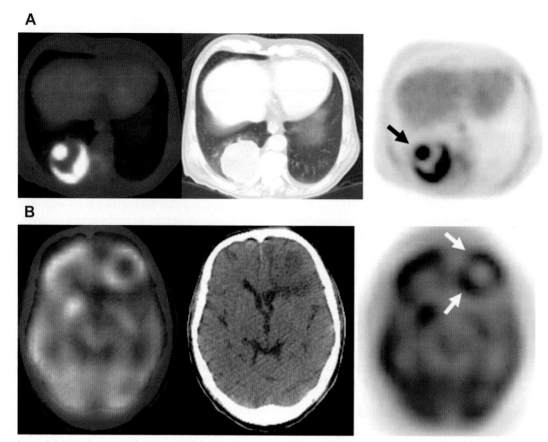

Fig. 1. (*A*) Axial image, right lower lobe squamous cell carcinoma of lung (*arrow*); Maximum standardized uptake value (SUV$_{max}$) = 16.2. (*B*) Axial image through brain shows a mass lesion in left frontal lobe showing increased ^{18}F-fluorodeoxyglucose (^{18}F-FDG) uptake, and associated mass effect, in keeping with a solitary metastatic deposit. No other metastases were seen on the whole-body scan.

analysis of the nodules. However, given the same exposure parameters, thinner image reconstructions incur an increase in image noise. As a primary lung adenocarcinoma may contain a mixed attenuation of solid and ground-glass densities, the contrast to noise ratio (CNR) in such a lesion needs to be maintained to ensure satisfactory evaluation of the ground-glass density component. Therefore, a slice thickness/reconstruction interval of 2.5 to 3/2 mm provides a useful compromise between accurate demarcation of the tumor margin and image noise. Low-dose CT (1 mGy)

Table 1
Basic MR imaging protocol of the lung parenchyma for nodule and lymph node detection

Sequence	Comments	Duration
Localizer based on steady-state free precession (SSFP)	Free breathing, 3 orientations	3 × 40 s
Single-shot turbo spin echo (HASTE)	Breath-hold or respiratory gated, 2 orientations	2 × 30 s
T1-weighted 3-dimensional gradient echo (VIBE) without fat saturation	Breath-hold, 2 orientations	2 × 30 s
T1-weighted 3-dimensional gradient echo (VIBE) with fat saturation	Breath-hold, 2 orientations	2 × 30 s
T2-weighted turbo spin echo (TSE) with fat saturation	Respiratory gated, 2 orientations	2 × approx. 4 min

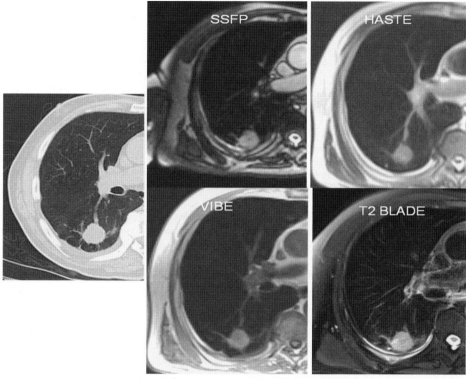

Fig. 2. Typical MR imaging scan sequences for lung nodule visualization and characterization. Lung nodules are characterized based on demonstrable signal intensity with T1- and T2-weighted sequences and on lesion enhancement with intravenous gadolinium-based contrast agent.

is shown to be adequate for detection of small solid nodules (1.6–12.7 mm) in phantom[12] and human studies[24]; it is a useful imaging tool for the follow-up of indeterminate solid nodules. ^{18}F-FDG PET is increasingly being used to characterize solitary pulmonary nodules (SPN) as small as 1 cm in diameter. Smaller lesions may be difficult to categorize because of low count rates with low tumor volume. False-negative results can also occur with low-grade malignancies such

as neuroendocrine tumors of the lung, well-differentiated tumors (**Fig. 3**), or tumors exhibiting purely ground-glass morphology, as seen in bronchoalveolar carcinomas. Two systematic reviews of the literature with meta-analysis report an overall sensitivity of PET for detection of malignant SPN ranging from 96% to 97% with specificity of 78% to 86%.[25,26] Specificity of PET depends on the patient population, and in locations where there is a high prevalence of active granulomatous

Table 2
Extended MR protocol for functional characterization of lung/hilar lesions

Sequence	Comments	Duration
Diffusion-weighted imaging	Respiratory gated, 1 orientation	Approx. 4 min
First-pass perfusion	Breath-hold, contrast media application using an automatic injector	3 min
T1-weighted 3-dimensional gradient echo (VIBE) with fat saturation	Breath-hold, 2 orientations	2 × 30 s
Steady-state free precession CINE	Chest wall invasion: free breathing Mediastinal/vascular/cardiac invasion: ECG gated	N × 20 s

Number of CINE slices depends on size of the lesion; the complete contact area of the lesion with the region of invasion in question needs to be covered.

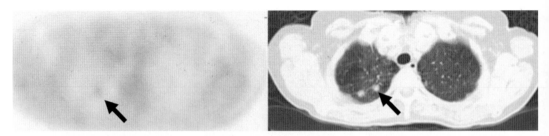

Fig. 3. Axial CT image (*right*) through upper chest shows 2 discrete nodules. The more medial 0.9-cm nodule shows focal uptake of ^{18}F-FDG (SUV$_{max}$ = 1.2), and given its small size, the degree of uptake is suggestive of a malignant nodule. Surgical pathology revealed a moderately differentiated adenocarcinoma, predominantly acinar type. The lateral 0.8-cm nodule is not associated with appreciable ^{18}F-FDG uptake (uptake similar to background). Surgical pathology revealed clear cell carcinoma of lung (a rare, but relatively indolent tumor type).

disease, the false-positive rate of PET may be high, as active granulomas may be ^{18}F-FDG avid. Nodules with ^{18}F-FDG uptake greater than blood pool have a high likelihood of being cancerous.

Recently, Fletcher and colleagues[27] reported that nodules with no increased uptake in comparison with reference lung have a 97% likelihood of being benign, and can be safely followed with repeat imaging, whereas a nodule that has visible uptake but less than blood pool was found to have a 13% likelihood of malignancy. There is little role for PET in patients with a very low or high risk of lung cancer or in characterizing nodules less than 1 cm in diameter. PET appears most useful in patients who have a low or intermediate risk of lung cancer as determined by an evaluation of symptoms, risk factors, and radiographic appearance.[28] The degree of ^{18}F-FDG uptake within the primary tumor can be semiquantitatively assessed using the standardized uptake value (SUV). The SUV of the primary tumor appears to be the strongest prognostic factor for disease-free survival and overall survival among patients treated by curative surgery or radiotherapy.[29] A further analysis of 170 patients who underwent PET/CT showed that even when adjusting for tumor stage and performance status, SUV is prognostic of survival in patients with early-stage NSCLC.[30]

On MR imaging, many pulmonary nodules, including lung cancers and pulmonary metastases, demonstrate low or intermediate signal intensities (SI) on T1-weighted (T1w) images and slightly high intensity on T2-weighted (T2w) images when spin-echo or turbo spin-echo (TSE) sequences are used.[19] MR imaging provides accurate assessment of lesion size in an artificial porcine model using 3-dimensional (3D) and 2-dimensional (2D) gradient-echo (GRE) sequences to achieve a sensitivity of 88% for 4-mm nodules.[31] T2w fast spin-echo (T2-FSE) and T2w half-Fourier single-shot sequences (T2-HASTE)

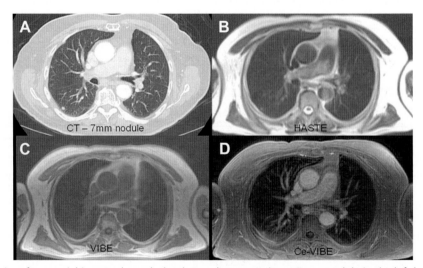

Fig. 4. A series of transaxial images through the thorax demonstrating a 7-mm nodule in the left lower lobe on CT (*A*), half-Fourier single-shot sequences (HASTE) (*B*), and ultrafast gradient-echo (VIBE) sequences before (*C*) and after (*D*) administration of intravenous gadolinium-based contrast agent.

are slightly inferior. For lesions larger than 5 mm, the sensitivity, specificity, and positive and negative predictive values of all sequences except T2-HASTE were close to 100% (**Fig. 4**). These results were reproduced in a patient study, with respiratory triggered T2-FSE and volumetric interpolated 3D gradient-echo (VIBE) outperforming the HASTE sequences.[32] Respiratory triggered T2-FSE required 20 to 30 minutes of scan time, whereas HASTE images were faster to acquire and demonstrated the fewest artifacts. A comparison of ECG-gated axial and coronal breath-hold HASTE acquisitions with CT in 30 patients with pulmonary metastasis or primary lung tumors demonstrated sensitivity values for the HASTE MR imaging sequence of 73% for lesions smaller than 3 mm, 86.3% for lesions between 3 and 5 mm, 95.7% for lesions between 6 and 10 mm, and 100% for lesions larger than 10 mm. The overall sensitivity of the HASTE sequence for the detection of all pulmonary lesions was 85.4%.[33] A subsequent evaluation of different MR imaging techniques used for detection of pulmonary nodules in 28 patients with various primary malignancies revealed mean sensitivities for triggered short-tau inversion recovery (STIR), FSE, and STIR of 72.0%, 69.0%, and 63.4%, respectively.[34] In this study, HASTE, IR-HASTE, and pre- and postcontrast VIBE were inferior to conventional FSE sequences.

A more recent study compared the assessment of 200 (103 malignant) nodules in 161 patients using CT and non–contrast-enhanced MR imaging sequences.[35] Although CT outperformed MR imaging in overall nodule detection (97% vs 82.5%), there was no significant difference in the detection rate for malignant nodules.

One of the largest studies evaluating MR imaging for lung-nodule detection involved 11,766 people in a large screening cohort, examined using 2D-HASTE sequences and T1w 3D VIBE.[36] Forty-six individuals had primary lung cancers with a mean size of 1.98 cm (median, 1.5 cm; range, 0.5–8.2 cm) with a predominance of adenocarcinoma (38/46, 77.6%). The scanning time was only 5 minutes.

DW imaging is a new MR imaging technique for lung nodule characterization that yields information such as the integrity of microscopic structures. Compared with CT, detection of pulmonary nodules using a DW imaging sequence yields a sensitivity of 86.4% for nodules ranging from 6 to 9 mm and 97% for nodules larger than 10 mm.[37] DW imaging has been explored as a new method for evaluation of nodules including subtype classification of pulmonary adenocarcinoma.[38–40] From the few available studies, it can be concluded that basic signal intensity measurements, in combination with comparison of MR imaging signal from other structures such as the spinal cord, demonstrate superior differentiation of malignant from benign lesions in comparison with apparent diffusion coefficient values.

TUMOR (T) STAGING: INVASION OF ADJACENT TISSUES

Glazer and colleagues[41] evaluated 3 CT features to assess mediastinal tumor invasion: (1) less than 3 cm of mediastinal contact, (2) integrity of fat plane, and (3) less than 90° of circumferential contact with the thoracic aorta. The presence of any one of the features confirmed resectability in 36 of 37 cases where mediastinal invasion was a concern. However, irresectability is harder to judge, as in this series 21 of 48 resectable tumors had greater than 3 cm of mediastinal contact. Subsequent studies have not confirmed these results.[42] More than 90° of circumferential contact demonstrates only 40% sensitivity for tumor invasion,[43] and the loss of a fat plane has a sensitivity of only 27% for mediastinal invasion.[44] These figures are not surprising, as the apparent loss of a fat plane may be due to blur from motion artifact or from volume averaging. Therefore, ultrafast image acquisition with in-plane temporal resolution of 83 milliseconds, improved spatial resolution with detector elements of 0.5-mm thickness, along with cardiac and respiratory triggering have addressed many of these issues and are being used to clarify issues of tissue invasion in challenging cases. The advent of true isotropic image acquisition facilitates multiplanar interrogation of volumetric data and evaluation of anatomic regions that are difficult to fully assess on orthogonal planes, and helps to redress the advantage of MR in this area.[45] The use of 1-mm section thickness CT coronal reconstructions for evaluating mediastinal invasion have superior performance sensitivity (86%), specificity (96%) and accuracy (95%) compared with 5-mm axial (71%, 93%, and 90%, respectively) and 1-mm axial (specificity 93%, accuracy 90%) section thickness.[46] Recent introduction of ultrafast cardiac-gated CT acquisitions with functional review on cine loops has proved to be extremely useful in the evaluation of cardiac tumors[47] and is a providing a dynamic assessment of the integrity of anatomic tissue planes compatible with MR techniques, with improved spatial resolution over MR for the assessment of mediastinal invasion.

Although PET is advantageous to CT in delineating tumors associated with extensive atelectasis and may detect subtle areas of invasion not seen on CT, in many patients with NSCLC, PET alone lacks the anatomic resolution to correctly predict the T stage. Integrated PET/CT enables assessment of both metabolism and morphology and more accurately determines local tumor extent, as compared with either PET or CT alone.[48] In a meta-analysis, PET/CT accurately determined the T stage in 82% of cases compared with 55% and 68% with PET alone and CT alone, respectively.[49]

MR imaging has demonstrated utility for evaluation of invasion of mediastinal structures, especially the pericardium or myocardium (**Fig. 5**).[50] As in CT, MR depends on visualization of the tumor within the mediastinal fat. In a study in 170 patients, T1w images (without cardiac or respiratory gating) were compared with CT images regarding mediastinal invasion. No difference between CT and MR was found for distinguishing between T3-T4 and T1-T2 tumors. However, MR imaging showed mediastinal invasion in 11 patients, which resulted in a small but significantly higher accuracy than CT.

ECG-gated sequences are recommended to evaluate invasion of vascular and cardiac structures.[51] Using the presence of sliding motion of adjacent structures as a sign of noninvasion, CINE MR revealed an accuracy, sensitivity, and specificity of 94.4%, 100%, and 92.9%.[52] Also, evaluation of chest-wall invasion benefits from dynamic CINE imaging whereby the tumor moves along the parietal pleura during respiration if there is no invasion.[53] In case of invasion, the tumor is attached to the wall and shows little or no movement. In this study of 25 patients, sensitivity, specificity, and accuracy of dynamic CINE imaging for the detection of chest-wall invasion were 100%, 70%, and 76%, respectively, and those of conventional CT and MR imaging were 80%, 65%, and 68%. The negative predictive value in this study was 100%.

A series of 50 NSCLC patients with suspected mediastinal and hilar invasion were visualized with contrast-enhanced CT scans, and noncardiac and cardiac-gated contrast-enhanced MR angiographies.[54] The ECG-gated MR angiography showed higher sensitivity, specificity, and accuracy than the nongated angiography for detection of mediastinal and hilar invasion.

NODAL DISEASE

A short axis greater than 10 mm is widely used as the frame of reference for enlarged mediastinal and hilar lymph nodes on CT.[55,56] However, size criteria provide poor specificity for nodal

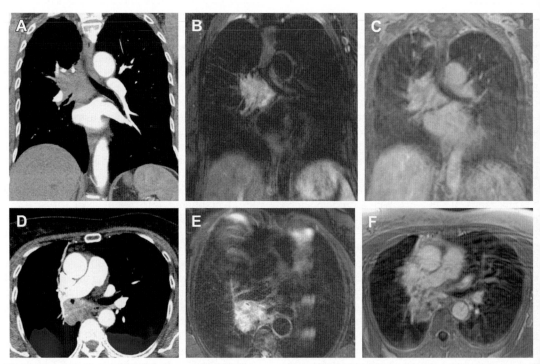

Fig. 5. A series of coronal (*A–C*) and transaxial (*D–F*) images through the thorax demonstrating the appearance of mediastinal and hilar lymph nodes on CT (*A*, *D*), T2-weighted inversion recovery (SPAIR) (*B*, *F*), and gadolinium-enhanced gradient-echo (VIBE) (*C*, *E*) sequences.

metastases, as significant lymph node enlargement occurs in the absence of metastatic involvement,[57] 37% of 2- to 4-cm lymph nodes are tumor free,[58] and nonenlarged nodes contain tumor deposits, particularly adenocarcinoma.[59] More recent evaluation of maximum iodine-related attenuation during dual-energy CT for the staging of lung cancer in 37 patients has demonstrated a moderate correlation ($r = 0.570$; $P = .047$) with ^{18}F-FDG PET/CT SUVs for nodal involvement.[60]

PET/CT is more sensitive than CT alone in mediastinal nodal staging. A meta-analysis of the literature reveals that PET/CT has a sensitivity of 81% and a specificity of 90% for detection of mediastinal lymph node metastasis (**Fig. 6**). Even though the specificity is relatively high, using PET to guide therapy would deny a significant number of patients a chance at curative therapy.[61] Furthermore, there remains an unacceptably high false-negative rate for nodal metastases with both modalities. In one study, patients with clinical N1 disease suggested by integrated PET/CT had a relatively high incidence (17.6% after mediastinoscopy and 23.5% after endoscopic ultrasound-guided fine-needle aspiration [EBUS-FNA]) of unsuspected N2 disease.[62] These findings were validated prospectively as well in a trial comparing PET/CT with histologic sampling of nodes. This study found an overall sensitivity, specificity, positive predictive value, and negative predictive value of 70%, 94%, 64%, and 95%, respectively.[63] The explanation for the relatively low positive predictive value is that interpretation of PET may be confounded by false-positive results; this may be a significant confounding factor in interpreting PET in areas endemic for granulomatous disease. The specificity of PET/CT nodal staging may be increased when incorporating morphologic data regarding the metabolically active nodes. Specifically, calcified nodes or nodes with attenuation higher than the surrounding great vessels on unenhanced CT are likely to be benign; the increased uptake of ^{18}F-FDG within these nodes may be attributed to follicular hyperplasia at the cortex and macrophage infiltration of the medulla at histologic evaluation (**Fig. 7**).[64]

Like CT, MR has a short-axis threshold of 10 mm for evaluating benignancy in mediastinal lymph nodes. Yi and colleagues[65] assessed 174 patients with NSCLC for nodal involvement, comparing MR (breath-hold, cardiac-gated T2-weighted triple-inversion black-blood TSE sequence) and ^{18}F-FDG PET/CT. It was found that high signal intensity and eccentric cortical thickening or obliteration of a fatty hilum can be reliable indicators of malignancy, even in normal-sized nodes. Ohno and colleagues[66] compared MR imaging with STIR TSE sequences with ^{18}F-FDG PET/CT in 115 patients with NSCLC. The signal intensity of each lymph node on MR was normalized to a saline phantom. By doing so, the MR-based sensitivity (90.1%) and accuracy (92.2%) was higher than that of PET/CT (76.7% sensitivity and 83.5% accuracy). In general, on STIR TSE metastatic nodes

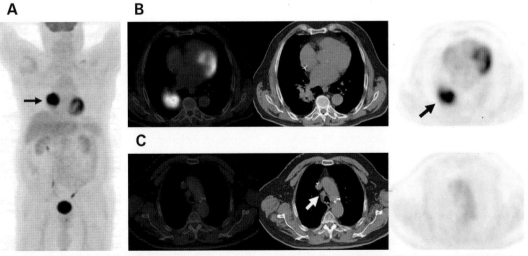

Fig. 6. (*A*) Maximum-intensity projection whole-body image shows focal uptake of ^{18}F-FDG in a right lower lobe lung mass, in keeping with malignancy. No other abnormal ^{18}F-FDG uptake is seen. (*B*) Axial CT image shows corresponding 6.6-cm metabolically active mass (SUV$_{max}$ = 12.4) whose surgical pathology represents a moderately differentiated squamous cell carcinoma (*arrow*). (*C*) On CT, below the level of the aortic arch, there is a borderline station 4R node (*white arrow*), which is not associated with increased ^{18}F-FDG uptake. This node was also negative on surgical pathology.

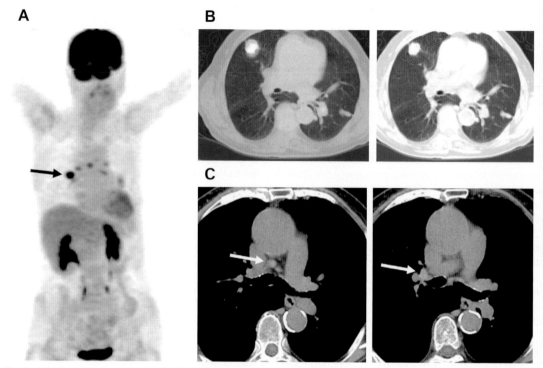

Fig. 7. (A) Maximum-intensity projection whole-body image shows marked focal uptake of ^{18}F-FDG in a right upper lobe moderately differentiated adenocarcinoma of lung (*arrow*). There is also symmetric increased uptake of ^{18}F-FDG in mediastinal nodes. (B) Axial fused and CT image shows primary tumor. (C) Axial non–contrast-enhanced CT shows that the metabolically active nodes are of higher attenuation than mediastinal vessels (*arrows*). Fine-needle aspiration under endobronchial ultrasonography revealed no evidence of metastatic disease.

have a high signal, whereas nonmetastatic nodes present with a low signal. In a later study by the same group using the same MR sequence, MR imaging achieved a sensitivity of 82.8% and accuracy of 86.8%.[67] In this study, MR outperformed ^{18}F-FDG PET/CT significantly, which showed a sensitivity of 74.2%. DW images were also obtained, showing a sensitivity and accuracy of 74.2% and 84.4%, respectively. Therefore, the investigators concluded that quantitative STIR TSE is the best method for differentiation of metastatic and nonmetastatic lymph nodes.[68] However, a more recent study including 70 patients with NSCLC demonstrated no significant difference between quantitative analyses of DW-MR images and STIR-MR images.[69]

DISTANT METASTASIS

Postmortem data reveal that metastatic disease from primary lung cancer involves several body organs; the liver is involved in 33% to 39%, the adrenal glands in 20% to 33%, the brain in 16% to 26%, the kidney in 14% to 18%, and bone metastases in 15% to 21%.[70] Metastases from a primary lung cancer are typically hypovascular

and best demonstrated on a venous phase of enhancement,[71] which is typically 70 seconds after initiation of contrast injection in abdominal tissues.

One of the main advantages of PET/CT over conventional imaging is its higher sensitivity in identifying extrathoracic metastases. A limitation of PET in staging of NSCLC is in identification of cranial metastases, owing to the high physiologic uptake of ^{18}F-FDG in the brain. However, PET is superior to conventional imaging in detecting noncranial distant metastases. A meta-analysis performed by the Health Technology Board for Scotland included 19 studies evaluating distant metastases in NSCLC. The investigators concluded that ^{18}F-FDG PET may be useful in staging patients believed to be free of distant metastases. PET seemed to have incremental value in identifying occult metastatic disease in the skeleton and adrenal glands.[72] A more recent review by the National Institute for Clinical Excellence (NICE) calculated a summary sensitivity of 93% and specificity of 96% for staging with PET. NICE also found that in an average of 15% of patients, unexpected extrathoracic metastases may be detected by ^{18}F-FDG PET (**Fig. 8**).[73] Furthermore, in a recent randomized, controlled

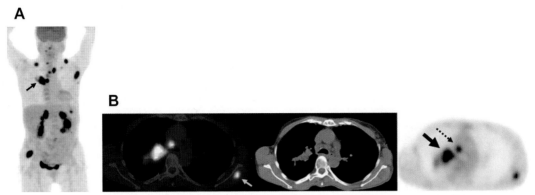

Fig. 8. (*A*) Maximum-intensity projection whole-body image shows marked focal uptake of ^{18}F-FDG in a right upper lobe tumor (*arrow*). Uptake of ^{18}F-FDG is also seen in multiple mediastinal and supraclavicular nodes, bilateral adrenal glands, and several soft-tissue sites. (*B*) Axial image at level of tumor (*arrow*) shows abnormal metabolism in mediastinal nodes (*dotted arrow*) and a deposit in left infraspinatous muscle (further skeletal muscle deposits were seen on the whole-body scan including in right gluteus maximus muscle).

multicenter trial including 320 patients who were randomized to a PET/CT plus cranial imaging arm (n = 163) and conventional imaging arm (n = 157; CT abdomen, bone scan, and cranial imaging), 23 (14%) of 163 patients in the PET/CT arm were correctly upstaged and avoided inappropriate surgery compared with 11 (7%) of 157 in the conventional imaging arm (*P* = .046).[74] The investigators concluded that in NSCLC, staging with PET/CT better identifies those patients with extrathoracic disease, sparing some from stage-inappropriate surgery. It was also concluded that PET/CT can replace conventional imaging in the staging of early-stage NSCLC.

The introduction of multichannel MR systems, parallel imaging technology, and moving tables have enabled whole-body MR examinations to become possible on a routine basis. Examinations from head to toe within 60 minutes are possible and are thus shorter than a PET/CT examination. In this context it has to be mentioned that in approximately 20% of patients who undergo surgical treatment, PET/CT missed metastases.[75] The overall experience is that whole-body MR imaging is better for detecting brain and liver metastases, whereas PET/CT is better for detecting bone and soft-tissue metastases or extrathoracic nodal metastases.[65] In an early study comprising 41 patients, lymph nodes were detected with a sensitivity/specificity of 98%/83% for PET/CT and 80%/75% for whole-body MR imaging, respectively.[76] Distant lesions were detected with a sensitivity/specificity of 82% for PET/CT and 96%/82% for whole-body MR imaging. Accuracy for correct TNM staging was 96% for PET/CT and 91% for whole-body MR imaging.

In a large comparison study, 203 patients with NSCLC were included.[77] Including evaluation of

brain metastasis sensitivities, specificities, and accuracy of whole-body MR imaging with DW imaging (70%, 92%, and 87.7%) yielded the same results as PET/CT (62.5%, 94.5%, and 88.2%). In 65 patients whole-body MR imaging was done using a 3-T system.[65] Primary tumors were correctly staged in 82% at PET/CT and 86% at whole-body MR imaging. N stages were correctly determined in 70% at PET/CT and in 68% at whole-body MR imaging. Accuracy for detecting metastases was 86% at PET/CT and 86% at whole-body MR imaging. Thus overall, whole-body MR imaging is as accurate as PET/CT for M staging in patients with lung cancer.

IMAGING ALGORITHM

There has been considerable interest in the utility of conventional imaging, PET/CT, and interventional procedures for the accurate staging of lung cancer. Fischer and colleagues[78] performed a randomized controlled trial to compare the role of conventional staging alone and conventional staging with PET/CT in compiling the rate of futile thoracotomies in patients with lung cancer. Futile thoracotomy was defined as any thoracotomy for a benign lung lesion, pathologically proven mediastinal lymph node involvement (N2), stage IIIB or IV disease, inoperable T3 or T4 disease, or recurrent disease or death from any cause within 1 year after randomization. A lower rate of thoracotomies was reported in the PET/CT arm as well as a lower rate of futile thoracotomies, but there was no survival benefit. A further prospective, randomized multicenter trial including 337 patients compared staging with conventional imaging versus PET/CT. Inappropriate surgery was avoided in 14% of patients upstaged by

PET/CT, compared with 7% in the conventional imaging group (P = .046). PET/CT and cranial imaging identified more precisely those patients with mediastinal and extrathoracic disease. The investigators also concluded that PET/CT can replace conventional imaging in staging of early NSCLC.[79]

After a detailed clinical history and physical examination, a patient suspected of having a primary lung cancer will have a 2-view chest radiograph and a CT scan of the thorax and upper abdomen. Chest radiography is easy to perform, accessible, and of low cost, and provides a useful baseline for disease surveillance. If a patient has disseminated malignancy based on chest radiography, this will necessitate careful consideration regarding the need for further imaging investigations and the requirement for obtaining tissue confirmation of disease. Occasionally in this scenario, the patient presents with palpable lymphadenopathy, and a fine-needle aspiration biopsy is performed. Whenever possible, a tissue diagnosis is required to confirm the diagnosis and to delineate potential treatment options. Thoracic and upper abdominal CT is helpful to confirm the presence of a lung mass or the presence of any complications, metastasis, or synchronous lung cancers. If the CT appearances suggest localized disease, a PET/CT scan is performed to confirm absence of mediastinal nodal disease in nonenlarged lymph nodes, and the absence of occult distant metastases. Guidelines of the American Association of Chest Physicians do not recommend invasive mediastinal staging in cases of normal-sized mediastinal nodes on CT, negative nodes on PET/CT, a peripheral clinical stage 1A tumor (T1N0M0), and a negative clinical examination. Mediastinoscopy with lymph node sampling is recommended in patients with tumors within the central third of the hemithorax, or T2 tumors regardless of CT or PET/CT findings or if there are abnormal mediastinal nodes on either CT or PET/CT.[80] Positive nodes on ^{18}F-FDG PET should be confirmed histologically by mediastinoscopy or EBUS-FNA before curative surgery is excluded as a treatment option. Negative ^{18}F-FDG PET/CT should be interpreted in light of the patient's pretest probability of mediastinal metastases (as per location and size of tumor) and whether there are morphologically abnormal mediastinal nodes on CT.

MR imaging is performed to exclude brain metastases in asymptomatic patients who have potentially curable disease, particularly patients with a diagnosis of lung adenocarcinoma; and patients who present with signs or symptoms suggestive of brain metastases but in whom cranial CT is nondiagnostic. Targeted MR imaging can also be performed to answer specific questions, for example, to exclude brachial plexus invasion.

The use of dedicated imaging algorithms for the staging of SCLC and NSCLC has become less differentiated in many centers because of the drive to minimize the wait time between initial patient assessment and treatment. Therefore, once the patient is clinically assessed and the chest radiograph evaluated, the patient is further assessed with CT of the thorax and upper abdomen. Further evaluation is determined by the results of these scans. Specific imaging guidelines for the staging of lung cancer incorporate a multimodality approach as outlined in this article[81]; however, the protocol is tailored to the specific circumstances of individual patients and institutional resources.

REFERENCES

1. Doria-Rose VP, Szabo E. Screening and prevention of lung cancer. In: Kernstine KH, Reckamp KL, editors. Lung cancer: a multidisciplinary approach to diagnosis and management. New York: Demos Medical Publishing; 2010. p. 53–72.

2. Dalrymple NC, Prasad SR, El-Merhi FM, et al. Price of isotropy in multidetector CT. Radiographics 2007;27:49–62.

3. Brenner DJ, Hall EJ. Computed tomography—an increasing source of radiation exposure. N Engl J Med 2007;357:2277–84.

4. Singh S, Kalra MK, Gilman MD, et al. Adaptive statistical iterative reconstruction technique for radiation dose reduction in chest CT: a pilot study. Radiology 2011;259:565–73.

5. Kinahan PE, Hasegawa BH, Beyer T. X-ray-based attenuation correction for positron emission tomography/computed tomography scanners. Semin Nucl Med 2003;33:166–79.

6. Webb WR, Jensen BG, Sollitto R, et al. Bronchogenic carcinoma: staging with MR compared with staging with CT and surgery. Radiology 1985;156:117–24.

7. Patz EF Jr, Erasmus JJ, McAdams HP, et al. Lung cancer staging and management: comparison of contrast – enhanced and nonenhanced helical CT of the thorax. Radiology 1999;212:56–60.

8. Swensen SJ, Viggiano RW, Midthun DE, et al. Lung nodule enhancement at CT: multicentre study. Radiology 2000;214:73–80.

9. Jackson R, Schlarman TC, Hubble WL, et al. Prevalence and patterns of physiologic muscle uptake detected with whole body ^{18}F-FDG PET. J Nucl Med Technol 2006;34(1):29–33.

10. ACR practice guidelines: ACR Practice Guideline for Performing FDG-PET/CT in Oncology. Accessed April 19, 2012.

11. McCullough C, Bruesewitz MR, Kofler JM, et al. Tools: overview of available options. Radiographics 2006;26:503–12.

12. Sieren JC, Ohno Y, Koyama H, et al. Recent technological and application developments in computed tomography and magnetic resonance imaging for improved pulmonary nodule detection and lung cancer staging. J Magn Reson Imag 2010;32(6): 1353–69.

13. Heyer CM, Mohr P, Lemburg SP, et al. Image quality and radiation exposure at pulmonary CT angiography with 100- or 120-kVp protocol: prospective randomized study. Radiology 2007;245:577–83.

14. Goerres GW, Burger C, Schwitter MR, et al. PET/CT of the abdomen: optimizing the patient breathing pattern. Eur Radiol 2003;13(4):734–9.

15. Beyer T, Antoch G, Muller SP, et al. Acquisition protocol considerations for combined PET/CT Imaging. J Nucl Med 2004;45:25s–35s.

16. Puderbach M, Hintze C, Ley S, et al. MR imaging of the chest: a practical approach at 1.5T. Eur J Radiol 2007;64:345–55.

17. Biederer J, Hintze C, Fabel M. MRI of pulmonary nodules: technique and diagnostic value. Cancer Imaging 2008;8:125–30.

18. Hochhegger B, Marchiori E, Sedlaczek O, et al. MRI in lung cancer: a pictorial essay. Br J Radiol 2011; 84:661–8.

19. Sieren JC, Ohno Y, Koyama H, et al. Recent technological and application developments in computed tomography and magnetic resonance imaging for improved pulmonary nodule detection and lung cancer staging. J Magn Reson Imaging 2010;32: 1353–69.

20. MacMahon H, Austin JH, Gamsu G, et al. Guidelines for management of small pulmonary nodules detected on CT scans: a statement from the Fleischner Society. Radiology 2005;237:395–400.

21. Yankelevitz DF, Gupta R, Zhao B, et al. Small pulmonary nodules: evaluation with repeat CT—preliminary experience. Radiology 1999;212:561–6.

22. Yankelevitz DF, Reeves AP, Kostis WJ, et al. Small pulmonary nodules: volumetrically determined growth rates based on CT evaluation. Radiology 2000;217:251–6.

23. Petrou M, Qunit LE, Nan B, et al. Pulmonary nodule volumetric measurement variability as a function of CT slice thickness and nodule morphology. AJR Am J Roentgenol 2007;188:306–12.

24. Aberle DR, Adams AM, Berg C, et al. Reduced lung-cancer mortality with low-dose Computed Tomographic Screening. N Engl J Med 2011;365: 395–409.

25. Fischer BM, Mortensen J, Hojgaard L. Positron emission tomography in the diagnosis and staging of lung cancer: a systematic, quantitative review. Lancet Oncol 2001;2(11):659–66.

26. Gould MK, Maclean CC, Kuschner WG, et al. Accuracy of positron emission tomography for diagnosis of pulmonary nodules and mass lesions: a meta-analysis. JAMA 2001;285(7):914–24.

27. Fletcher JW, Kymes SM, Gould M, et al. A comparison of the diagnostic accuracy of ^{18}F-FDG PET and CT in the characterization of solitary pulmonary nodules. J Nucl Med 2008;49:179–85.

28. Detterbeck FC, Falen S, Rivera MP, et al. Seeking a home for a PET, part 1: defining the appropriate place for positron emission tomography imaging in the diagnosis of pulmonary nodules or masses. Chest 2004;125:2294–9.

29. Downey RJ, Akhurst T, Gonen M, et al. Preoperative F-18 fluorodeoxyglucose-positron emission tomography maximal standardized uptake value predicts survival after lung cancer resection. J Clin Oncol 2004;22:3255–60.

30. Gulenchyn KY, Farncombe TH, Maziak DE, et al. Survival of non-small cell lung cancer (NSCLC) patients in a randomized trial as predicted by the FDG-PET standardized uptake value (SUV). 2010 ASCO Annual Meeting abstract. Chicago (IL), June 4–8, 2010.

31. Biederer J, Schoene A, Freitag S, et al. Simulated pulmonary nodules implanted in a dedicated porcine chest phantom: sensitivity of MR imaging for detection. Radiology 2003;227:475–83.

32. Both M, Schultze J, Reuter M, et al. Fast T1- and T2-weighted pulmonary MR-imaging in patients with bronchial carcinoma. Eur J Radiol 2005;53: 478–88.

33. Schroeder T, Ruehm SG, Debatin JF, et al. Detection of pulmonary nodules using a 2D HASTE MR sequence: comparison with MDCT. AJR Am J Roentgenol 2005;185:979–84.

34. Bruegel M, Gaa J, Woertler K, et al. MRI of the lung: value of different turbo spin-echo, single-shot turbo spin-echo, and 3D gradient-echo pulse sequences for the detection of pulmonary metastases. J Magn Reson Imaging 2007;25:73–81.

35. Koyama H, Ohno Y, Kono A, et al. Quantitative and qualitative assessment of non-contrast-enhanced pulmonary MR imaging for management of pulmonary nodules in 161 subjects. Eur Radiol 2008;18: 2120–31.

36. Wu NY, Cheng HC, Ko JS, et al. Magnetic resonance imaging for lung cancer detection: experience in a population of more than 10,000 healthy individuals. BMC Cancer 2011;11:242.

37. Regier M, Schwarz D, Henes FO, et al. Diffusion-weighted MR-imaging for the detection of pulmonary nodules at 1.5 Tesla: intraindividual comparison with multidetector computed tomography. J Med Imaging Radiat Oncol 2011;55:266–74.

38. Satoh S, Kitazume Y, Ohdama S, et al. Can malignant and benign pulmonary nodules be

differentiated with diffusion-weighted MRI? AJR Am J Roentgenol 2008;191:464–70.

39. Uto T, Takehara Y, Nakamura Y, et al. Higher sensitivity and specificity for diffusion-weighted imaging of malignant lung lesions without apparent diffusion coefficient quantification. Radiology 2009;252:247–54.

40. Koyama H, Ohno Y, Aoyama N, et al. Comparison of STIR turbo SE imaging and diffusion-weighted imaging of the lung: capability for detection and subtype classification of pulmonary adenocarcinomas. Eur Radiol 2010;20:790–800.

41. Glazer HS, Kaiser LR, Anderson DJ, et al. Indeterminate mediastinal invasion in bronchogenic carcinoma: CT evaluation. Radiology 1989;173:37–42.

42. Scott IR, Muller NL, Miller RR, et al. Resectable stage III lung cancer: CT, surgical and pathological correlation. Radiology 1988;166:75–9.

43. Herman SJ, Winton TI, Weisbrod GL, et al. Mediastinal invasion by bronchogenic carcinoma: CT signs. Radiology 1994;190:841–6.

44. White PG, Admas H, Crane MD, et al. Preoperative staging of carcinomas of the bronchus: can computed tomography scanning reliably identify stage III tumours? Thorax 1994;49:951–7.

45. Laurent F, Drouillard J, Dorcier F. Bronchogenic carcinoma staging: CT vs MR imaging—assessment with surgery. Eur J Cardiothorac Surg 1988;2:31–6.

46. Higashino T, Ohno Y, Takenaka D, et al. Thin-section multiplanar reformats from multidetector-row CT data; utility for assessment of regional tumour extent in non-small cell lung cancer. Eur J Radiol 2005;56: 48–55.

47. Wintersperger BJ. Imaging of cardiac and paracardiac masses and pseudotumors. In: Schoepf UJ, editor. CT of the heart: principles and applications. Humana Press: New Jersey 2005. part IV. p. 171–82.

48. Halpern BS, Schiepers C, Weber WA, et al. Presurgical staging of non-small cell lung cancer: positron emission tomography, integrated positron emission tomography/CT, and software image fusion. Chest 2005;128:2289–97.

49. De Wever W, Stroobants S, Coolen J, et al. Integrated PET/CT in the staging of non-small cell lung cancer: technical aspects and clinical integration. Eur Respir J 2009;33:201–12.

50. Webb WR, Gatsonis C, Zerhouni EA, et al. CT and MR imaging in staging non-small cell bronchogenic carcinoma: report of the Radiologic Diagnostic Oncology Group. Radiology 1991;178:705–13.

51. White CS. MR evaluation of the pericardium and cardiac malignancies. Magn Reson Imaging Clin N Am 1996;4:237–51.

52. Seo JS, Kim YJ, Choi BW, et al. Usefulness of magnetic resonance imaging for evaluation of cardiovascular invasion: evaluation of sliding motion between thoracic mass and adjacent structures on cine MR images. J Magn Reson Imaging 2005;22:234–41.

53. Sakai S, Murayama S, Murakami J, et al. Bronchogenic carcinoma invasion of the chest wall: evaluation with dynamic cine MRI during breathing. J Comput Assist Tomogr 1997;21:595–600.

54. Ohno Y, Adachi S, Motoyama A, et al. Multiphase ECG-triggered 3D contrast-enhanced MR angiography: utility for evaluation of hilar and mediastinal invasion of bronchogenic carcinoma. J Magn Reson Imaging 2001;13:215–24.

55. Glazer GM, Gross BH, Quint LE, et al. Normal mediastinal lymph nodes: number and size according to American Thoracic Society mapping. AJR Am J Roentgenol 1985;144:261–5.

56. Kiyono K, Sone S, Sakai F, et al. The number and size of normal mediastinal lymph nodes: a post mortem study. AJR Am J Roentgenol 1985;150: 771–6.

57. Kerr KM, Lamb D, Wathen CG, et al. Pathological assessment of mediastinal lymph nodes in lung cancer: implications for non invasive staging. Thorax 1992;47:337–41.

58. McCloud TC, Bourgouin PM, Greenberg RW, et al. Bronchogenic carcinoma: analysis of staging in the mediastinum with CT by correlative lymph node mapping and sampling. Radiology 1992;182:319–23.

59. Gross BH, Glazer GM, Orringer MB, et al. Bronchogenic carcinoma metastatic to normal sized lymph nodes: frequency and significance. Radiology 1986;166:71–4.

60. Schmid-Bindert G, Henzler T, Chu TQ, et al. Functional Imaging of lung cancer using dual energy CT: how does iodine related attenuation correlate with standardized uptake value of ^{18}FDG-PET-CT? Eur Radiol 2012;22:93–103.

61. Ung Y, Walker-Dilks C. Program in evidence-based care. PET recommendation report 9. PET imaging in small cell lung cancer. Available at: https://www.cancercare.on.ca/. Accessed April 22, 2012.

62. Cerfolio RJ, Bryant AS, Eloubeidi MA. Routine mediastinoscopy and esophageal ultrasound fine-needle aspiration in patients with non-small cell lung cancer who are clinically N2 negative: a prospective study. Chest 2006;130(6):1791–5.

63. Darling GE, Maziak DE, Incluet RI, et al. Positron emission tomography-computed tomography compared with invasive mediastinal staging in non-small cell lung cancer: results of mediastinal staging in the early lung positron emission tomography trial. J Thorac Oncol 2011;6(8):1367–72.

64. Shim SS, Lee KS, Kim BT, et al. Non-small cell lung cancer: prospective comparison of integrated FDG PET/CT and CT alone for preoperative staging. Radiology 2005;236:1011–9.

65. Yi CA, Shin KM, Lee KS, et al. Non-small cell lung cancer staging: efficacy comparison of integrated PET/CT versus 3.0-T whole-body MR imaging. Radiology 2008;248:632–42.

66. Ohno Y, Koyama H, Nogami M, et al. STIR turbo SE MR imaging vs. coregistered FDG-PET/CT: quantitative and qualitative assessment of N-stage in non-small-cell lung cancer patients. J Magn Reson Imaging 2007;26:1071–80.

67. Ohno Y, Koyama H, Yoshikawa T, et al. N stage disease in patients with non-small cell lung cancer: efficacy of quantitative and qualitative assessment with STIR turbo spin-echo imaging, diffusion-weighted MR imaging, and fluorodeoxyglucose PET/CT. Radiology 2011;261:605–15.

68. Takenaka D, Ohno Y, Hatabu H, et al. Differentiation of metastatic versus non-metastatic mediastinal lymph nodes in patients with non-small cell lung cancer using respiratory-triggered short inversion time inversion recovery (STIR) turbo spin-echo MR imaging. Eur J Radiol 2002;44:216–24.

69. Nakayama J, Miyasaka K, Omatsu T, et al. Metastases in mediastinal and hilar lymph nodes in patients with non-small cell lung cancer: quantitative assessment with diffusion-weighted magnetic resonance imaging and apparent diffusion coefficient. J Comput Assist Tomogr 2010;34:1–8.

70. Spencer H. Pathology of the lung. 4th edition. Oxford (United Kingdom): Pergamon Press; 1985. p. 924.

71. Sica GT, Ji H, Ros PR. CT and MR imaging of hepatic metastases. AJR Am J Roentgenol 2000;174:691–8.

72. Bradbury I, Bonnell E, Boynton J, et al. Positron emission tomography (PET) imaging in cancer management. Glasgow (Scotland): Health Technology Board for Scotland; 2002. Health Technology Assessment Report No.: 2.

73. The diagnosis and treatment of lung cancer (CG121). In: Clinical Guidelines April 2011. Available at: http://www.nice.org.uk/nicemedia/pdf/CG024niceguideline.pdf. Accessed April 25, 2012.

74. Maziuk D, Darling GE, Inculet RI, et al. A randomized controlled trial (RCT) of ^{18}F-fluorodeoxyglucose (FDG) positron emission tomography (PET) versus conventional imaging (CI) in staging potentially resectable non-small cell lung cancer (NSCLC). J Clin Oncol 2008;26(Suppl):739s [abstract: 7502].

75. Ohno Y, Koyama H, Dinkel J, et al. Lung cancer. In: Kauczor H-U, editor. MRI of the lung. Springer; 2009;179–216.

76. Schmidt GP, Baur-Melnyk A, Herzog P, et al. High-resolution whole-body magnetic resonance image tumor staging with the use of parallel imaging versus dual-modality positron emission tomography-computed tomography: experience on a 32-channel system. Invest Radiol 2005;40:743–53.

77. Ohno Y, Koyama H, Onishi Y, et al. Non-small cell lung cancer: whole-body MR examination for M-stage assessment—utility for whole-body diffusion-weighted imaging compared with integrated FDG PET/CT. Radiology 2008;248:643–54.

78. Fischer B, Lassen U, Mortensen J, et al. Preoperative staging of lung cancer with combined PET-CT. N Engl J Med 2009;361:32–9.

79. Maziak DE, Darling GE, Inculet RI, et al. Positron emission tomography in staging early lung cancer: a randomized trial. Ann Intern Med 2009;151:221–8 W-48.

80. Detterbeck FC, Jantz MA, Wallace M, et al. Invasive mediastinal staging of lung cancer: ACCP evidence-based clinical practice guidelines (2nd edition). Chest 2007;132(Suppl 3):202S–20S.

81. Silvestri GA, Gould MK, Margolis ML, et al. Noninvasive staging of non-small cell lung cancer*: ACCP evidenced-based clinical practice guidelines (2nd edition). Chest 2007;132:178S–201S.

Lung Cancer
Multidisciplinary Approach to Tissue Sampling

Andrew C. Chang, MD[a],
Baskaran Sundaram, MBBS, MRCP, FRCR[b],
Douglas A. Arenberg, MD[c],*

KEYWORDS

- Lung • Nodule • Biopsy • Bronchoscopy • Computed tomography • Surgery • Multidisciplinary

KEY POINTS

- Patients with lung nodules suspicious for malignancy should not have a biopsy (as opposed to surgery) if it won't change the treatment.
- Whenever possible, any biopsy done for suspected cancer should provide both a diagnosis, and an unambiguous stage, as well as tissue for molecular analysis.
- The choice of biopsy approach should balance certainty (accuracy), safety, the patients' preferences, and account for local expertise.

With the spreading use of computed tomography (CT) imaging for ever-widening indications and the potential for widespread screening for lung cancer among those perceived to be at risk, lung nodules that raise varying degrees of suspicion for cancer are an increasingly relevant problem in radiology practice. The care of patients with known or suspected lung cancer has become increasingly complex. As management of lung cancer evolves, the majority of patients now receive, at some time during the course of their disease, multiple modes of treatment, for example, surgery, chemotherapy, radiotherapy, and/or palliative treatment. In line with this, evidence-based guidelines from the American College of Chest Physicians (ACCP)[1] and the National Comprehensive Cancer Network (NCCN)[2] advocate that patient care and treatment planning be managed by multidisciplinary teams.[1] The term multidisciplinary implies that teams combining individuals with diverse expertise in surgical, medical, and radiologic subspecialties provide efficient, evidence-based care and achieve optimal outcomes of complex diseases. Individuals with

at least a special interest, if not a career focus, in thoracic malignancies should comprise such teams. In the context of tissue sampling, the goal of multidisciplinary care should be to establish a seamless, efficient, and coordinated approach to diagnosis, staging, and treatment of patients with suspected lung cancer. The goal should be to first determine which patients require a biopsy, then to select the one biopsy approach that provides both a diagnosis and an accurate stage, balancing certainty for treating physicians and safety for the patient. Accurate staging of patients with lung cancer is of paramount importance because of the prognostic importance of disease stage, as well as the fact that treatment of lung cancer varies widely across stages (Table 1). Finally, it is increasingly important that tissue be obtained for both pathologic diagnosis and selected molecular analyses to guide treatment decisions. The greatest impact of the multidisciplinary team may be the coordinated efforts of multiple specialists to stage the patient's lung cancer accurately, to provide reliable prognostic

[a] Section of Thoracic Surgery, University of Michigan, 2120 Taubman Center, SPC 5344, 1500 East Medical Center Drive, Ann Arbor, MI 48109, USA; [b] Department of Radiology, University of Michigan Health System, 1500 East Medical Center Drive, Cardiovascular Center-Room 5481, Ann Arbor, MI 48109, USA; [c] Pulmonary & Critical Care Medicine, 6301 MSRB III, SPC 5642, 1150 West Medical Center Drive, Ann Arbor, MI 48109, USA
* Corresponding author.
E-mail address: darenber@umich.edu

Radiol Clin N Am 50 (2012) 951–960
http://dx.doi.org/10.1016/j.rcl.2012.05.001
0033-8389/12/$ – see front matter © 2012 Elsevier Inc. All rights reserved.

Table 1
Variation in the treatment options for lung cancer according to stage

Anatomic Stage	Acceptable Physiologic Reserve	Poor Physiologic Reserve
I	Surgery (certain patients with stage IB *may* be candidates for adjuvant chemotherapy)	Biopsy[a]
		EBRT
		SBRT
II	Surgery and adjuvant chemotherapy	RFA
		Other (cryotherapy, wedge resection, or brachytherapy)
	Performance status[b] 0 to ~2	Performance status[b] 3 to 4
III	Biopsy[a]	Biopsy[a]
	Definitive chemo-RT	Palliative RT
	Surgery[c]	Chemotherapy if feasible
	Adjuvant chemotherapy	
IV	Biopsy[a]	Biopsy[a] for diagnosis and molecular testing
	Palliative chemotherapy	Palliative chemotherapy (cytotoxic or targeted)
	CNS and/or skeletal radiation	Palliative radiation

The paramount importance of accurate staging can be appreciated best by understanding how stage (both physiologic and anatomic, ie, TNM stage) affects treatment and prognosis, which vary greatly depending on the stage. For stages I to III, the treatment goal is given with curative intent.

Abbreviations: CNS, central nervous system; EBRT, external beam radiotherapy; RFA, radiofrequency ablation; RT, radiotherapy; SBRT, stereotactic body radiotherapy.

[a] Biopsy indicates situations whereby pretreatment biopsy is indicated. Note the absence of a role for routine biopsy of patients with suspected lung cancer who are good surgical candidates.

[b] Eastern Cooperative Oncology Group (ECOG) performance status scale (http://ecog.dfci.harvard.edu/general/perf_stat.html).

[c] Surgery for clinical stage IIIA (bulky or multiple station mediastinal lymph nodes) is currently not indicated, but stage IIIA disease discovered at the time of surgical resection (pathologic stage IIIA) should be followed by adjuvant chemotherapy.

information to and guide therapy.[3,4] This article addresses the questions: in whom is a tissue diagnosis necessary, and what is the best means of obtaining that diagnosis?

EVALUATION OF THE PATIENT WITH A LUNG NODULE OR MASS

A safe rule of thumb regarding the patient with a lung nodule or mass is to assume that all such findings are lung cancer until proven otherwise. This assumption seems extreme in light of the fact that the more than 95% of lesions discovered on screening CT scans are not in fact lung cancer.[5] However, the urgency of obtaining proof and the level of evidence needed to support that proof differs greatly from patient to patient, and this distinction should govern the approach. The degree of urgency and burden of evidence required is informed by estimating the pretest probability that any given nodule or mass is a lung cancer. For patients with lung nodules, ACCP evidence-based guidelines recommend starting the evaluation by estimating the probability of lung cancer.[6] Experienced clinicians intuitively estimate this

pretest probability with good accuracy,[7] but a quantitative tool was developed for this purpose by Swensen and colleagues.[8] The likelihood of malignancy in the Swensen model is based on 3 radiologic features of the lesion (location, size, and border character) and 3 clinical characteristics of the patient (tobacco use, age, and history of prior malignancy). A simple calculator that provides this quantitative estimate is available online (http://www.chestx-ray.com/SPN/SPNProb.html). This tool is very useful to both practitioners and educators working with trainees in this area. Once a pretest probability is in mind, most patients will require further evaluation. Only those with very low pretest probability of cancer (<5%) or those with extenuating circumstances (refusal of more invasive procedures, competing risks for mortality) should be considered for more conservative follow-up. For very small, indeterminate nodules, the Fleischner Society Guidelines have served clinicians and patients very well, and should continue to guide recommendations for follow-up.[9] When pursuing follow-up imaging, serial comparisons of nodule size are best made with CT scans, because small but important changes in size are not easily detected on plain chest radiographs.

A second rule of thumb is that there is a limited number of means to prove that a nodule is benign. One is to find a benign radiologic pattern (eg, benign calcification or fatty attenuation) and a second is to remove the nodule. Long-term radiologic follow-up is appropriate in patients with nodules with a very low likelihood of malignancy, and this risk for malignancy can be informed by characteristics of both nodule and patient, as well as with ^{18}F-fluorodeoxyglucose (FDG) positron emission tomography (PET) imaging. In general, a biopsy (CT-guided or transbronchial) with a high negative predictive value cannot prove something is benign. For most patients with moderate- to high-risk lesions, the next test to determine the likelihood of malignancy in a lung nodule should be an integrated PET/CT scan. Where PET scans are not available, dynamic contrast-enhanced CT has excellent sensitivity (although lesser specificity than PET) for identifying malignant nodules.[10] Although FDG-PET scans can be falsely negative in several situations (eg, small size, ground-glass, part solid, and highly mobile lower lobe lesions), for those patients with solid lung nodules in a size range large enough to be imaged with FDG-PET, the finding of low FDG avidity can justify conservative follow-up without further invasive workup. Although this is the practice at the authors' institution, data from an article by Gould and colleagues,[11] in which they examined the cost-effectiveness of varying strategies for managing indeterminate lung nodules, found that one of several cost-effective strategies was to offer biopsy for nodules where the pretest and posttest probability were discordant, and the PET scan was negative. In such a situation, the low probability of cancer in an FDG-negative nodule makes the negative predictive value of the biopsy sufficient to discontinue the workup if the biopsy yields a benign diagnosis.[11] In the multidisciplinary clinic the authors most often choose long-term radiographic follow-up of most indeterminate, FDG-negative nodules. In patients considered to be at risk for lung cancer, lesions that show significant uptake of FDG should be considered for tissue confirmation by biopsy or pulmonary resection.

Determining whether a given suspicious lesion is surgically resectable requires accurately estimating both the clinical stage of the tumor and the physiologic stage of the patient (**Fig. 1**). The approach to non–small cell lung cancer staging is based on the T, N, and M system, not covered in detail in this review.[12–16] From a staging standpoint, malignant involvement of mediastinal lymph

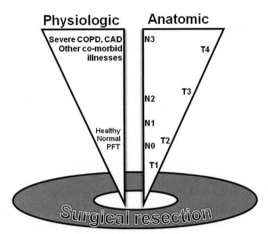

Fig. 1. The trade-off between the burden of lung cancer and the physiologic burden required to withstand pulmonary resection for lung cancer. As an example, patients with small peripheral nodules can withstand surgery with a greater burden of comorbid illness than can a patient with a large mass requiring a pneumonectomy or chest wall resection. CAD, coronary artery disease; COPD, chronic obstructive pulmonary disease; PFT, pulmonary function test.

nodes most often determines whether pulmonary resection is appropriate. Patients having clinically evident nodal involvement do not benefit from surgical resection alone. From a physiologic perspective, adequate pulmonary function and an acceptable burden of comorbid illness are major elements of determining whether a patient is medically fit for surgery. Arguably the best person to determine whether a patient can withstand surgical resection is a surgeon who specializes in thoracic malignancy.[4,17,18]

Noninvasive methods of mediastinal staging include CT and PET/CT. Invasive mediastinal staging approaches include transbronchial needle aspiration, with or without endobronchial ultrasonography (EBUS), esophageal endoscopic ultrasonography (EUS), mediastinoscopy, mediastinotomy, and video-assisted thoracic surgery (VATS). In many centers EBUS and/or EUS are becoming the first choice for mediastinal staging, given their high sensitivity, acceptable negative predictive value, and lower costs compared with mediastinoscopy.[19–22] The authors always advocate for FDG-PET scanning in the setting of abnormally enlarged mediastinal nodes on CT because of the higher risk of clinically silent distant metastases when there is CT evidence of mediastinal node involvement. In cases where FDG-PET suggests metastases outside of the chest, pathologic confirmation of stage IV disease should be sought whenever feasible. If clinical staging based on CT and CT/PET suggests stage III disease, biopsy efforts should be directed at the suspicious mediastinal nodes, not at the primary tumor. The rationale for this dictum is the rate of false positivity for FDG-PET in characterizing malignant mediastinal nodes. False-positive rates can be as high as 25% in selected populations, especially if sarcoid and granulomatous infections are prevalent. Likewise, fibrotic interstitial lung disease is another common condition in which the risk of lung cancer is high, and enlarged reactive mediastinal nodes that show uptake on PET are not uncommon.

The choice of approach to confirm stage III disease pathologically should be based on the anatomy (nodal station), local expertise, and the consideration of potential treatment options (chemotherapy with definitive radiation, chemotherapy and radiation therapy for neoadjuvant intent followed by surgery, or, for those with poor performance status, palliative therapy). In centers where users are experienced in endoscopic or endobronchial ultrasonography, nodal stations 2, 4, and 7 to 12 are accessible with either the bronchoscope (2, 4, 7, 10, 11, and 12), the endoscope (2, 7, 8, and 9), or both. Both EBUS and EUS are most commonly performed with moderate-consciousness sedation, avoiding the higher risk associated with general anesthesia. A good estimation rule for radiologists when considering whether EBUS is capable of reaching a node is to ask whether an airway of significant caliber (8 mm) is adjacent to the node. EUS is similarly restricted to nodes adjacent to the esophagus, but has the added advantage of being able to visualize (and biopsy) suspicious left adrenal or even hepatic lesions. All of these stations except for hilar nodes (11–12) and deep paraesophageal lymph nodes (8–9) are accessible to the surgeon with experience in mediastinoscopy, although 10R nodes can be difficult to reach. In general, prevascular nodes (stations 3 and 5) require a surgical approach, although in some larger individuals the apical-posterior segment of the left upper lobe bronchus is adjacent to an aortopulmonary window node (station 5). If this airway is large enough to enable approaching this station with an EBUS bronchoscope, transbronchial needle aspiration biopsy with direct ultrasound visualization is feasible. It must be noted that even mediastinoscopy can result in false-negative findings in patients with malignant involvement of their mediastinal nodes, and experience in this technique is just as important in achieving the optimum sensitivity and specificity.[23] Anterior mediastinal lymph nodes (stations 3, 5, and 6) can be assessed by several surgical techniques: anterior mediastinotomy (Chamberlain) or VATS, although VATS approaches typically require single-lung ventilation and may disrupt tissue planes for subsequent pulmonary resection.[24] More advanced techniques of minimally invasive surgery, transcervical extended mediastinal lymphadenectomy (TEMLA) or video-assisted mediastinoscopic lymphadenectomy (VAMLA), may provide more extensive evaluation of mediastinal lymph node status, including the prevascular and periesophageal lymph nodes.[25–27] These techniques have yet to be validated or incorporated broadly into clinical practice.[23]

If clinical staging evaluation (including a PET scan) suggests an early stage of disease (stage I–II), the question that must be asked before obtaining pathologic confirmation of the diagnosis is whether a diagnosis is required, and whether it will change the ultimate management. Patients who (1) are good surgical candidates with (2) a mass or nodule suspicious for lung cancer, and (3) a thorough staging evaluation suggesting no metastatic or locally advanced (N2) disease should be referred directly to surgery. For patients meeting these criteria, obtaining a tissue diagnosis before surgery offers little or no benefit to the patient or the surgeon. It follows logically, then, that pretreatment tissue diagnosis is necessary for patients at high risk for surgery, or (for example) patients requiring pneumonectomy (a more morbid procedure), in whom a definitive preoperative diagnosis informs the surgeon's discussion of risk and benefit with the patient. In such scenarios, discussion of these issues in the multidisciplinary setting facilitates prompt referral and diagnosis using the most appropriate preoperative means (eg, CT-guide or electromagnetic navigation–guided biopsy in centers with experience in this procedure). There are other common situations whereby a biopsy of a suspicious lung nodule is necessary, which include, but are not limited to: (1) a patient whose risk for surgery is high, and a definitive diagnosis of lung cancer facilitates the discussion of risks, benefits, and alternatives to surgery; (2) a patient who is a surgical candidate, but has no identifiable risk for cancer (based on age, and minimal or no history of tobacco use); and (3) a patient who is medically unresectable, in whom a pathologic diagnosis is required for treatment (almost always radiotherapy, but this also can imply radiofrequency ablation, or other thermal ablative techniques). Once a multidisciplinary team has determined that a biopsy is indicated, the choice of biopsy approach is made, weighing several factors that include local experience and expertise with various biopsy techniques, characteristics of the nodule, patient's preference, and the possible need for placement of fiducial markers near the tumor for stereotactic radiotherapy. For patients with early-stage disease but who are deemed medically unresectable because of poor functional status or comorbid diseases, biopsy of a lung nodule or mass is indicated to allow for consideration of radiotherapy (which has a high success rate for local control). In the past CT-guided biopsies were considered the gold standard, because of their accuracy in sampling peripheral lesions when compared with bronchoscopy; this still remains largely true in most centers, and this has become the standard for medically inoperable patients with suspected lung cancer. The recent development of electromagnetic guidance bronchoscopy (ENB) has resulted in the availability of additional biopsy options for patients with suspected early-stage lung cancer who are not surgical candidates. Experience with ENB is gaining wider acceptance, and the lower risk of pneumothorax associated with bronchoscopic biopsy makes this preferable in centers with experienced users.

CHOOSING AMONG OPTIONS FOR A TISSUE DIAGNOSIS

There are multiple options for obtaining a tissue diagnosis of a lesion suspected to be lung cancer, each with strengths and drawbacks to be considered when developing an approach that allows a clinician to determine the best balance between diagnostic certainty, risk, and cost. These diagnostic options, including fiberoptic bronchoscopy, percutaneous CT-guided biopsy, and surgical resection, are discussed here, with each successive option associated with increasing accuracy (sensitivity and negative predictive value) but also with increased risk of morbidity and greater cost.

Bronchoscopy

Fiberoptic bronchoscopy is particularly useful for accessing centrally located lesions and mediastinal lymph nodes. Transbronchial needle aspiration of enlarged mediastinal lymph nodes is safe and has a reasonable diagnostic accuracy in cases of malignant mediastinal lymph node metastasis. The development of bronchoscopes with real-time linear probe EBUS increases sensitivity and permits the biopsy of much smaller lymph nodes in both the mediastinum and hilar lymph node stations. EBUS technology has diminished or eliminated the role of blind transbronchial needle aspiration. The accuracy of traditional bronchoscopy for lung parenchymal lesions declines rapidly as the distance between the lesion and the mainstem bronchi increases, such that traditional transbronchial sampling techniques have less than 20% sensitivity when evaluating peripheral lung nodules.[28] Recently, a newer technique using 3-dimensional CT reconstruction combined with electromagnetic navigation of an extended working channel has facilitated biopsy of small peripheral lung nodules with significantly greater accuracy. Experienced users of this newer approach report a 69% to 80% sensitivity for the diagnosis of small peripheral lung nodules (as small as 7 mm, ranging up to 8 cm, and average size less than 2 cm).[29,30] Combining this technique with real-time imaging using a radial-probe ultrasound catheter to confirm the location suggested by virtual images further increased the accuracy of transbronchial biopsy to 88% in one series.[31] Using navigational bronchoscopy, multiple samples can be taken from one area or from multiple different nodules in a single procedure without an appreciable increase in the risk for pneumothorax. An added advantage of navigational bronchoscopy is the ability to implant fiducial markers around the tumor, which either facilitates or is required for delivery of stereotactic radiotherapy, depending on which system is used. Given the low risk of pneumothorax (<5%) and major bleeding (<1%), the chief risk of bronchoscopic biopsy, even when combined with electromagnetic navigation and real-time radial-probe ultrasonography, is that of a false-negative biopsy. The most experienced users still have false-negative or nondiagnostic biopsy specimens in up to 25% of procedures.[29,30,32] A visible airway passing through the lesion may be associated with a higher likelihood of success.[33] Navigational bronchoscopy requires CT formatted with no more than 3-mm slice thickness, with 50% overlap between slices. Images acquired at 1.25-mm slice thickness and 0.625-mm intervals (which is routine at the authors' institution) generally produce excellent 3-dimensional airway reconstructions with the navigational system used.

CT-Guided Biopsy

The first transcutaneous lung sampling was performed in 1883,[34] even before the development of radiographic imaging. Peripheral lung lesions and other intrathoracic lesions that are inaccessible by transbronchial or transesophageal routes may be sampled under imaging guidance.[35–37] Peripheral lesions may also be sampled using ultrasound guidance. Large lesions that are easily visible on fluoroscopy and not surrounded by vital structures may be sampled under fluoroscopy. Also, there are sporadic case reports of lung biopsies using magnetic resonance (MR) imaging as guidance. However, lung biopsies are most routinely done under CT guidance. Fine-needle aspirate (FNA) and core biopsy of lung lesions are performed in various combinations[38]; core biopsy is preferred over FNA, because of the need for a large amount tissue samples for molecular analysis of the tumors.[39,40] Core biopsy is done in a coaxial fashion through an introducer needle. The typical size of the coaxial introducer needles is 19-gauge. A core-biopsy needle is 20-gauge and an FNA needle is 22-gauge. Typically lung nodules of 1 cm or larger are sampled under imaging guidance. However, nodules located in the lower lobes, especially those adjacent to the diaphragm, can move significantly with respiratory motion, making them difficult or impossible to sample under imaging guidance. With different patient positions on the scanner table, gantry tilting, respiratory gating, and creative procedure techniques, almost all intrathoracic lesions may be accessible to needle biopsy under image guidance. The decision to sample a lung lesion should be made following a discussion in a multidisciplinary fashion with experts in radiology, pulmonary medicine, and thoracic surgery, with specific considerations of the patient's safety, proper staging (not merely the diagnosis) of the suspected malignancy, and therapeutic options.

The accuracy of lung biopsies in making a definitive benign or malignant diagnosis varies across reported series. At the authors' institution the accuracy of CT-guided lung biopsies over the last 5 years has been approximately 80%. Hence, it is critical to recall that a negative biopsy result (ie, the negative predictive value) does not exclude malignancy. The most common complication of CT-guided lung biopsy is pneumothorax (0%–61%) for which a proportion (3.3%–15%) of patients will require chest-tube drainage.[41] The wide range of reported pneumothorax incidence in the literature probably reflects the use of postprocedure imaging modalities with varied sensitivity in detecting pneumothorax. Precautionary measures such as postbiopsy blood/saline patches, not traversing through large bulla, emphysematous lung, and pleural fissures may help to reduce the risk of pneumothorax.[42–44] At the authors' institution, pneumothorax rates over the last 5 years ranged from 24% to 36% with 1% to 4% of all biopsies requiring chest-drain insertion. The second most common complication is internal hemorrhage (5%–16.7%) and hemothorax (1.5%).[41] Other rare complications are also reported in the literature, ranging from systemic embolism to death. The American College of Radiology and Society of Interventional Radiology suggested thresholds as a national benchmark for the sampling procedure of: accuracy 70% to 90%, major complications 20%, routine management

with chest tube following a lung biopsy less than 20%, complicated chest tube management after lung biopsy 3%, and hemoptysis requiring hospitalization of specific therapy 2%.[45]

The factors correlated with postprocedure pneumothorax are poor pulmonary function, needle gauge, lesions closer to the diaphragm, lung nodules that are 1 cm or smaller, and the deeper (more than 1.8 cm) lung lesions.[46–48] Tumor seeding along the needle track is exceedingly rare,[49] even when 12-gauge biopsy needles are used.[50] Radiation doses during lung biopsies should be monitored and every effort should be made to reduce the dose. At present the radiation dose for a CT-guided lung biopsy at the authors' institution is approximately 1 mSv. Limiting the number of images, scan coverage zone, respiratory gating devices, and altering scan parameters (kV and mA) may help to decrease radiation exposure for both the patient and practitioner.[51,52]

Surgery

Resection of a nodule provides the greatest sensitivity in determining the nature of the lesion(s), and makes it possible to diagnose and to treat the lesions definitively in a single procedure. The sensitivity of surgery for diagnosis is as close to 100% as any test can get, given that it is the accepted gold standard for tissue diagnosis of lung lesions. However, very small lung lesions can be difficult for the surgeon to palpate and may be missed. Approaches that use radiographic or bronchoscopic marking of the nodule such as ink dye staining,[53] radionuclide tracer,[54,55] or implantable fiducial markers[56] allow surgeons to locate and resect small and nonpalpable nodules that typically are located peripherally, within 1 to 2 cm of the visceral pleura. In addition to small tumor size and increasing depth from the visceral pleural surface, lesions with nonsolid morphology can be localized with these techniques for subsequent excisional biopsy. The risks of surgery for diagnosis include those for general anesthesia in addition to the risks associated with lung resection. **Fig. 2** shows a general outline of factors considered by a multidisciplinary team when selecting among biopsy options for a patient with a lung nodule.

A guiding principle in thoracic oncology that governs the choice of biopsy is to subject the patient to the least invasive approach that provides both the diagnosis and the stage in one procedure. For example, in a patient whose evaluation of clinical staging shows suspicious mediastinal nodes, a CT-guided biopsy of the parenchymal lung nodule or mass associated

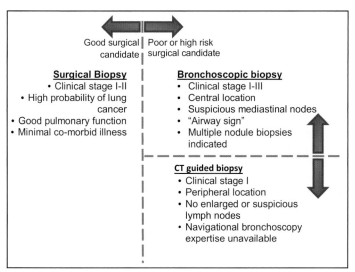

Fig. 2. A general set of guidelines for considering the best approach for tissue confirmation in a patient with findings suspicious for lung cancer.

with the enlarged node(s) still leaves unanswered the question of whether the nodes are reactive or metastatic. In such patients, the PET scan must never serve as the equivalent of a tissue biopsy. The authors advocate for the PET scan to be viewed as a road map toward the most informative biopsy. A single invasive procedure that provides both a diagnosis and an unequivocal stage is always the best option. An exception to this is the patient with a lung mass and suspected intracerebral metastasis. In these patients, the least invasive approach is usually the most appropriate, but enlarged mediastinal lymph nodes should not be assumed to indicate nodal metastasis, because aggressive therapy including lung resection and metastasectomy may be appropriate for patients with localized (N0) thoracic disease and a resectable intracranial metastasis.

Once it is clear that a patient requires a tissue diagnosis, and the team has chosen a method of obtaining that diagnosis, a final emphasis must be on the acquisition of enough tissue to allow both a definitive histologic diagnosis and selected molecular diagnostic studies. The latter is particularly true for the large percentage of patients with metastatic lung cancer. A study comparing pemetrexed with gemcitabine as the second agent in a platinum-based regimen for patients with metastatic cancer was the first to demonstrate a histology-specific benefit to a cytotoxic chemotherapy drug in lung cancer.[57,58] This study showed that in patients with metastatic nonsquamous lung cancer, pemetrexed was superior to gemcitabine in terms of overall survival. Likewise, the modest benefit identified in studies of the

angiogenesis inhibitor bevacizumab (anti–vascular endothelial growth factor monoclonal antibody) was associated with an unacceptably high risk of hemorrhage in patients with squamous histology, contraindicating the use of this targeted drug in patients with advanced (metastatic) squamous lung cancer. These findings highlight the importance of providing pathologists enough tissue to distinguish, via light microscopy–level immunohistochemistry, between squamous carcinoma and adenocarcinoma. The use of "non–small cell lung cancer, not otherwise specified" is strongly discouraged, and it behooves those of us who perform biopsies to provide samples of sufficient size and quantity that permit pathologists to make this distinction whenever it is possible.

Perhaps more importantly, recent studies demonstrating improved outcomes with targeted tyrosine kinase inhibitors for those bearing specific mutations of the epidermal growth factor receptor (EGFR) or gene rearrangements of the anaplastic lymphoma kinase (ALK) gene have opened the door to an era in the treatment of lung cancer. As more targeted agents are made available, the emerging paradigm is that any one agent may be useful for only a small proportion of patients whose tumors demonstrate activation of a specific oncogenic pathway; this is sometimes referred to as oncogene addiction. Targeted agents such as erlotinib (for mutant EGFR) and crizotinib (for ALK-mutant fusion proteins) have led to remarkable responses when used in patients harboring tumors with the appropriate activating mutations.[59,60] Moreover, these responses, while dramatic in some instances, are almost always short lived. As resistance emerges, further studies are emerging to provide an understanding of resistance mechanisms that might also lend themselves to specific targeted agents currently in development.[61–64] Erlotinib targets the tyrosine kinase domain of EGFR, and in patients with tumors bearing specific activating mutations in this domain, it is first-line therapy for metastatic lung cancer. Recently the US Food and Drug Administration granted approval for crizotinib, a targeted agent that acts to inhibit ALK, which is activated most commonly through a gene rearrangement. These findings now dictate that tissue acquisition takes into account the need for specific molecular studies that include either DNA sequencing (for EGFR mutations) or fluorescent in situ hybridization (FISH) probes that allow for detection of specific chromosome-level rearrangements that drive oncogene addiction. The approach of multidisciplinary care teams depends on communication between the ultimate providers of treatment and those involved in obtaining tissue biopsies, as well as the pathologists, to assure that the proper information is available to make critical decisions concerning individualized targeted therapy.

REFERENCES

1. Alberts WM. Introduction: diagnosis and management of lung cancer. Chest 2007;132(Suppl 3): 20S–2S.

2. Ettinger D, Johnson B. Update: NCCN small cell and non-small cell lung cancer clinical practice guidelines. J Natl Compr Canc Netw 2005;3(Suppl 1): S17–21.

3. Farjah F, Flum DR, Ramsey SD, et al. Multimodality mediastinal staging for lung cancer among Medicare beneficiaries. J Thorac Oncol 2009;4(3): 355–63.

4. Farjah F, Flum DR, Varghese TK Jr, et al. Surgeon specialty and long-term survival after pulmonary resection for lung cancer. Ann Thorac Surg 2009; 87(4):995–1004 [discussion: 1005–6].

5. Aberle DR, Adams AM, Berg CD, et al. Reduced lung-cancer mortality with low-dose computed tomographic screening. N Engl J Med 2011;365(5): 395–409.

6. Gould MK, Fletcher J, Iannettoni MD, et al. Evaluation of patients with pulmonary nodules: when is it lung cancer?: ACCP evidence-based clinical practice guidelines (2nd edition). Chest 2007; 132(Suppl 3):108S–30S.

7. Swensen SJ, Silverstein MD, Edell ES, et al. Solitary pulmonary nodules: clinical prediction model versus physicians. Mayo Clin Proc 1999;74(4):319–29.

8. Swensen SJ, Silverstein MD, Ilstrup DM, et al. The probability of malignancy in solitary pulmonary nodules. Application to small radiologically indeterminate nodules. Arch Intern Med 1997;157(8):849–55.

9. MacMahon H, Austin JHM, Gamsu G, et al. Guidelines for management of small pulmonary nodules detected on CT scans: a statement from the Fleischner Society. Radiology 2005;237(2):395–400.

10. Swensen S, Viggiano R, Midthun D, et al. Lung nodule enhancement at CT: multicenter study. Radiology 2000;214(1):73–80.

11. Gould MK, Sanders GD, Barnett PG, et al. Cost-effectiveness of alternative management strategies for patients with solitary pulmonary nodules. Ann Intern Med 2003;138(9):724–35.

12. Goldstraw P, Crowley J, Chansky K, et al. The IASLC Lung Cancer Staging Project: proposals for the revision of the TNM stage groupings in the forthcoming (seventh) edition of the TNM Classification of malignant tumours. J Thorac Oncol 2007;2(8):706–14.

13. Groome PA, Bolejack V, Crowley JJ, et al. The IASLC Lung Cancer Staging Project: validation of the proposals for revision of the T, N, and M descriptors and consequent stage groupings in the forthcoming (seventh) edition of the TNM classification of malignant tumours. J Thorac Oncol 2007;2(8):694–705.

14. Postmus PE, Brambilla E, Chansky K, et al. The IASLC Lung Cancer Staging Project: proposals for revision of the M descriptors in the forthcoming (seventh) edition of the TNM classification of lung cancer. J Thorac Oncol 2007;2(8):686–93.

15. Rami-Porta R, Ball D, Crowley J, et al. The IASLC Lung Cancer Staging Project: proposals for the revision of the T descriptors in the forthcoming (seventh) edition of the TNM classification for lung cancer. J Thorac Oncol 2007;2(7):593–602.

16. Rusch VW, Crowley J, Giroux DJ, et al. The IASLC Lung Cancer Staging Project: proposals for the revision of the N descriptors in the forthcoming seventh edition of the TNM classification for lung cancer. J Thorac Oncol 2007;2(7):603–12.

17. Kohman LJ. What constitutes success in cancer surgery? Measuring the value of specialist care. Chest 1998;114(3):663–4.

18. Silvestri GA, Handy J, Lackland D, et al. Specialists achieve better outcomes than generalists for lung cancer surgery. Chest 1998;114(3):675–80.

19. Annema JT, van Meerbeeck JP, Rintoul RC, et al. Mediastinoscopy vs endosonography for mediastinal nodal staging of lung cancer. JAMA 2010; 304(20):2245–52.

20. Yasufuku K, Pierre A, Darling G, et al. A prospective controlled trial of endobronchial ultrasound-guided transbronchial needle aspiration compared with mediastinoscopy for mediastinal lymph node staging of lung cancer. J Thorac Cardiovasc Surg 2011;142(6): 1393–400.e1.

21. Wallace MB, Pascual JM, Raimondo M, et al. Minimally invasive endoscopic staging of suspected lung cancer. JAMA 2008;299(5):540–6.

22. Ernst A, Anantham D, Eberhardt R, et al. Diagnosis of mediastinal adenopathy-real-time endobronchial ultrasound guided needle aspiration versus mediastinoscopy. J Thorac Oncol 2008;3(6):577–82.

23. Little AG, Rusch VW, Bonner JA, et al. Patterns of surgical care of lung cancer patients. Ann Thorac Surg 2005;80(6):2051–6.

24. Nechala P, Graham AJ, McFadden SD, et al. Retrospective analysis of the clinical performance of anterior mediastinotomy. Ann Thorac Surg 2006;82(6): 2004–9.

25. Kuzdzal J, Zielinski M, Papla B, et al. The transcervical extended mediastinal lymphadenectomy versus cervical mediastinoscopy in non-small cell lung cancer staging. Eur J Cardiothorac Surg 2007;31(1): 88–94.

26. Witte B, Messerschmidt A, Hillebrand H, et al. Combined videothoracoscopic and videomediastinoscopic approach improves radicality of minimally invasive mediastinal lymphadenectomy for early stage lung carcinoma. Eur J Cardiothorac Surg 2009;35(2):343–7.

27. Witte B, Wolf M, Huertgen M, et al. Video-assisted mediastinoscopic surgery: clinical feasibility and accuracy of mediastinal lymph node staging. Ann Thorac Surg 2006;82(5):1821–7.

28. Baaklini WA, Reinoso MA, Gorin AB, et al. Diagnostic yield of fiberoptic bronchoscopy in evaluating solitary pulmonary nodules. Chest 2000;117(4):1049–54.

29. Gildea TR, Mazzone PJ, Karnak D, et al. Electromagnetic navigation diagnostic bronchoscopy: a prospective study. Am J Respir Crit Care Med 2006;174(9):982–9.

30. Schwarz Y, Mehta A, Ernst A, et al. Electromagnetic navigation during flexible bronchoscopy. Respiration 2003;70(5):516.

31. Eberhardt R, Anantham D, Ernst A, et al. Multimodality bronchoscopic diagnosis of peripheral lung lesions: a randomized controlled trial. Am J Respir Crit Care Med 2007;176(1):36–41.

32. Eberhardt R, Anantham D, Herth F, et al. Electromagnetic navigation diagnostic bronchoscopy in peripheral lung lesions. Chest 2007;131(6):1800–5.

33. Sethi S, Bansal S, Gildea TR. Impact of the airway-nodule relationship on electromagnetic navigational bronchoscopy yield [abstract]. Chest 2007;132: 452a.

34. Leyden I. Uber infectiose pneumonie. Deutsche Medizinische Wochenschrift 1883;9:52–4.

35. Matsui Y, Hiraki T, Mimura H, et al. Role of computed tomography fluoroscopy-guided cutting needle biopsy of lung lesions after transbronchial examination resulting in negative diagnosis. Clin Lung Cancer 2011;12(1):51–5.

36. Hur J, Lee HJ, Byun MK, et al. Computed tomographic fluoroscopy-guided needle aspiration biopsy as a second biopsy technique after indeterminate transbronchial biopsy results for pulmonary lesions: comparison with second transbronchial biopsy. J Comput Assist Tomogr 2010;34(2):290–5.

37. Milman N, Faurschou P, Grode G. Diagnostic yield of transthoracic needle aspiration biopsy following negative fiberoptic bronchoscopy in 103 patients with peripheral circumscribed pulmonary lesions. Respiration 1995;62(1):1–3.

38. Yamagami T, Iida S, Kato T, et al. Combining fine-needle aspiration and core biopsy under CT fluoroscopy guidance: a better way to treat patients with lung nodules? AJR Am J Roentgenol 2003;180(3):811–5.

39. Solomon SB, Zakowski MF, Pao W, et al. Core needle lung biopsy specimens: adequacy for EGFR and KRAS mutational analysis. AJR Am J Roentgenol 2010;194(1):266–9.

40. Cheung YC, Chang JW, Hsieh JJ, et al. Adequacy and complications of computed tomography-guided core needle biopsy on non-small cell lung cancers for epidermal growth factor receptor mutations demonstration: 18-gauge or 20-gauge biopsy needle. Lung Cancer 2010;67(2):166–9.

41. Manhire A, Charig M, Clelland C, et al. Guidelines for radiologically guided lung biopsy. Thorax 2003; 58(11):920–36.

42. Billich C, Muche R, Brenner G, et al. CT-guided lung biopsy: incidence of pneumothorax after instillation of NaCl into the biopsy track. Eur Radiol 2008; 18(6):1146–52.

43. Wu CC, Maher MM, Shepard JA. Complications of CT-guided percutaneous needle biopsy of the chest: prevention and management. AJR Am J Roentgenol 2011;196(6):W678–82.

44. Wagner JM, Hinshaw JL, Lubner MG, et al. CT-guided lung biopsies: pleural blood patching reduces the rate of chest tube placement for post-biopsy pneumothorax. AJR Am J Roentgenol 2011; 197(4):783–8.

45. ACR-SIR practice guideline for the performance of image-guided percutaneous needle biopsy (PNB) in adults (Resolution 14). 2008. Available at: http://www.acr.org/SecondaryMainMenuCategories/ quality_safety/guidelines/iv/pnb.aspx. Accessed December 16, 2011.

46. Geraghty PR, Kee ST, McFarlane G, et al. CT-guided transthoracic needle aspiration biopsy of pulmonary nodules: needle size and pneumothorax rate. Radiology 2003;229(2):475–81.

47. Kazerooni EA, Lim FT, Mikhail A, et al. Risk of pneumothorax in CT-guided transthoracic needle aspiration biopsy of the lung. Radiology 1996;198(2):371–5.

48. Rizzo S, Preda L, Raimondi S, et al. Risk factors for complications of CT-guided lung biopsies. Radiol Med 2011;116(4):548–63.

49. Sano Y, Date H, Toyooka S, et al. Percutaneous computed tomography-guided lung biopsy and pleural dissemination: an assessment by intraoperative pleural lavage cytology. Cancer 2009;115(23): 5526–33.

50. Izumi Y, Nakatsuka S, Asakura K, et al. Feasibility of CT-guided large-bore biopsy of lung tumors with the use of an outer sheath. J Vasc Interv Radiol 2011; 22(5):699–701.

51. Smith JC, Jin DH, Watkins GE, et al. Ultra-low-dose protocol for CT-guided lung biopsies. J Vasc Interv Radiol 2011;22(4):431–6.

52. Carlson SK, Felmlee JP, Bender CE, et al. CT fluoroscopy-guided biopsy of the lung or upper abdomen with a breath-hold monitoring and feedback system: a prospective randomized controlled clinical trial. Radiology 2005;237(2): 701–8.

53. Endo M, Kotani Y, Satouchi M, et al. CT fluoroscopy-guided bronchoscopic dye marking for resection of small peripheral pulmonary nodules. Chest 2004; 125(5):1747–52.

54. Bellomi M, Veronesi G, Trifiro G, et al. Computed tomography-guided preoperative radiotracer localization of nonpalpable lung nodules. Ann Thorac Surg 2010;90(6):1759–64.

55. Stiles BM, Altes TA, Jones DR, et al. Clinical experience with radiotracer-guided thoracoscopic biopsy of small, indeterminate lung nodules. Ann Thorac Surg 2006;82(4):1191–7.

56. Lizza N, Eucher P, Haxhe JP, et al. Thoracoscopic resection of pulmonary nodules after computed tomographic-guided coil labeling. Ann Thorac Surg 2001;71(3):986–8.

57. Syrigos KN, Vansteenkiste J, Parikh P, et al. Prognostic and predictive factors in a randomized phase III trial comparing cisplatin-pemetrexed versus cisplatin-gemcitabine in advanced non-small-cell lung cancer. Ann Oncol 2010;21(3):556–61.

58. Scagliotti GV, Parikh P, von Pawel J, et al. Phase III study comparing cisplatin plus gemcitabine with cisplatin plus pemetrexed in chemotherapy-naive patients with advanced-stage non-small-cell lung cancer. J Clin Oncol 2008;26(21):3543–51.

59. Mok T, Wu YL, Zhang L. A small step towards personalized medicine for non-small cell lung cancer. Discov Med 2009;8(43):227–31.

60. Kwak EL, Bang YJ, Camidge DR, et al. Anaplastic lymphoma kinase inhibition in non-small-cell lung cancer. N Engl J Med 2010;363(18):1693–703.

61. Engelman JA, Zejnullahu K, Gale CM, et al. PF00299804, an irreversible pan-ERBB inhibitor, is effective in lung cancer models with EGFR and ERBB2 mutations that are resistant to gefitinib. Cancer Res 2007;67(24):11924–32.

62. Bean J, Brennan C, Shih JY, et al. MET amplification occurs with or without T790M mutations in EGFR mutant lung tumors with acquired resistance to gefitinib or erlotinib. Proc Natl Acad Sci U S A 2007; 104(52):20932–7.

63. Pao W, Miller VA, Politi KA, et al. Acquired resistance of lung adenocarcinomas to gefitinib or erlotinib is associated with a second mutation in the EGFR kinase domain. PLoS Med 2005;2(3):e73.

64. Engelman JA, Zejnullahu K, Mitsudomi T, et al. MET amplification leads to gefitinib resistance in lung cancer by activating ERBB3 signaling. Science 2007;316(5827):1039–43.

Treatment of Lung Cancer

Shirish M. Gadgeel, MD[a], Suresh S. Ramalingam, MD[b],
Gregory P. Kalemkerian, MD[c],*

KEYWORDS

- Lung cancer • Small cell • Non–small cell • Chemotherapy • Radiotherapy • Surgery
- Molecular therapy

KEY POINTS

- Early-stage non–small cell lung cancer (NSCLC) is managed primarily by surgical resection, with adjuvant chemotherapy for selected patients.
- Stage III NSCLC is treated with combined modality therapy, usually concurrent chemotherapy plus radiotherapy, with curative intent.
- Advanced NSCLC remains an incurable disease treated primarily with chemotherapy and/or radiotherapy with palliative intent.
- Molecularly targeted therapy can greatly benefit selected patients with advanced NSCLC with specific genetic mutations.
- Limited-stage small cell lung cancer (SCLC) is treated with concurrent chemoradiotherapy with curative intent. Chemotherapy can prolong survival in patients with extensive-stage SCLC.

NON–SMALL CELL LUNG CANCER

Non–small cell lung cancer (NSCLC), which accounts for 85% of all cases of lung cancer, includes the histologic subtypes of adenocarcinoma, squamous cell carcinoma, and large cell carcinoma. The goals of therapy for patients with NSCLC depend on the stage of disease: for patients with stage I to III disease, the goal is cure, whereas, for those with stage IV disease, the goals are palliation of symptoms and prolongation of life. Initial staging procedures need to answer 3 questions to adequately guide therapeutic decision making: (1) is the primary tumor confined to the lung with or without involvement of the hilar or peribronchial lymph nodes (stage I/II)? (2) Is the primary tumor invading the mediastinum or has the cancer spread to mediastinal lymph nodes (stage III)? (3) Are there distant metastases (stage IV)?

Stage I/II NSCLC

Surgery

About 25% of patients with NSCLC have stage I or II disease, with tumor confined to the lung (T1–T2) with (N1) or without (N0) metastases to hilar or peribronchial lymph nodes. The goal of therapy in these patients is cure, which is achievable in 60% to 80% and 40% to 50% with stage I and stage II disease, respectively. The primary curative modality is surgical resection with either lobectomy or pneumonectomy, depending on the extent of disease, along with mediastinal lymph node sampling or dissection (**Box 1**). When the chest wall or diaphragm is involved, an en bloc resection of these structures along with the lung may be required. An older randomized trial found that sublobar resections, such as wedge resection or segmentectomy, are inferior to lobectomy, with a higher rate of local/regional recurrence and lower

[a] Department of Hematology and Oncology, Wayne State University - Karmanos Cancer Institute, 4HWCRC, 4100 John R Street, Detroit, MI 48201, USA; [b] Department of Hematology and Medical Oncology, Emory University - Winship Cancer Institute, Atlanta, GA, USA; [c] Division of Hematology/Oncology, University of Michigan, C350 Med Inn - SPC 5848, 1500 East Medical Center Drive, Ann Arbor, MI 48109-5848, USA
* Corresponding author.
E-mail address: kalemker@umich.edu

Radiol Clin N Am 50 (2012) 961–974
http://dx.doi.org/10.1016/j.rcl.2012.06.003
0033-8389/12/$ – see front matter © 2012 Elsevier Inc. All rights reserved.

Box 1
Treatment of stage I/II NSCLC

Local therapy

Lobectomy with mediastinal lymph node sampling (pneumonectomy if required to achieve negative margins)

Local therapy options in high-risk patients

Sublobar resection (wedge, segmentectomy)

Conventional external-beam radiation therapy

Stereotactic body radiation therapy

Radiofrequency ablation

Adjuvant chemotherapy

Stage IB (consider if tumor ≥4 cm)

Stage IIA/B (recommended)

Platinum-based, 2-drug regimen × 4 cycles

5-year survival rate.[1] However, because of improved imaging techniques and the trend toward the diagnosis of smaller, more peripheral tumors, lung-sparing procedures are currently being reevaluated. A retrospective analysis of 784 patients who underwent either sublobar resection or lobectomy for stage IA tumors (<3 cm) noted no differences in efficacy outcomes.[2] However, other retrospective analyses have shown that sublobar resections result in lower survival rates than lobectomy in patients with tumors greater than or equal to 3 cm. Prospective, nonrandomized trials have suggested that, for patients with small tumors, limited resections may provide the same outcomes as lobectomy, particularly in older patients and those with limited lung function.[3] Based on these observations, an ongoing, phase III, Cancer and Leukemia group B (CALGB) trial is randomizing patients with tumors less than or equal to 2 cm and no evidence of lymph node metastases to undergo either sublobar resection or lobectomy.

Thoracic surgical techniques have improved markedly in the past decade, with the major advance being video-assisted thoracoscopic surgery (VATS). VATS lobectomy is associated with reduced acute postoperative pain, less impairment in pulmonary function, and shorter hospital stays. A recent meta-analysis reported no difference in the locoregional recurrence, but a significant decrease in systemic recurrence and improvement in 5-year survival with VATS lobectomy compared with open lobectomy.[4] The lower rate of pulmonary morbidity with VATS has opened up the surgical option for patients who are not considered candidates for open thoracotomy.[5] However, a recent

retrospective analysis found a higher intraoperative complication rate with VATS versus open lobectomy, and no differences in in-hospital mortality, length of stay, wound infection rate, or pulmonary and cardiovascular complication rates.[6] There are, as yet, no specific guidelines to assist in deciding between VATS versus open thoracotomy. Recent reports have shown the feasibility and safety of robotic lobectomy, but it remains to be determined whether this technology offers any significant advantages compared with conventional VATS or open approaches.[7]

Before surgery, patients need appropriate preoperative assessment to ensure that they can tolerate the predicted reduction in lung volume, especially because most patients with lung cancer are current or former smokers with impaired baseline pulmonary function. At a minimum, patients need full pulmonary function testing, including diffusion capacity (carbon monoxide diffusion in the lung [DLCO]), with further evaluations, such as quantitative V/Q scans or exercise capacity testing, conducted if pulmonary function is impaired. Cardiac status should also be assessed before surgery. All patients should be encouraged to stop smoking before surgery because complication rates and postoperative mortality are both substantially higher among patients who are active smokers.[8]

Nonsurgical therapy

Conventional radiotherapy Some patients with stage I/II NSCLC are not candidates for surgical resection, primarily because of impaired lung function. In such situations, the standard of care is radiation therapy (RT) to the primary tumor and any involved lymph nodes (see **Box 1**). Clinical trial RTOG 73-01, in which patients with inoperable NSCLC were randomized to various doses of RT, concluded that a total dose of 60 Gy administered in daily fractions of 2 Gy over 6 weeks resulted in the best local control and 2-year survival rates.[9] The 5-year survival rates for patients with medically inoperable stage I NSCLC treated with conventional RT range from 15% to 48%, with a local failure rate of about 50%.[10] Although these outcomes are clearly inferior to those of patients who undergo surgical resection, it is not clear whether these differences are caused by the inadequacy of conventional RT or patient selection.

A major limitation of RT is the occurrence of normal lung injury with higher radiation doses. The incorporation of specialized computed tomography (CT) scanners and software that allows three-dimensional delineation of the tumor and adjacent normal structures has greatly improved the safety of thoracic RT. Other advances, including intensity-modulated radiotherapy, respiratory gating and control, and the use of positron emission tomography (PET) to guide target volume, have allowed radiation oncologists to maximize the delivery of radiation to the tumor and minimize damage to normal surrounding tissues.

Stereotactic body RT Stereotactic body RT (SBRT) incorporates multiple photon beams to deliver a high dose of radiation to a defined volume of tumor with a high level of precision in a small number of fractions. In addition to the potential for improved tumor kill caused by higher dose therapy, SBRT also allows a significant decrease in the dose received by surrounding normal tissue. SBRT is applicable to small (<5 cm) tumors and requires the minimization and/or tracking of tumor motion with radiation delivery at specific points in the respiratory cycle. The total dose and fractionation for SBRT varies between 30 Gy in 1 fraction to 60 Gy in 3 to 5 fractions. The biologic effective dose of these treatments is higher than the absolute value of the dose, with 60 Gy in 3 fractions being roughly equivalent to 150 Gy delivered in conventional 2 Gy daily fractions. For patients with medically inoperable stage I NSCLC, SBRT has achieved excellent local control rates of 85% to 96% and 5-year survival rates of more than 50%.[11] In addition, patients do not need to meet a minimum threshold of pulmonary function to undergo SBRT.

Toxicity associated with SBRT is generally limited, with severe adverse events reported in less than 5% of patients.[12] The major side effects are pulmonary injury, chest wall pain, and rib fractures. Toxicity rates are higher when SBRT is applied to tumors near the major bronchi, with an 11-fold increase in the risk of severe toxicity in patients with central tumors compared with those with peripheral tumors.[12]

Thus far, SBRT has been used primarily in patients with medically inoperable stage I NSCLC (see **Box 1**), although ongoing trials are comparing SBRT with sublobar resections in patients with marginal lung function (forced expiratory volume in 1 second or DLCO <50%), and even with lobectomy in patients who are deemed fit for optimal resection.

Radiofrequency ablation Radiofrequency ablation (RFA) involves imparting thermal injury through electromagnetic energy generated from a probe emitting high-frequency alternating current. The probe is placed with CT guidance, usually under conscious sedation. Pathologic studies have shown that a well-circumscribed region of coagulative necrosis develops around the RFA probe. An important limiting factor to the adequacy of tumor ablation by RFA is heat loss through convection by means of nearby blood circulation, the heat-sink effect. This effect is particularly problematic if the target tumor sits close to blood vessels larger than 3 mm in diameter. The major complications of RFA are pneumothorax requiring chest tube placement in 11% of patients, pleural effusion, and intrapulmonary hemorrhage. No significant decline in post-RFA lung function has been reported.

RFA can be used as primary treatment of stage I NSCLC in patients who are not surgical candidates, or as salvage therapy for recurrent lung tumors (see **Box 1**). A recent prospective study of RFA in patients with either primary lung cancer or lung metastases from other primary sites reported that the complete ablation rate by imaging was 80% for tumors less than or equal to 3.5 cm, with 1-year and 2-year survival rates of 70% and 48%, respectively, in patients with NSCLC.[13] Another study of 75 patients with stage I NSCLC reported a 27% 5-year survival rate.[14] Overall, these results seem to be comparable with those achieved with external-beam RT. All reports on RFA have shown that outcomes vary based on tumor size, with declining rates of complete response in tumors greater than 3 cm in diameter. A recent report on 64 patients with stage I NSCLC who were not candidates for lobectomy and were treated with either sublobar resection, cryotherapy, or RFA found that all outcomes, including overall and cancer-specific survival, were similar with each of these treatment modalities.[15] Although this was not a randomized study, these results suggest that RFA is a reasonable option for medically inoperable patients with stage I NSCLC. The value of nonsurgical treatments in patients with localized NSCLC remains to be determined in prospective clinical trials.

Adjuvant therapy

Distant relapse is the primary cause of death in patients with NSCLC who die within 5 years of a complete surgical resection. Thus, even when the cancer seems to be limited to the lung, undetected micrometastases remain a common problem. Randomized clinical trials have recently shown an absolute improvement of 5% to 15% in the 5-year survival rate for patients with stage II and III NSCLC who receive adjuvant platinum-based chemotherapy after complete surgical resection (see **Box 1**).[16] However, there is no clear benefit for adjuvant chemotherapy in patients with stage I disease. Secondary analyses have shown that patients with stage IB NSCLC who have tumors greater than or equal to 4 cm may derive a survival benefit from adjuvant chemotherapy.[17,18]

Any of the platinum-based, 2-drug chemotherapy regimens that are currently used in patients with advanced NSCLC are considered reasonable options for treatment in the adjuvant setting. Adjuvant chemotherapy should be started within 2 to 3 months of surgical resection, so only patients with good performance status who have an uncomplicated surgical recovery within that timeframe should be considered for adjuvant treatment. Although standard adjuvant therapy consists of 4 cycles of an appropriate regimen, the toxicity of chemotherapy after lung resection can be challenging and only 60% to 70% of patients are able to complete all 4 cycles of therapy. Toxicities vary based on the agents used, but common toxicities include neutropenia, anemia, nausea, vomiting, fatigue, and neuropathy.[19]

Stage III NSCLC

Up to 35% of patients with NSCLC present with stage III disease in which the primary tumor has directly invaded local structures outside the lung (T3–T4) and/or the cancer has spread to mediastinal lymph nodes (N2–N3). These locally advanced tumors are generally not amenable to primary surgical resection. In addition, they are usually associated with systemic micrometastases that frequently result in distant relapse. In the past, RT or surgical resection were used to treat patients with locally advanced NSCLC, yielding 5-year survival rates less than 5% because of frequent systemic recurrences. Patients with locally advanced disease are now most commonly treated with combined modality therapy incorporating chemotherapy and RT in an effort to control both local and distant disease (**Box 2**). Initial studies of sequential chemotherapy followed by RT reported improved 5-year survival rates of 10% to 15%.[20]Concurrent administration of chemotherapy and radiotherapy subsequently further increased long-term survival rates to 20% to 30%, with median survival times of 18 to 24 months.[21,22] Standard chemotherapy regimens used during chemoradiotherapy include cisplatin or carboplatin plus etoposide, paclitaxel or, more recently, pemetrexed. Definitive RT is given 5 d/wk for 6 to 7 weeks to a total dose of 60 to 70 Gy.[23–25] The increase in survival with concurrent therapy is mirrored by increased toxicity, primarily esophagitis and pneumonitis. Many patients with locally advanced NSCLC are not able to tolerate concurrent chemoradiotherapy because of poor performance status, substantial weight loss, or comorbid conditions. In such patients, the treatment plan needs to be individualized to optimize control of symptoms and the disease, without

---

Box 2
Treatment of stage III NSCLC

Standard therapy

Concurrent chemotherapy plus definitive radiotherapy

Induction chemoradiotherapy followed by surgical resection (selected patients with non-bulky mediastinal lymph nodes who do not require pneumonectomy for adequate resection)

Options in poor-risk patients

Sequential chemotherapy followed by radiotherapy

Radiotherapy alone

Pathologic stage III following surgical resection

Adjuvant chemotherapy: platinum-based, 2-drug regimen × 4 cycles

Consider adjuvant radiotherapy after completion of chemotherapy

---

inducing excessive therapy-related complications (see **Box 2**).

Several trials have evaluated trimodality therapy, using induction chemotherapy or chemoradiotherapy before surgical resection with further chemotherapy or RT after surgery. Patients enrolled in such studies must be fit and have non-bulky mediastinal disease. Thus far, these trials have failed to show a clear survival benefit for trimodality therapy compared with standard, definitive chemoradiotherapy for patients with stage III NSCLC.[26] However, secondary analyses suggest that some patients may benefit from this approach. Therefore, induction chemoradiotherapy followed by surgery should be considered in a select subgroup of patients to maximize the possibility of cure (see **Box 2**).

Some patients who undergo surgery for clinical stage I or II NSCLC have microscopic involvement of mediastinal lymph nodes on pathologic review following apparent complete resection. These patients have a high risk of systemic relapse and should receive adjuvant chemotherapy. Although adjuvant RT does increase local control rates, it has not resulted in a clear survival benefit in patients with completely resected NSCLC. However, based on retrospective analyses suggesting an improvement in overall survival with adjuvant RT in patients with microscopic mediastinal lymph node involvement (N2), mediastinal RT, given after the completion of adjuvant chemotherapy, is a reasonable option in such patients.[19]

Stage IV NSCLC

NSCLC is diagnosed at an advanced stage in more than 40% of patients. The widespread use of PET has contributed to a recent increase in the proportion of patients being diagnosed with advanced, or metastatic, disease.[27] Common metastatic sites include the contralateral lung, brain, bone, liver, and adrenal glands. In patients with advanced disease, clinical and molecular differences between adenocarcinoma and squamous cell carcinoma are increasingly being used in therapeutic decision making. The outcome of patients with advanced NSCLC has steadily improved in the past 2 decades as a result of more effective therapeutic options, improved supportive care measures, and stage migration because of advanced imaging technology.[28]

First-line chemotherapy

Platinum-based chemotherapy is the cornerstone of treatment of patients with advanced NSCLC.[29] The superiority of platinum-based chemotherapy compared with best supportive care was conclusively established in randomized studies that noted improvements in both overall survival and quality of life.[30] Combination chemotherapy results in higher response rates and better overall survival than single-agent therapy.[31] Combination regimens consisting of cisplatin or carboplatin plus a third-generation chemotherapeutic agent, such as paclitaxel, docetaxel, vinorelbine, gemcitabine, or pemetrexed, have all shown similar efficacy, but varying toxicity, when used as first-line therapy, suggesting that an efficacy plateau had been reached with standard cytotoxic chemotherapy in patients with advanced NSCLC.[32,33] For patients with a good performance status (Eastern Cooperative Oncology Group [ECOG] scale 0–1), platinum-based chemotherapy remains the standard of care (**Box 3**). For patients with a marginal performance status (ECOG 2), single-agent therapy may be a more reasonable option based on the poor overall prognosis in these patients. Cytotoxic chemotherapy does not benefit patients with a poor performance status (ECOG 3–4).

Given that advanced NSCLC is an incurable disease in which the overall goal of care is palliation, carboplatin-based regimens have become a more popular alternative than cisplatin-based regimens in the United States because of their more favorable toxicity profile. Randomized studies have established that 4 cycles of combination chemotherapy is optimal for first-line therapy.[34] Continuation of chemotherapy beyond 4 cycles often leads to excessive toxicity without improvement in overall survival. Modern, platinum-based chemotherapy

---

Box 3
Treatment of advanced-stage NSCLC

First-line therapy (combination chemotherapy)

Carboplatin/cisplatin + paclitaxel

Carboplatin/cisplatin + docetaxel

Carboplatin/cisplatin + pemetrexed (nonsquamous)

Carboplatin/cisplatin + gemcitabine

Bevacizumab (nonsquamous)[a]

Erlotinib (EGFR-mutant tumor)

Crizotinib (ALK-mutant tumor)

Second-line therapy (single-agent therapy)

Docetaxel

Pemetrexed (nonsquamous)

Erlotinib

Crizotinib (ALK-mutant tumor)

Third-line therapy (single-agent therapy)

Erlotinib

Maintenance therapy (single-agent therapy)

Pemetrexed (nonsquamous)

Erlotinib

Bevacizumab (nonsquamous)[b]

[a] In combination with platinum-based chemotherapy.
[b] Only in patients who received bevacizumab plus chemotherapy as first-line therapy.

---

regimens result in objective response rates of 30% to 40%, median overall survival of 8 to 10 months, and 1-year and 2-year survival rates of 30% to 40% and 20% to 25%, respectively.

Maintenance therapy

Maintenance therapy, or early second-line therapy, refers to the continued treatment of patients with an active therapeutic agent after achieving an objective response or stable disease with 4 cycles of first-line chemotherapy. The purpose of maintenance therapy is to delay disease progression, improve overall survival, and maintain the period of symptomatic benefits achieved with first-line therapy. The US Food and Drug Administration (FDA) has approved both pemetrexed and erlotinib as maintenance therapy in patients with advanced NSCLC.

In a randomized, phase III study, pemetrexed was compared with placebo in patients who had achieved disease control with a platinum-based first-line regimen.[35] Pemetrexed maintenance resulted in modest improvements in both progression-free and overall survival, particularly for patients with adenocarcinoma who garnered a 5-month improvement in median survival. Another randomized study compared maintenance erlotinib with placebo.[36] In the overall study population, erlotinib led to a modest, but statistically significant, improvement in both progression-free and overall survival. Patients whose tumors had an activating EGFR mutation had a more robust benefit. However, both of these studies were flawed in that less than 20% of patients in the placebo arms received either pemetrexed or erlotinib, respectively, on disease progression, which likely exaggerated the observed clinical benefits of maintenance therapy.[35,36] In addition, patients in the maintenance therapy arms received more active therapy overall than those in the placebo arms. These issues are underscored by a study that randomized patients to receive docetaxel as either maintenance therapy or salvage therapy and reported similar overall survival in those patients who received docetaxel in both arms.[37] Proponents of maintenance therapy have argued that maintenance therapy may be beneficial precisely because it ensures that patients receive a greater number of active agents.[38] The use of maintenance therapy is currently considered an option for patients without progression of disease after the completion of first-line chemotherapy (see **Box 3**). The decision on whether or not to use maintenance therapy is based on multiple factors, including disease burden, patient preference, performance status, disease-related symptoms, treatment-related side effects, and cost.

Salvage chemotherapy

Most patients who receive first-line chemotherapy develop progression of disease within 4 to 6 months. Docetaxel and pemetrexed are both approved by the FDA as second-line chemotherapy in patients with advanced NSCLC (see **Box 3**). Docetaxel has shown superiority compared with best supportive care in relapsed NSCLC based on modest improvements in overall survival and symptom control.[39] Pemetrexed was directly compared with docetaxel in a large, randomized study of patients with relapsed, advanced NSCLC and had similar efficacy, but less toxicity.[40] The benefits of pemetrexed seem to be restricted to patients with nonsquamous histology.[41] Both docetaxel and pemetrexed yield a response rate of less than 10% and a median survival of approximately 8 months in the second-line setting.

Erlotinib, an EGFR inhibitor, is also approved for therapy for relapsed, advanced NSCLC. In a large phase III study, patients with progressive NSCLC following 1 or 2 prior chemotherapy regimens were randomized to receive either erlotinib or placebo.[42] Erlotinib resulted in a response rate of 9%, greater symptom relief, and a modest improvement in overall survival (6.7 months vs 4.7 months; $P<.001$). Although approved for use in unselected patients, erlotinib has been most effective in the subset of patients whose tumors harbor activating mutations of the EGFR gene.[43,44]

Targeted therapy

In the past decade, there has been a large increase in knowledge regarding critical cell-signaling pathways that affect carcinogenesis, cellular proliferation, evasion of apoptosis, and metastasis. As a result, numerous therapeutic agents that interact with specific molecular targets have been developed to improve outcomes for patients with many types of cancer, including NSCLC.

EGFR mutation EGFR is part of a critical cell-signaling pathway in NSCLC. Activation of EGFR results in phosphorylation of downstream proteins that then promote cancer proliferation and metastasis. EGFR tyrosine kinase inhibitors (TKI), such as erlotinib and gefitinib, were initially evaluated without molecular selection in patients with relapsed NSCLC.[42,45] In 2004, it was recognized that robust clinical responses to EGFR TKIs were linked to activating mutations in exons 19 or 21 of the EGFR gene and that these mutations are associated with certain clinical characteristics, such as female sex, adenocarcinoma histology, never smokers, and east Asian ethnicity.[43,44] In patients with tumors harboring EGFR-activating mutations, EGFR TKIs are superior to chemotherapy with response rates of 60% to 80% and median progression-free survivals of 9 to 11 months (see **Box 3, Table 1**).[46–50] In the white population, EGFR mutations are observed in 10% to 15% of patients with advanced NSCLC. These agents are associated with a favorable toxicity profile, with the main toxicities being rash and diarrhea. Molecular testing for EGFR mutations has now become a standard approach for patients with advanced lung adenocarcinoma.

ALK gene rearrangement Rearrangement of the ALK gene is observed in 4% to 5% of tumors from patients with advanced NSCLC, and is associated with never-smoking status and adenocarcinoma histology.[51] The resulting fusion protein acts as a dominant oncogenic signal.[52] Crizotinib, an inhibitor of the ALK kinase, has recently received accelerated approval by the FDA for the treatment of patients with ALK mutation–positive NSCLC. Crizotinib results in an objective response rate of nearly 60% and a median progression-free survival of 10 months in patients with relapsed NSCLC with an ALK gene rearrangement

Table 1
Randomized trials of EGFR inhibitors versus chemotherapy in EGFR-mutant NSCLC

Study	Regimens	N	Response Rate %	P	Progression-free Survival Median	HR (P)	Overall Survival Median	HR (P)
IPASS[46]	Gefitinib	132	71	<.001	NR	0.48 (<.001)	21.6 mo	1.00 (.99)
	Carboplatin + paclitaxel	129	47		NR		21.9 mo	
NEJSG[47]	Gefitinib	114	74	<.001	10.8 mo	0.30 (<.001)	30.5 mo	(.31)
	Carboplatin + paclitaxel	114	31		5.4 mo		23.6 mo	
WJTOG[48]	Gefitinib	86	62	<.0001	9.2 mo	0.49 (<.0001)	Not reported	
	Cisplatin + docetaxel	86	32		6.3 mo			
OPTIMAL[49]	Erlotinib	82	83	<.0001	13.7 mo	0.16 (<.0001)	Not reported	
	Carboplatin + gemcitabine	72	36		4.6 mo			
CTONG[50]	Erlotinib	77	58	<.0001	9.7 mo	0.37 (<.0001)	22.9 mo	0.80 (.42)
	Platinum + docetaxel or Platinum + gemcitabine	76	15		5.2 mo		18.8 mo	

Abbreviations: CTONG, China thoracic oncology group; EURTAC, European Erlotinib Versus Chemotherapy; IPASS, Iressa Pan-Asia study; NEJSG, North-East Japan study group; WJTOG, West Japan thoracic oncology group.

(see **Box 3, Table 2**).[53–55] Daily oral administration of crizotinib is well tolerated, and is now being compared with standard chemotherapy in randomized studies of patients with ALK mutation–positive NSCLC.

Antiangiogenic therapy Angiogenesis is a critical event for tumor formation and metastasis. The vascular endothelial growth factor (VEGF) is an important regulator of angiogenesis and has been extensively evaluated as a target for anticancer therapy. Bevacizumab is a monoclonal antibody that binds to VEGF and inhibits new vessel formation. Bevacizumab is approved by the FDA for use in combination with chemotherapy as first-line treatment in patients with advanced NSCLC based on a randomized trial in which bevacizumab plus chemotherapy resulted in a higher response rate and improved overall survival (12.3 months vs 10.3 months, $P = .003$) compared with

chemotherapy alone (see **Box 3**).[56] Common side effects of bevacizumab include hypertension, bleeding, arterial thrombosis, and proteinuria. The use of bevacizumab is not recommended for patients with squamous cell histology because of a high risk of pulmonary hemorrhage.[57] Several other antiangiogenic agents have been evaluated in patients with advanced NSCLC, with disappointing results. Thus far, efforts to identify biomarkers to aid patient selection for antiangiogenic therapy have been unsuccessful.

Future Directions

There are some novel targeted agents and predictive biomarkers for the treatment of advanced NSCLC. In a recent study analyzing NSCLCs for mutations in several relevant genes, including EGFR, HER2, KRAS, MET, BRAF, PI3K, and PTEN, a dominant, activating mutation

Table 2
ALK inhibition in ALK mutation–positive NSCLC

Trial	Agent	N	Response Objective Response Rate (%)[a]	Disease Control Rate (%)[b]	Median Progression-Free Survival
Phase I[53,54]	Crizotinib 250 mg by mouth twice daily	119	61	88	10 mo
Phase II[55]	Crizotinib 250 mg by mouth twice daily	76	54	91	Not reported

[a] Objective response rate = complete response rate + partial response rate.
[b] Disease control rate = complete response rate + partial response rate + stable disease rate.

was found in tumors from 54% of patients with advanced lung adenocarcinoma.[58] Efforts are now underway to study specific targeted agents in these molecularly distinct patient subsets with the overall goal of selecting appropriate therapy based on the mutational profile of the individual patient's tumor. In patients with squamous cell histology, amplification of the fibroblast growth factor receptor was recently noted in nearly 25% of tumors.

Given the growing number of molecular targets and therapeutic agents available for specific subgroups of patients with NSCLC, it is important to obtain sufficient tissue specimens to allow an accurate diagnosis and molecular studies. Core biopsies are preferable to aspiration biopsies in patients with suspected lung cancer to maximize the diagnostic yield of the specimens. The shift toward individualized therapy for NSCLC has begun to yield significant improvements in patient outcomes during the past decade.

SMALL CELL LUNG CANCER

Small cell lung cancer (SCLC) is an aggressive malignancy characterized by neuroendocrine differentiation, early metastases, and initial responsiveness to therapy. The overall incidence of SCLC peaked in the 1980s and has been declining since then, with SCLC now comprising about 15% of all cases of lung cancer.[59,60]

The Veterans' Administration Lung Group classification scheme is routinely used to stage SCLC.[61] Limited stage (LS) is defined as tumor confined to 1 hemithorax, with or without regional lymph node involvement, which can be safely encompassed in a single radiotherapy port. Extensive stage (ES) is defined as disease that has spread beyond this point, including malignant pleural effusion and hematogenous metastases. At presentation, two-thirds of patients have ES disease.[60] The tumor-node-metastasis (TNM) staging system for lung cancer can be applied to SCLC because the T and N descriptors, and the overall stage I to IV groupings, are discriminatory for survival in SCLC, as well as NSCLC.[62]

Treatment

Radiotherapy
The goal of therapy in patients with LS-SCLC is cure, which can be achieved through combined modality therapy with chemotherapy plus radiation (**Box 4**). Two meta-analyses have concluded that the addition of definitive thoracic RT to

---

> **Box 4**
> **Stage-specific treatment of SCLC**
>
> *LS*
>
> Cisplatin + etoposide × 4 cycles (substitute carboplatin if cisplatin is contraindicated)
>
> Early, concurrent thoracic radiotherapy
>
> Prophylactic cranial irradiation for responders
>
> Surgical resection followed by adjuvant chemotherapy (stage I only)
>
> *ES*
>
> Platinum-based chemotherapy (eg, carboplatin + etoposide) × 4 to 6 cycles
>
> Prophylactic cranial irradiation for responders
>
> *Recurrent disease*
>
> Single-agent chemotherapy
>
> Palliative radiotherapy, as indicated for symptoms
>
> Clinical trials of investigational agents

---

chemotherapy significantly improves 2-year to 3-year overall survival in patients with LS-SCLC by 5.4% ($P = .001$).[63,64] In addition, initiating thoracic RT early in the course of chemotherapy yields a 5% 2-year overall survival benefit compared with late RT ($P = .03$).[65] The optimal fractionation schedule of thoracic RT remains unclear, with discrepant findings in 2 large randomized trials. Turrisi and colleagues[66] randomized 417 patients with LS-SCLC to receive standard cisplatin plus etoposide with 45 Gy of early, concurrent RT given either once daily over 5 weeks or twice daily over 3 weeks. There was a significant improvement in overall survival in patients receiving twice-daily RT compared with those receiving once-daily RT (5-year survival, 26% vs 16%; $P = .04$). The primary criticism of this trial is a the lack of biologic equivalence between the radiation doses administered on the 2 arms caused by the low total dose given to patients receiving once-daily RT. A second trial randomized 262 patients with LS-SCLC to receive standard cisplatin plus etoposide with either once-daily RT to 50.4 Gy in 28 fractions or twice-daily RT to 48 Gy in a split course of 32 fractions.[67] This trial found no significant differences in overall survival between the 2 arms (3 years: once-daily arm, 34%, vs twice-daily arm, 29%; $P = .49$). However, late initiation of RT with the third cycle of chemotherapy and the use of split-course therapy in the twice-daily arm may have compromised the outcome of this study. It is hoped that the role of hyperfractionated RT in LS-SCLC will be more clearly defined in ongoing, well-designed trials.

Up to 60% of patients with SCLC develop brain metastases during the course of their illness. A meta-analysis of studies evaluating prophylactic cranial irradiation (PCI) reported a 25% decrease in the incidence of brain metastases (58.6% vs 33.3%, P<.001) and a 5.4% increase in 3-year overall survival (15.3% vs 20.7%, P = .01) with the addition of PCI after primary treatment.[68] Most patients included in this meta-analysis had LS-SCLC. To determine the role of PCI in patients with ES-SCLC, a European Organisation for Research and Treatment of Cancer (EORTC) trial randomized 286 patients with ES-SCLC to receive PCI or not to receive PCI after response to initial chemotherapy.[69] The investigators reported that PCI decreased the incidence of symptomatic brain metastases (14.6% vs 40.4%, P<.001) and increased the 1-year survival rate (27.1% vs 13.3%, P = .003) without a long-term decrement in global quality of life. Based on these trials, PCI is now recommended for patients with either LS-SCLC or ES-SCLC who have a good performance status after achieving a response to initial therapy (see **Box 4**).

Chemotherapy

Without treatment, patients with SCLC have a poor prognosis, with median survival times of 7 to 14 weeks depending on stage. Early trials with single agents revealed high rates of partial response of brief duration. Subsequent clinical trials of combination chemotherapy regimens, such as cyclophosphamide, doxorubicin, and vincristine (CAV) or etoposide and cisplatin (EP), yielded significant improvements with response rates of 60% to 80%, complete response rates of 15% to 25%, and median survival times of 7 to 10 months.[70,71] A recent phase III study comparing EP with cyclophosphamide, epirubicin, and vincristine (CEV) reported that overall survival was significantly better in patients receiving EP (10.2 vs 7.8 months, P = .0004).[72] In addition, 2 meta-analyses have shown a modest survival advantage for cisplatin-based therapy.[73,74] EP is now the preferred regimen in both ES-SCLC and LS-SCLC (see **Box 4**).

Several newer combinations of drugs have shown promising efficacy in early phase trials. Among these, the combination of irinotecan plus cisplatin (IP) has garnered the most interest, and 3 randomized trials comparing IP with EP in patients with ES-SCLC have been completed (**Table 3**). The first study, from Japan, reported that IP resulted in significantly better response rate, progression-free survival, and overall survival.[75] However, 2 randomized trials in Western patients have failed to confirm these findings, with both reporting no significant differences in response rate or survival between patients receiving IP or EP.[76,77] A large, phase III trial comparing EP with the combination of cisplatin plus topotecan, a drug related to irinotecan, also failed to show any significant differences in the efficacy of these 2 regimens (see **Table 3**).[78] Therefore, EP remains the standard of care for non-Japanese patients with SCLC.

A variety of chemotherapy-based strategies, including dose intensification, weekly administration, 3-drug regimens, high-dose consolidation with stem cell rescue, alternating or sequential non–cross-resistant regimens, and maintenance therapy, have failed to yield substantial improvements in survival, and many of these approaches have resulted in unacceptable toxicity.

Table 3
Randomized trials of cisplatin plus irinotecan or topotecan in ES-SCLC

Trial	Arm	N	Response Rate %	P	Overall Survival Median (mo)	1 y (%)	2 y (%)	P
Noda et al,[75] 2002	IP	77	84	.02	12.8	58.4	19.5	.002
	EP	77	68		9.4	37.7	5.2	
Hanna et al,[76] 2006	IP	221	48	NS	9.3	35	8	.74
	EP	110	44		10.2	35	8	
Lara et al,[77] 2009	IP	324	60	.56	9.9	41	NR	.71
	EP	327	57		9.1	34	NR	
Eckardt et al,[78] 2006	TP	389	63	NS	9.0	31	NR	.48
	EP	395	69		9.2	31	NR	

Abbreviations: EP, etoposide + cisplatin; IP, irinotecan + cisplatin; NR, not reported; NS, not significant; TP, oral topotecan + cisplatin.

Recurrent disease

Most patients with LS-SCLC, and nearly all with ES-SCLC, develop recurrence of disease. Recurrent SCLC is categorized as either resistant (primary progression or recurrence within 3 months of initial therapy) or sensitive (recurrence more than 3 months after initial therapy), with lower response rates to second-line therapy noted in those with resistant disease. For patients whose initial response lasts for more than 6 to 8 months, the reinitiation of the initial chemotherapy regimen may be the favored approach, with reported response rates of up to 60%.[79] For patients relapsing within 6 months of initial therapy, treatment with a second-line agent seems to be a more appropriate strategy.

The benefit of second-line therapy in patients with recurrent SCLC was shown in a randomized trial that compared oral topotecan with best supportive care and reported that overall survival was significantly better in patients receiving chemotherapy (median survival, 26 vs 14 weeks; 6-month survival, 49% vs 26%; $P = .01$).[80] Many single agents and combination regimens .have been evaluated in noncomparative phase II trials of patients with relapsed SCLC. Although response rates seem to be higher with combination therapy, overall survival does not seem to be improved and the toxicity of combination regimens can be excessive. One randomized phase III trial compared single-agent topotecan with the combination of CAV in patients with relapsed SCLC and found no significant differences in response rate (24% vs 18%, $P = .29$), time to progression (13 vs 12 weeks, $P = .55$), or overall survival (median, 25 vs 25 weeks, $P = .79$).[81] However, hematologic toxicity was significantly greater with CAV. Based on these results, single-agent chemotherapy is the preferred approach for patients with recurrent SCLC who have maintained a good performance status (see **Box 4**).

Future Directions

The investigational drug amrubicin has shown promising activity in patients with SCLC. Single-agent amrubicin has yielded response rates of up to 79% in chemotherapy-naive patients with ES-SCLC and up to 52% in patients with recurrent disease.[82,83] However, a randomized, phase III trial comparing amrubicin with topotecan in patients with recurrent SCLC reported a significant improvement in response rate with amrubicin (31% vs 17%, $P = .0002$), but no significant differences in progression-free or overall survival.[84]

Numerous molecular pathways that drive the progression of cancer have been identified and many therapeutic agents that target these pathways have been developed. Many such molecularly targeted strategies have been evaluated in clinical trials in patients with SCLC. Thus far all of them, including antiangiogenic agents, metalloproteinase inhibitors, growth factor inhibitors, and proapoptotic agents, have failed to show promising clinical activity. Despite these setbacks, more molecular strategies are now being evaluated in preclinical and clinical studies in SCLC, including those targeting apoptotic pathways (small-molecule Bcl-2 inhibitors) and cancer stem cells (Notch and hedgehog inhibitors).[85]

From 1973 to 2002, the 2-year survival rate for patients with LS-SCLC improved incrementally from 15% to 22%, whereas little improvement was noted for patients with ES-SCLC (3.4%–5.6%).[56] It is clear that new, more effective therapeutic strategies are needed if there are going to be any further substantial gains in the treatment of patients with SCLC.

ACKNOWLEDGMENTS

We appreciate Dr Mary Varterasian's critical review of the article.

REFERENCES

1. Ginsberg RJ, Rubinstein LV. Randomized trial of lobectomy versus limited resection for T1 N0 non-small cell lung cancer. Ann Thorac Surg 1995;60: 615–23.
2. El-Sherif A, Gooding WE, Santos R, et al. Outcomes of sublobar resection versus lobectomy for stage I non-small cell lung cancer: a 13-year analysis. Ann Thorac Surg 2006;82:408–15.
3. Okada M, Yoshikawa K, Hatta T, et al. Is segmentectomy with lymph node assessment an alternative to lobectomy for non-small cell lung cancer of 2 cm or smaller? Ann Thorac Surg 2001;71:956–60.
4. Yan TD, Black D, Bannon PG, et al. Systematic review and meta-analysis of randomized and non-randomized trials on safety and efficacy of video-assisted thoracic surgery lobectomy for early-stage non-small-cell lung cancer. J Clin Oncol 2009;27: 2553–62.
5. Cattaneo SM, Park BJ, Wilson AS, et al. Use of video-assisted thoracic surgery for lobectomy in the elderly results in fewer complications. Ann Thorac Surg 2008;85:231–6.
6. Gopaldas RR, Bakaeen FG, Dao TK, et al. Video-assisted thoracoscopic versus open thoracotomy lobectomy in a cohort of 13,619 patients. Ann Thorac Surg 2010;89:1563–70.
7. Gharagozloo F, Margolis M, Tempseta B, et al. Robot-assisted lobectomy for early-stage lung cancer: report

of 100 consecutive cases. Ann Thorac Surg 2009;88: 380–4.

8. Agostini P, Cieslik H, Rathinam S, et al. Postoperative pulmonary complications following thoracic surgery: are there any modifiable risk factors? Thorax 2010;65:815–8.

9. Salazar OM, Slawson RG, Poussin-Rosillo H, et al. A prospective randomized trial comparing once-a-week vs daily radiation therapy for locally-advanced, non-metastatic, lung cancer: a preliminary report. Int J Radiat Oncol Biol Phys 1986;12:779–87.

10. Qiao X, Tullgren O, Lax I, et al. The role of radiotherapy in treatment of stage I non-small cell lung cancer. Lung Cancer 2003;41:1–11.

11. Timmerman R, Paulus R, Galvin J, et al. Stereotactic body radiation therapy for inoperable early stage lung cancer. JAMA 2010;303:1070–6.

12. Timmerman R, McGarry R, Yiannoutsos C, et al. Excessive toxicity when treating central tumors in a phase II study of stereotactic body radiation therapy for medically inoperable early-stage lung cancer. J Clin Oncol 2006;24:4833–9.

13. Lencioni R, Crocetti L, Cioni R, et al. Response to radiofrequency ablation of pulmonary tumours: a prospective, intention-to-treat, multicentre clinical trial (the RAPTURE study). Lancet Oncol 2008;9: 621–8.

14. Simon CJ, Dupuy DE, DiPetrillo TA, et al. Pulmonary radiofrequency ablation: long-term safety and efficacy in 153 patients. Radiology 2007;243: 268–75.

15. Zemlyak A, Moore WH, Bilfinger TV. Comparison of survival after sublobar resections and ablative therapies for stage I non-small cell lung cancer. J Am Coll Surg 2010;211:68–72.

16. NSCLC Meta-analyses Collaborative Group. Adjuvant chemotherapy, with or without postoperative radiotherapy, in operable non-small-cell lung cancer: two meta-analyses of individual patient data. Lancet 2010;375:167–77.

17. Butts CA, Ding K, Seymour L, et al. Randomized phase III trial of vinorelbine plus cisplatin compared with observation in completely resected stage IB and II non-small-cell lung cancer: updated survival analysis of JBR-10. J Clin Oncol 2010;28:29–34.

18. Strauss GM, Herndon JE, Maddaus MA, et al. Adjuvant paclitaxel plus carboplatin compared with observation in stage IB non-small-cell lung cancer: CALGB 9633 with the Cancer and Leukemia Group B, Radiation Therapy Oncology Group, and North Central Cancer Treatment Group Study Groups. J Clin Oncol 2008;26:5043–51.

19. Douillard JY, Rosell R, De Lena M, et al. Impact of postoperative radiation therapy on survival in patients with complete resection and stage I, II, or IIIA non-small-cell lung cancer treated with adjuvant chemotherapy: the Adjuvant Navelbine International

Trialist Association (ANITA) randomized trial. Int J Radiat Oncol Biol Phys 2008;72:695–701.

20. Dillman RO, Seagren SL, Propert KJ, et al. A randomized trial of induction chemotherapy plus high-dose radiation versus radiation alone in stage III non-small-cell lung cancer. N Engl J Med 1990; 323:940–5.

21. Curran WJ, Paulus R, Langer CJ, et al. Sequential vs. concurrent chemoradiation for stage III non-small cell lung cancer: randomized phase III trial RTOG 9410. J Natl Cancer Inst 2011;103:1452–60.

22. O'Rourke N, Roque IF, Farre BN, et al. Concurrent chemoradiotherapy in non-small cell lung cancer. Cochrane Database Syst Rev 2010;(6):CD002140.

23. Hanna N, Neubauer M, Yiannoustos C, et al. Phase III study of cisplatin, etoposide, and concurrent chest radiation with or without consolidation docetaxel in patients with inoperable stage III non-small-cell lung cancer: the Hoosier Oncology Group and U.S. Oncology. J Clin Oncol 2008;26:5755–60.

24. Belani CP, Choy H, Bonomi P, et al. Combined chemoradiotherapy regimens of paclitaxel and carboplatin for locally advanced non-small-cell lung cancer: a randomized phase II locally advanced multi-modality protocol. J Clin Oncol 2005;23: 5883–91.

25. Govindan R, Bogart J, Stinchcombe T, et al. Randomized phase II study of pemetrexed, carboplatin, and thoracic radiation with or without cetuximab in patients with locally advanced unresectable non-small-cell lung cancer: Cancer and Leukemia Group B trial 30407. J Clin Oncol 2011;29:3120–5.

26. Albain KS, Swann RS, Rusch VW, et al. Radiotherapy plus chemotherapy with or without surgical resection for stage III non-small-cell lung cancer: a phase III randomised controlled trial. Lancet 2009;374:379–86.

27. Morgensztern D, Ng SH, Gao F, et al. Trends in stage distribution for patients with non-small cell lung cancer: a National Cancer Database survey. J Thorac Oncol 2010;5:29–33.

28. Ramalingam S, Belani CP. State-of-the-art chemotherapy for advanced non-small cell lung cancer. Semin Oncol 2004;31(Suppl 1):68–74.

29. Azzoli CG, Baker S, Temin S, et al. American Society of Clinical Oncology Clinical Practice Guideline update on chemotherapy for stage IV non-small-cell lung cancer. J Clin Oncol 2009;27:6251–66.

30. Rapp E, Pater JL, Willan A, et al. Chemotherapy can prolong survival in patients with advanced non-small-cell lung cancer–report of a Canadian multicenter randomized trial. J Clin Oncol 1988;6: 633–41.

31. Wozniak AJ, Crowley JJ, Balcerzak SP, et al. Randomized trial comparing cisplatin with cisplatin plus vinorelbine in the treatment of advanced

non-small-cell lung cancer: a Southwest Oncology Group study. J Clin Oncol 1998;16:2459–65.

32. Schiller JH, Harrington D, Belani CP, et al. Comparison of four chemotherapy regimens for advanced non-small-cell lung cancer. N Engl J Med 2002; 346:92–8.

33. Scagliotti GV, Parikh P, von Pawel J, et al. Phase III study comparing cisplatin plus gemcitabine with cisplatin plus pemetrexed in chemotherapy-naive patients with advanced-stage non-small-cell lung cancer. J Clin Oncol 2008;26:3543–51.

34. Socinski MA, Schell MJ, Peterman A, et al. Phase III trial comparing a defined duration of therapy versus continuous therapy followed by second-line therapy in advanced-stage IIIB/IV non-small-cell lung cancer. J Clin Oncol 2002;20:1335–43.

35. Ciuleanu T, Brodowicz T, Zielinski C, et al. Maintenance pemetrexed plus best supportive care versus placebo plus best supportive care for non-small-cell lung cancer: a randomised, double-blind, phase 3 study. Lancet 2009;374:1432–40.

36. Cappuzzo F, Ciuleanu T, Stelmakh L, et al. Erlotinib as maintenance treatment in advanced non-small-cell lung cancer: a multicentre, randomised, placebo-controlled phase 3 study. Lancet Oncol 2010;11:521–9.

37. Fidias PM, Dakhil SR, Lyss AP, et al. Phase III study of immediate compared with delayed docetaxel after front-line therapy with gemcitabine plus carboplatin in advanced non-small-cell lung cancer. J Clin Oncol 2009;27:591–8.

38. Owonikoko TK, Ramalingam SS, Belani CP. Maintenance therapy for advanced non-small cell lung cancer: current status, controversies, and emerging consensus. Clin Cancer Res 2010;16:2496–504.

39. Shepherd FA, Dancey J, Ramlau R, et al. Prospective randomized trial of docetaxel versus best supportive care in patients with non-small-cell lung cancer previously treated with platinum-based chemotherapy. J Clin Oncol 2000;18:2095–103.

40. Hanna N, Shepherd FA, Fossella FV, et al. Randomized phase III trial of pemetrexed versus docetaxel in patients with non-small-cell lung cancer previously treated with chemotherapy. J Clin Oncol 2004;22:1589–97.

41. Scagliotti G, Hanna N, Fossella F, et al. The differential efficacy of pemetrexed according to NSCLC histology: a review of two phase III studies. Oncologist 2009;14:253–63.

42. Shepherd FA, Rodrigues-Pereira J, Ciuleanu T, et al. Erlotinib in previously treated non-small-cell lung cancer. N Engl J Med 2005;353:123–32.

43. Lynch TJ, Bell DW, Sordella R, et al. Activating mutations in the epidermal growth factor receptor underlying responsiveness of non-small-cell lung cancer to gefitinib. N Engl J Med 2004;350: 2129–39.

44. Paez JG, Janne PA, Lee JC, et al. EGFR mutations in lung cancer: correlation with clinical response to gefitinib therapy. Science 2004;304:1497–500.

45. Kris MG, Natale RB, Herbst RS, et al. Efficacy of gefitinib, an inhibitor of the epidermal growth factor receptor tyrosine kinase, in symptomatic patients with non-small cell lung cancer: a randomized trial. JAMA 2003;290:2149–58.

46. Mok TS, Wu YL, Thongprasert S, et al. Gefitinib or carboplatin-paclitaxel in pulmonary adenocarcinoma". N Engl J Med 2009;361:947–57.

47. Maemondo M, Inoue A, Kobayashi K, et al. Gefitinib or chemotherapy for non-small-cell lung cancer with mutated EGFR. N Engl J Med 2010;362: 2380–8.

48. Mitsudomi T, Morita S, Yatabe Y, et al. Gefitinib versus cisplatin plus docetaxel in patients with non-small-cell lung cancer harbouring mutations of the epidermal growth factor receptor (WJTOG3405): an open label, randomised phase 3 trial. Lancet Oncol 2010;11:121–8.

49. Zhou C, Wu YL, Chen G, et al. Updated efficacy and quality-of-life analyses in OPTIMAL, a phase III, randomized, open-label study of first-line erlotinib versus gemcitabine/carboplatin in patients with EGFR-activating mutation-positive advanced non-small cell lung cancer. J Clin Oncol 2011; 29(Suppl 15):480s.

50. Rosell R, Gervais R, Vergnenegre B, et al. Erlotinib versus chemotherapy in advanced non-small cell lung cancer patients with epidermal growth factor receptor mutations: interim results of the European Erlotinib Versus Chemotherapy (EURTAC) phase III randomized trial. J Clin Oncol 2011;29(Suppl 15): 476s.

51. Shaw AT, Yeap BY, Mino-Kenudson M, et al. Clinical features and outcome of patients with non-small-cell lung cancer who harbor EML4-ALK. J Clin Oncol 2009;27:4247–53.

52. Soda M, Choi YL, Enomoto M, et al. Identification of the transforming EML4-ALK fusion gene in non-small-cell lung cancer. Nature 2007;448:561–6.

53. Kwak EL, Bang YJ, Camidge R, et al. Anaplastic lymphoma kinase inhibition in non-small-cell lung cancer. N Engl J Med 2010;363:1693–703.

54. Camidge DR, Bang Y, Kwak EL, et al. Progression-free survival from a phase I study of crizotinib (PF-02341066) in patients with ALK-positive non-small cell lung cancer. J Clin Oncol 2001;29(Suppl 15): 165s.

55. Crino L, Kim DW, Riely GJ, et al. Initial phase II results with crizotinib in advanced ALK-positive non-small cell lung cancer (NSCLC): profile 1005. J Clin Oncol 2011;29(Suppl 15):479s.

56. Sandler A, Gray R, Perry MC, et al. Paclitaxel-carboplatin alone or with bevacizumab for non-small-cell lung cancer. N Engl J Med 2006;355:2542–50.

57. Johnson DH, Fehrenbacher L, Novotny WF, et al. Randomized phase II trial comparing bevacizumab plus carboplatin and paclitaxel with carboplatin and paclitaxel alone in previously untreated locally advanced or metastatic non-small-cell lung cancer. J Clin Oncol 2004;22:2184–91.

58. Kris MG, Johnson BE, Kwiatkowski DJ, et al. Identification of driver mutations in tumor specimens from 1,000 patients with lung adenocarcinoma: The NCI's Lung Cancer Mutation Consortium (LCMC). J Clin Oncol 2011;29(Suppl 18):787s.

59. Navada S, Lai P, Schwartz AG, et al. Temporal trends in small cell lung cancer: analysis of the national surveillance, epidemiology, and end-results database. J Clin Oncol 2006;24(Suppl 18):384s.

60. Govindan R, Page N, Morgensztern D, et al. Changing epidemiology of small-cell lung cancer in the United States over the last 30 years: analysis of the Surveillance, Epidemiologic, and End-Results database. J Clin Oncol 2006;24:4539–44.

61. Zelen M. Keynote address on biostatistics and data retrieval. Cancer Chemother Rep 3 1973;4:31–42.

62. Shepherd FA, Crowley J, Van Houtte P, et al. The IASLC Lung Cancer Staging Project: proposals regarding the clinical staging of small cell lung cancer in the forthcoming (seventh) edition of the tumor, node, metastasis classification for lung cancer. J Thorac Oncol 2007;2:1067–77.

63. Pignon JP, Arriagada R, Ihde DC, et al. A meta-analysis of thoracic radiotherapy for small-cell lung cancer. N Engl J Med 1992;327:1618–24.

64. Warde P, Payne D. Does thoracic irradiation improve survival and local control in limited-stage small-cell carcinoma of the lung? A meta-analysis. J Clin Oncol 1992;10:890–5.

65. Fried DB, Morris DE, Poole C, et al. Systematic review evaluating the timing of thoracic radiation therapy in combined modality therapy for limited-stage small cell lung cancer. J Clin Oncol 2004;22:4785–93.

66. Turrisi AT, Kim K, Blum R, et al. Twice-daily compared with once-daily thoracic radiotherapy in limited small-cell lung cancer treated concurrently with cisplatin and etoposide. N Engl J Med 1999; 340:265–71.

67. Bonner JA, Sloan JA, Shanahan TG, et al. Phase III comparison of twice-daily split-course irradiation versus once-daily irradiation for patients with limited-stage small-cell lung carcinoma. J Clin Oncol 1999;17:2681–91.

68. Auperin A, Arriagada R, Pignon JP, et al. Prophylactic cranial irradiation for patients with small-cell lung cancer in complete remission. Prophylactic Cranial Irradiation Overview Collaborative Group. N Engl J Med 1999;341:476–84.

69. Slotman B, Faivre-Finn C, Kramer G, et al. Prophylactic cranial irradiation in extensive small-cell lung cancer. N Engl J Med 2007;357:664–72.

70. Lowenbraun S, Bartolucci A, Smalley RV, et al. The superiority of combination chemotherapy over single agent chemotherapy in small cell lung carcinoma. Cancer 1979;44:406–13.

71. Roth BJ, Johnson DH, Einhorn LH, et al. Randomized study of cyclophosphamide, doxorubicin, and vincristine versus etoposide and cisplatin versus alternation of these two regimens in extensive small-cell lung cancer: a phase III trial of the Southeastern Cancer Study Group. J Clin Oncol 1992;10: 282–91.

72. Sundstrøm S, Bremnes RM, Kaasa S, et al. Cisplatin and etoposide regimen is superior to cyclophosphamide, epirubicin, and vincristine regimen in small-cell lung cancer: results from a randomized phase III trial with 5 years' follow-up. J Clin Oncol 2002; 20:4665–72.

73. Pujol JL, Carestia L, Duares JP. Is there a case for cisplatin in the treatment of small-cell lung cancer? A meta-analysis of randomized trials of a cisplatin-containing regimen versus a regimen without this alkylating agent. Br J Cancer 2000;83:8–15.

74. Mascaux C, Paesmans M, Breghmans T, et al. A systematic review of the role of etoposide and cisplatin in the chemotherapy of small cell lung cancer with methodology assessment and meta-analysis. Lung Cancer 2000;30:23–36.

75. Noda K, Nishiwaki Y, Kawahara M, et al. Irinotecan plus cisplatin compared with etoposide plus cisplatin for extensive small-cell lung cancer. N Engl J Med 2002;346:85–91.

76. Hanna N, Bunn PA, Langer C, et al. Randomized phase III trial comparing irinotecan/cisplatin with etoposide/cisplatin in patients with previously untreated extensive-stage small-cell lung cancer. J Clin Oncol 2006;24:2038–43.

77. Lara PN, Natale R, Crowley J, et al. Phase III trial of irinotecan/cisplatin compared with etoposide/cisplatin in extensive-stage small-cell lung cancer: clinical and pharmacogenomic results from SWOG S0124. J Clin Oncol 2009;27:2530–5.

78. Eckardt JR, von Pawel J, Papai Z, et al. Open-label, multicenter, randomized, phase III study comparing oral topotecan/cisplatin versus etoposide/cisplatin as treatment for chemotherapy-naive patients with extensive-disease small-cell lung cancer. J Clin Oncol 2006;24:2044–51.

79. Giaccone G, Ferrati P, Donadio M, et al. Reinduction chemotherapy in small cell lung cancer. Eur J Cancer Clin Oncol 1987;23:1697–9.

80. O'Brien MER, Ciuleanu TE, Tsekov H, et al. Phase III trial comparing supportive care alone with supportive care with oral topotecan in patients with relapsed small-cell lung cancer. J Clin Oncol 2006; 24:5441–7.

81. Von Pawel J, Schiller JH, Shepherd FA, et al. Topotecan versus cyclophosphamide, doxorubicin, and

vincristine for the treatment of recurrent small-cell lung cancer. J Clin Oncol 1999;17:658–67.

82. Yana T, Negoro S, Takada M, et al. Phase II study of amrubicin in previously untreated patients with extensive-disease small cell lung cancer: West Japan Thoracic Oncology Group study. Invest New Drugs 2007;25:253–8.

83. Onoda S, Masuda N, Seto T, et al. Phase II trial of amrubicin for the treatment of refractory or relapsed small-cell lung cancer: Thoracic Oncology Research Group study 0301. J Clin Oncol 2006;24:5448–53.

84. Jotte R, von Pawel J, Spigel DR, et al. Randomized phase III trial of amrubicin versus topotecan as second-line treatment for small cell lung cancer. J Clin Oncol 2011;29(Suppl 15):453s.

85. Rudin CM, Hann CL, Peacock CD, et al. Novel systemic therapies for small cell lung cancer. J Natl Compr Canc Netw 2008;6:315–22.

Image-Guided Ablative Therapies for Lung Cancer

Amita Sharma, MD[a], Fereidoun Abtin, MD[b],
Jo-Anne O. Shepard, MD[a],*

KEYWORDS

- Ablation • Radiofrequency ablation • Cryoablation • Microwave ablation • Lung tumors • Thoracic
- Lung cancer • Treatment • Image-guided

KEY POINTS

- Image-guided ablation is an alternative treatment in stage 1 nonsmall cell lung cancer (NSCLC) in selected nonsurgical patients with comorbidities and recurrent disease after radiation or surgery.
- Application of radiofrequency, microwave energy, or cryotherapy can be used to destroy tumor cells.
- A multidisciplinary approach to patient selection and follow-up is desirable.
- The purpose of radiologic imaging after ablation is to identify any complications, to confirm the expected postablation appearances, and to exclude tumor progression.
- Ablative therapies offer the advantage of lung preservation, low morbidity, and mortality; further experience will define their role in the treatment algorithm for NSCLC.

INTRODUCTION

Lung cancer is the most common cause of cancer-related death in adults. Although surgical treatment remains the gold standard, only patients with localized, early-stage disease with or without involvement of regional lymph nodes (upto stage 3A) are eligible for lobectomy. Most patients have advanced-stage disease at presentation and are not surgical candidates. Some high-risk patients may still be candidates for limited surgical resection such as wedge resection or segmentectomy, which can be performed using video-assisted thoracoscopic surgery.[1–3] However, there are many patients who are considered nonsurgical candidates because of comorbidities or limited pulmonary reserve after evaluation with tests, including pulmonary function test, cardiac stress test, exercise stress test, or pulmonary stress test.[4]

Image-guided ablation has been accepted as an alternative treatment of localized disease. Application of electric currents, microwave energy, or cryotherapy can be used to destroy tumor cells. Image guidance allows precise placement of the percutaneous device within the tumor, and the technique has been shown to be well tolerated and safe. Ablation also has a role in the treatment of recurrent disease at the site of surgical resection, or within a radiation field. It has a limited role in palliation of tumors and in combination with radiation therapy. If there is local tumor progression, ablation can be repeated and does not preclude other treatment options. As a result, ablative therapies have become part of the spectrum of lung cancer management and should be considered as a viable treatment option in carefully selected patients. This article discusses the principles, technique, follow-up, and outcome of the 3 main ablative therapies currently used in the lung, radiofrequency ablation

The authors report no financial disclosures.
[a] Department of Radiology, Massachusetts General Hospital, Founders 202, 55 Fruit Street, Boston, MA 02114, USA; [b] Department of Radiology, UCLA Medical Center, 757 Westwood Plaza, Suite 1621, Los Angeles, CA 90095-1721, USA
* Corresponding author.
E-mail address: jshepard@partners.org

Radiol Clin N Am 50 (2012) 975–999
http://dx.doi.org/10.1016/j.rcl.2012.06.004
0033-8389/12/$ – see front matter © 2012 Elsevier Inc. All rights reserved.

(RFA), microwave ablation (MWA), and percutaneous cryotherapy (PCT).

RFA

The lung is an ideal tissue for RFA. A tumor can be easily distinguished from surrounding normal lung on computed tomography (CT), allowing precise placement of the electrode within the center of the lesion. Air in the lung acts as an excellent insulator, concentrating the energy delivered to the tumor and reducing dissipation of energy into the adjacent tissue.[5] In addition, the characteristic changes after ablation are immediately seen in the lung, allowing the radiologist to evaluate the success of the treatment at the time of the ablation and on subsequent studies. The main disadvantage of RFA of the lung is that the pulmonary vasculature can dramatically reduce the amount of heat that is concentrated within the tumor because of a heat sink effect. When the tumor is in contact with flowing blood, blood conducts heat away from the site of ablation, acting as a heat sink that reduces the potential temperature increase within the tumor.[6,7]

Mechanism of Action

During RFA a radiofrequency generator creates an alternating current in an electrode that is placed percutaneously into the tumor with the help of image guidance. Large, conductive grounding pads placed on the patient's thighs dissipate the heat and complete the electric circuit. An alternating current at the electrode tip leads to rapid oscillation of the ions in the adjacent tumor. Frictional heating caused by the rapid oscillation of the ions is then transferred through the tumor by means of conduction. Tissue temperatures greater than 57°C lead to instantaneous coagulation necrosis and irreversible cell death in the tumor.[8,9]

There are 3 different RFA electrode designs. The first design uses an internally cooled electrode (Covidien, Boulder, CO), which is available as a single electrode or 3 parallel electrodes that move as a single unit (**Fig. 1**). The 17-gauge electrode has an insulated shaft and a noninsulated 2-cm or 3-cm tip that deposits RF energy within the tumor. Ice-cold water is pumped through a closed channel within the electrode shaft to cool the tip of the electrode and prevent charring of tissue at the tip of the electrode, which may reduce the flow of current. The second design consists of a 14-gauge multitined electrode (Boston Scientific, Natick, MA and RITA Medical Systems, Fremont, CA). The retractable tines are deployed from the tip of the electrode once it is placed in the tumor, similar to opening an umbrella (**Fig. 2**). The tines are small

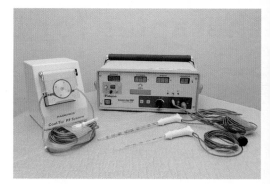

Fig. 1. Cool-tip system for RFA (Covidien, Boulder, CO) comprising a generator, perfusion pump, and internally cooled electrode.

electrodes that fan out within the tumor, each depositing radiofrequency current. The third design (Berchtold, Tuttlingen, Germany) consists of a single electrode with a side-hole, through which hypertonic saline is infused into the tissue around the tumor. The fluid that replaces the air within the lung allows for increased conductivity and subsequent enlargement of the ablation zone.

There are variable zones of ablation that can be created by the 3 different electrode designs. Typically, a spherical 3-cm zone is obtained with the cluster or multitined electrode and an ovoid 1-cm by 2-cm to 3-cm zone is seen with the single electrode. Repeated overlapping treatments are frequently used for the ablation of lesions larger than 2 cm. To enlarge the zone of ablation and reduce the time for treatment, multiple electrodes may be placed within a lesion and a switch box generator can switch the radiofrequency current between the electrodes.

Histologic Changes

After RFA, 3 concentric zones of histologic change are seen extending from the center of the electrode, corresponding to different temperatures achieved during ablation.[5,10–15] The central zone immediately adjacent to the electrode tip receives the greatest temperature increase and consists entirely of nonviable cells that are destroyed through coagulation necrosis. An intermediate zone lying beyond the central zone receives less heat from the electrode and comprises nonviable cells that complete the phase of necrosis over a few days. In the peripheral zone, where the least amount of heat is deposited, there is a mixture of viable and nonviable cells, which result in a zone of partial necrosis. To achieve complete ablation of a tumor, the tumor has to lie within the central and intermediate zones of ablation.

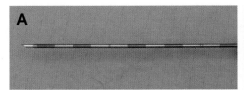 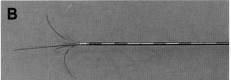

Fig. 2. Multitined expandable electrode consists of a 14-G electrode (*A*), from which multiple tines are deployed (*B*). Each tine acts as an individual electrode and thermocouple.

Immediately after RFA, focal ground-glass opacity is characteristically seen on the CT scan. The ground-glass opacity corresponds to the coagulation necrosis, congestion, inflammation, and pulmonary hemorrhage that occur in the tumor and the surrounding lung.[14,16,17] It is important to confirm that ground-glass opacity extends 5 to 10 mm beyond the margin of the tumor in all dimensions to achieve complete tumor necrosis. This goal may require multiple overlapping treatments after repositioning of the electrode within the tumor.

Patient Selection

Ablation should be performed only in patients with proven, localized malignancy. Appropriate patient selection is important to determine the best treatment of the patient and to maximize the success of RFA. A multidisciplinary approach is desirable, including radiologic assessment before RFA and evaluation of the patient by a thoracic surgeon to establish that the patient is nonresectable, as well as thoracic oncology assessment for long-term patient follow-up.

The choice to use 1 ablative technique over the other is dependent on the size, location, and proximity of the target lesion to vital structures. **Table 1** shows the factors to be considered on selection of ablative technique. Current RFA technology is most successful in smaller lesions, less than 3 cm. With lesions larger than 3 cm, local tumor progression occurs in up to 50% of cases.[18] Although repeat RFA is possible, combination treatment with RFA and radiotherapy may be desirable for larger lesions.[19] RFA is also best suited to tumors that are located in the peripheral two-thirds of the lung parenchyma, entirely surrounded by lung and not in contact with large vessels, pleural surfaces, or mediastinal structures. Adjacent vessels larger than 3 mm in diameter result in heat dissipation from the tumor during ablation, a phenomenon known as heat sink, resulting in incomplete ablation and local tumor progression.[7] Centrally located structures such as the esophagus, pericardium, and trachea can be damaged by the ablation and may be

a relative contraindication to ablation of an adjacent lesion. Local tumor progression has also been seen more frequently in lesions adjacent to the fissures or pleural surfaces, presumably because of the inability to create a safety margin of ablation around the tumor.

Relative contraindications to ablation include reduced pulmonary reserve (FEV$_1$ [forced expiratory volume in the first second of expiration] less than 0.6 L), severe pulmonary arterial hypertension, and pneumonectomy. The use of positive pressure ventilation, bilevel positive airway pressure or continuous positive airway pressure after RFA may be associated with increased incidence of pulmonary hemorrhage and bronchopleural fistula (BPF).[20] Although patients with pacemakers or automatic implantable cardioverter defibrillator devices can be safely ablated, evaluation by a cardiologist is recommended before and after RFA. A magnet can be placed over the control box of the pacemaker to shield the device from the radiofrequency current; however, the device should be checked at the end of the procedure.[21]

Confirmation of normal coagulation tests and platelet counts more than 50,000 is required and medications that effect bleeding, such as Coumadin (warfarin), Plavix (clopidogrel bisulfate), aspirin, and nonsteroidal antiinflammatory drugs, should be stopped for at least 5 days before RFA.[22] Immediately before RFA, antibiotic coverage is given to patients with prosthetic valves or joint prostheses. Prophylactic antibiotics are not routinely used.

Sedation

Most studies in the literature document a preference for conscious sedation in combination with local anesthesia, although use of general anesthesia, epidural anesthesia, and nerve blocks has also been reported.[23–29] Conscious sedation permits patient immobilization, provides excellent pain relief, and reduces respiratory excursions during RFA. Combination therapy with midazolam, fentanyl, and meperidine is often used, with incremental doses administered during placement of the electrode and during ablation. General

Table 1
Comparison of various factors that can influence the choice of ablative techniques, from + (least favorable) to + + + (most favorable).

Parameter(s)	Comparative Technologies		
	Radiofrequency	Microwave	Cryoablation
≤3 cm	+++	+++	+++
>3 cm	+ (up to 3)[a]	+++ (up to 3)[a]	++ (up to 8)[a]
≤1.5 cm from pleura	+ (pain)	+ (air leak)	+++
Proximity to chest wall and pleura	+	++	+++
Proximity to mediastinum	+	+	++
Thermal (heat or cold) sinks	+	+++	++
Pacer and automatic implantable cardioverter defibrillator	+	++	+++
Coagulopathies	+++	+++	+

[a] Represents the number of simultaneous electrodes in RFA, antennae in microwave, and cryoprobes in cryoablation.

anesthesia is indicated in patients who have airway compromise, high risk of bleeding, or severely limited cardiopulmonary reserve that does not allow the safe use of conscious sedation, including oxygen dependency, aortic stenosis, carotid stenosis, or severe coronary artery disease. Double-lumen endotracheal tubes are often used to isolate the lung and manage complications such as pulmonary hemorrhage. Single-lung ventilation can also be useful in small lesions or those close to the diaphragm to minimize respiratory motion.[30] When general anesthesia is used, small frequent ventilations are recommended to avoid large excursions and significant nodule movement during electrode placement. Complications related to general anesthesia may contribute to patient morbidity and increased length of hospital stay compared with conscious sedation.

Technique

The RFA procedure is similar to the technique used for percutaneous lung biopsy and has been described in detail.[31] The percutaneous electrode is incrementally advanced into the nodule. The electrode tip should pass through the distal end of the nodule to provide adequate ablation in all directions. With a multitined electrode, the positions of the tines radiating to the periphery of the nodule should be confirmed by CT. Some operators have used an induced pneumothorax to move a nodule away from the chest wall or mediastinum and decrease pain during ablation.[32] If a tandem approach is used with a second needle, the needle should be removed before RFA to prevent the current passing back along the tandem needle and causing skin burns.[25]

Adequate ablation is achieved when temperatures greater than 57°C are recorded by the thermocouple at the tip of the electrode. A repeat CT scan through the ablated lesion should show circumferential ground-glass opacity around the nodule (**Fig. 3**). This opacity should measure 5 to 10 mm in all directions. If the circumferential ground-glass opacity has not been shown, needle repositioning and repeat ablation are necessary. The presence of a large adjacent vessel may require repeated ablations, to try to overcome the heat sink from flowing blood within the vessel.

At the completion of the ablation session, recovery in the dependent position for several hours reduces complications. Uncomplicated cases may be sent home but overnight observation is often used, particularly in those with comorbidities or complications.

Complications

Most complications reported with RFA are similar to those that occur after percutaneous needle biopsy.[23–27] The most frequently seen complication is pneumothorax (11%–63%). Most pneumothoraces are small and treated conservatively, but a chest tube is required if a pneumothorax enlarges on serial chest radiographs or if the patient becomes symptomatic. Pleural effusions are reported in up to 50% of cases but are usually small and asymptomatic. BPF may develop in the weeks after ablation, because continuing necrosis of a peripheral postablation lesion leads to communication of an airway with the pleura (**Fig. 4**). Although most BPFs resolve spontaneously, they can persist for several months and show increased activity on positron emission

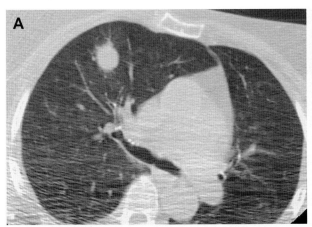
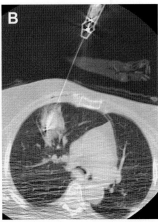

Fig. 3. 80-year-old man with a right upper lobe adenocarcinoma. (*A*) 2-cm right upper lobe nodule before RFA. (*B*) Ground-glass opacity surrounding nodule confirms adequate ablation zone. Single cool-tip electrode is in place.

tomography (PET) scan. Surgical evacuation and fibrin sealant obliteration of the necrotic cavity have been described for large, symptomatic cases.[20,33] Pulmonary hemorrhage and hemoptysis have been reported in up to 5.9% of RFA.[34] Pneumonia may be seen in up to 16% of cases and is more common in patients with underlying chronic lung disease and in central lesions, in which postobstructive pneumonia may occur from injury to the airways.[18] Hemothorax is often small and asymptomatic, but can progress, particularly if there is positive pressure ventilation.[20]

Complications specific to the radiofrequency technique may occasionally develop. Burns from the grounding pads are rare, but do occur more commonly if there are wrinkles within the metallic

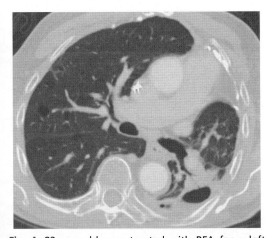

Fig. 4. 83-year-old man treated with RFA for a left lower lobe adenocarcinoma. CT performed 6 months after RFA shows an asymptomatic peripheral left lower lobe bronchopleural fistula, which resolved over 12 months without treatment.

portion of the pad, causing uneven heat dissipation. Ablation of adjacent nerves can lead to neuropathy, which may be transient or permanent. Neuropathy has occurred with the recurrent laryngeal and phrenic nerves during ablation of mediastinal lesions, intercostal nerves in peripheral lesions, and the brachial plexus in apical lesions.[25,35,36] A postablation flulike syndrome of fatigue, low-grade fever, and myalgia is common and may last for up to 2 weeks. It is believed to be caused by circulating toxins after tumor necrosis and can be relieved with nonsteroidal anti-inflammatory drugs.[37,38] Pneumomediastinum, rib necrosis (**Fig. 5**), air embolism, pulmonary artery pseudoaneurysm, acute respiratory distress syndrome (ARDS), organizing pneumonia, and renal failure have also been described in rare cases.[26,27,37–43] Death from RFA has been reported in patients with a single-lung and contralateral pneumonectomy, after delayed massive hemoptysis of an ablated central lesion, as a result of development of ARDS, and as a result of inadvertent puncture of the heart by the electrode.[24,27,41]

Follow-Up Imaging Protocol

The purpose of radiologic follow-up after RFA is to identify any complications, confirm the expected postablation appearances, and exclude local tumor progression. Contrast-enhanced chest CT has been most often used in follow-up, although some centers perform magnetic resonance (MR) imaging. The protocols for imaging after RFA may vary slightly between centers. A typical protocol includes an initial CT at 1 month after RFA to identify any complications of the procedure. Chest CT is repeated at 3, 6, 12, and 18 months and then annually for 5 years. Integrated

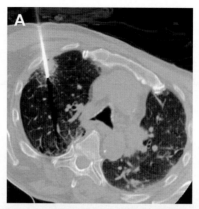

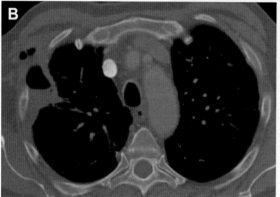
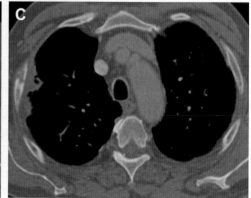

Fig. 5. Rib osteonecrosis in a 60-year-old man with subpleural right upper lobe adenocarcinoma treated with RFA. (*A*) CT image during RFA shows placement of electrode in the nodule and chest wall adjacent to a rib. (*B*) CT 2 months after RFA shows cavitary changes in the chest wall and periphery of the lung. (*C*) CT 6 months after RFA reveals necrosis of the adjacent rib because of osteonecrosis.

PET/CT may be performed at 1, 6, and 12 months to investigate the PET changes after RFA and detect potential distant metastatic disease.

CT Appearances

Immediately after RFA, there are characteristic CT findings in the tumor and the surrounding lung (**Fig. 6**).[14] In the first week after ablation, the ground-glass opacity within the surrounding lung and the continuing necrosis that occurs for several days after RFA lead to an increase in size of the postablation lesion from baseline.[10,26] Within 1 month, the ground-glass opacity becomes increasingly dense, usually starting from the periphery of the lesion. The increasing density progresses over the initial 3 months and the post-ablation lesion becomes solid. The increase in size of the post ablation lesion will plateau by 3 months and then decrease over the ensuing 6 months. The shape of the lesion also changes between 3 and 6 months from a spherical opacity to form a wedge-shaped or linear opacity, because of contraction and fibrosis within the ablated lung and tumor.

The postablation lesion forms a scar that may be larger than the baseline tumor and often retracts toward the pleura. This fibrotic scar may be associated with persistent focal pleural thickening and architectural distortion. Cavitation is seen in up to 50% of cases induced by devascularization of the tumor and lung and ensuing necrosis (**Fig. 7**).[24,26,27,44,45] Granulation tissue surrounding the cavity leads to a fibrous capsule. The cavity is sterile and its presence is not an indication for antibiotics, typically resolving within 6 months of ablation. Absence of contrast enhancement within the lesion is an expected finding on CT after RFA.[23,46] However, peripheral enhancement may be seen within the surrounding reactive lung, especially during the reparative phase.

The reactive changes in the adjacent lung are often associated with a reversible increase in size of regional hilar and mediastinal lymph nodes (see **Fig. 7**), initially seen at 1 and 3 months and subsequently decreased in size by 6 months.[47] In addition, a sympathetic pleural effusion is often apparent but usually small and asymptomatic. Reactive pleural thickening can enhance with

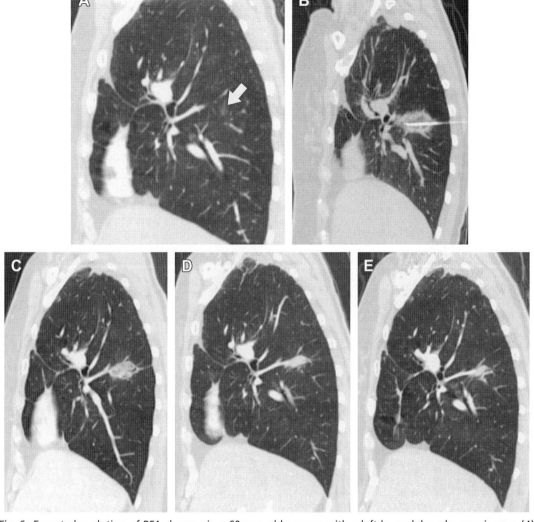

Fig. 6. Expected evolution of RFA changes in a 60-year-old woman with a left lower lobe adenocarcinoma. (*A*) 1-cm ground-glass nodule (*arrow*) in the left lower lobe on a sagittal multiplanar reconstruction. (*B*) Immediate post-RFA changes show ground-glass opacity. (*C*) 1 month after RFA the postablation lesion is more densely opacified. (*D*) 6 months postablation CT shows contraction of the ablated zone. (*E*) 12 months post-RFA CT shows a residual linear scar.

intravenous contrast and may show avid uptake on fluorodeoxyglucose (FDG)-PET.

MR Imaging Appearances

MR imaging is used in some centers to follow response to RFA; however, reports of typical MR imaging appearances after RFA are limited.[12,25,48,49] The signal intensity does not change on T1-weighted sequences; however, there is a central low signal on T2-weighted images after RFA, corresponding to coagulation necrosis. The peripheral high signal intensity on T2 weighting corresponds to the pulmonary congestion and inflammatory change in the surrounding lung.[12]

Changes in the apparent diffusion coefficient (ADC) on diffusion-weighted MR imaging after RFA of lung tumors has been studied to assess treatment response.[49] A pilot study reported a significantly higher ADC within 3 days of RFA in patients who showed local tumor progression compared with ADC in patients who did not show local tumor progression, suggesting that this may be a sensitive way to detect early response.

PET Appearances

The PET appearances after RFA have been reported in animal models.[50] In animals, an initial

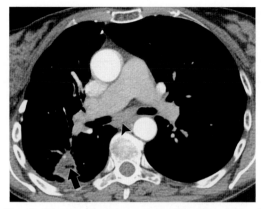

Fig. 7. 40-year-old woman 1 month after RFA of a 1-cm adenocarcinoma. CT shows a focal right lower lobe cavity at RFA site (*arrow*) and enlarged reactive subcarinal lymph nodes (*arrowhead*), which resolved at 6 months after RFA.

increase in peripheral lung activity clears after 4 weeks; the appearances are similar in humans but have a different time frame. PET reflects the changes in metabolic activity of the tumor and the surrounding lung (**Fig. 8**). Within the first month after RFA, the tumor should show decreased FDG uptake, corresponding to successful necrosis. However, a rim of activity is frequently present in the surrounding lung because of congestion and inflammatory change after ablation. This ring of activity may persist for up to 6 months after RFA, but resolves between 6 and 12 months. As the postablation lesion contracts and decreases in size with resorption of the central necrotic tumor, the increased activity seen in the peripheral ring collapses centrally, resulting in increased focal nodular activity in the center of the lesion at 6 months. We have documented this peripheral ring in patients treated successfully with RFA and it may be seen at 1 to 6 months after RFA. This ring should be recognized as a normal finding and not misinterpreted as local tumor progression. Posttreatment activity subsequently decreases at 12 months. Other investigators suggest that at follow-up between 3 and 9 months, maximum standardized uptake value (SUV_{max}) greater than 1.5 may indicate local tumor progression.[51]

Imaging Signs of Local Tumor Progression

Early post-RFA imaging may not detect residual disease because of the presence of reactive changes in the tumor and the surrounding lung. Local tumor progression is usually detected at 3 to 6 months after treatment, when reactive changes have decreased (**Fig. 9**). At this stage, it is expected that the postablation lesion will have

decreased in size. Signs of local tumor progression include increase in size after 3 months, eccentric nodular growth, or eccentric focal enhancement of the postablation lesion on CT. There may be corresponding eccentric activity on the PET scan at this time, although evaluation may be difficult. In suspicious cases, close-interval follow-up contrast-enhanced chest CT is helpful to document the focal increase in size or enhancement. In equivocal cases, CT-guided biopsy can also be performed.

Outcome

Reported local recurrence rate of 31.5% and average survival of 74% at median follow-up of 17 months has been reported.[18] Two-year and 4-year survival rates of 78% and 47% with median survival of 30 months were seen in patients with nonsmall cell lung cancer (NSCLC) treated with RFA. One-year and 2-year survival rates of 78% and 57% and 70% and 48% have been reported in 2 large studies.[24,52] Local tumor progression rates are reported between 9% and 62% in other studies.[24,26,27,53,54] The heterogeneity of the patient population and nonstandardized criteria for treatment make direct comparison between the studies difficult; however, a lesion larger than 3 cm in size is associated with greater local recurrence rate.

MWA
Introduction

MWA is another heat-based thermal ablative technique that has gained some momentum in recent years. Like RFA, it requires image-guided placement of antennae into the target lesion. An electromagnetic field is induced to create thermal injury in the lung. The benefits of microwave technology over RFA include higher intratumoral temperatures, faster ablation times, improved convection profile, and less procedural pain.[55–58] There is also less heat sink effect and proposed larger ablation volumes, because active microwave heating is not hampered by aerated, charred, or desiccated tissue. This situation may allow intratumoral temperatures to be driven higher, resulting in a larger ablation zone in a shorter time.[59–61]

Mechanism of Action

Microwave used for tissue ablation works on similar principles to a microwave oven. Medical technology uses microwaves oscillating in the 900-MHz to 2450-MHz range. The microwave energy induces excitation of water molecules or dipole excitation, which in turn causes the water

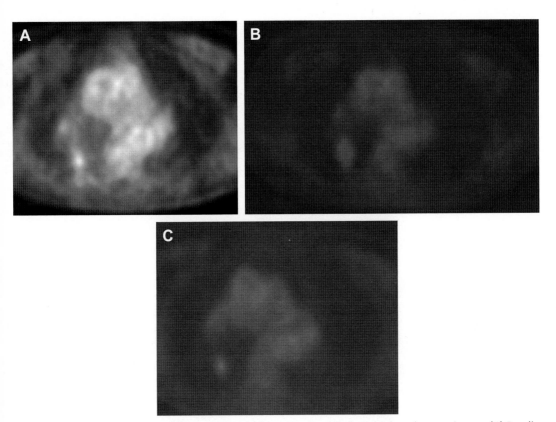

Fig. 8. Expected PET findings in a 57-year-old man after RFA of a right lower lobe adenocarcinoma. (A) Baseline PET shows focal activity in the right lower lobe tumor. (B) 1 month after RFA, a rim of activity is present in the surrounding lung with central photopenia. (C) 6 months after RFA, the central activity has increased because of retraction of the evolving ablation zone.

molecules to spin, creating friction. The transfer of some of their kinetic energy results in heat generation in tissue and coagulation necrosis.[61] The initial technologies for MWA used frequencies greater than 900 MHz for induction of heat; however, more recently higher frequencies have been used for more controlled and efficient ablation.

Patient Selection

MWA like other ablative techniques can either be used for curative or palliative management of lung carcinoma. Patients with advanced disease who are not surgical candidates can suffer from complications of local tumor invasion. Pain is the most common complication and up to 50% of patients dying from lung cancer are without adequate pain relief.[62] These advanced tumors are usually larger at time of diagnosis, which limits the use of RFA. One of the advantages of MWA is that it can be used for larger, peripheral, and central tumors.

MWA has been shown to induce larger ablation volumes[60] compared with RFA. MWA on porcine lung showed 25% larger mean diameter of ablation (3.32 cm $\pm$ 0.19 vs 2.70 cm $\pm$ 0.23, P <.001) and 50% larger mean cross-sectional area (8.25 cm^2 $\pm$ 0.92 vs 5.45 cm^2 $\pm$ 1.14, P <.001) compared with RF ablation. A larger volume of ablation allows ablation of larger tumors and satellite tumor deposits just beyond the periphery of the targeted tumor, in turn reducing recurrence rate and improving survival.[63]

MWA is also used in tumors at the periphery of the lung, because there is less pain associated with microwave for treatment of subpleural, juxtapleural, and chest wall lesions close to the somatically innervated parietal pleura and chest wall (Fig. 10). This situation is in part from lack of electric current conducted through intercostal nerves during the MWA procedure compared with RFA. Various studies describing the complications of MWA have shown limited pleuritic pain after the ablation.[64] However, in 1 study, skin burns were reported in 3% (2 of 66) of patients.[63]

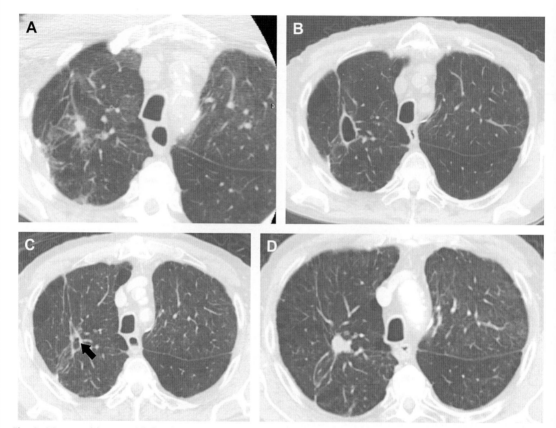

Fig. 9. 70-year-old man with focal recurrence 12 months after RFA of a right lung adenocarcinoma. (*A*) Baseline CT reveals a tumor in the right lung. (*B*) CT 3 months after RFA shows a thin-walled cavity. (*C*) CT 6 months after RFA shows a new nodule in the wall of the contracting cavity (*arrow*). (*D*) CT 12 months after RFA shows local nodular tumor progression, which was successfully treated with stereotactic body radiotherapy.

Central tumors are preferably ablated using MWA, because the heat sink effect is not as pronounced as with RFA. In a pilot lung study, patients with known lung cancer underwent MWA before elective lobar resection. Large blood vessels in the resection specimens did not create typical ablation zone distortion because of the minimal heat sink effect observed.[61]

The absolute contraindications for MWA remain the same as for RFA. Relative contraindications, although not unique to MWA, are mostly related to the interference of electromagnetic current with various implantable generators. This interference is seen less severely than with RFA.[21] Implantable cardiac devices, including pacemakers, and cardiac defibrillators may be susceptible to interference from electromagnetic energy in the microwave frequency range. Careful planning between radiology and cardiology staff is suggested, because it is recommended to reprogram pacemakers to automatic pacing modes and temporarily disable implanted defibrillators

during the procedure, during which external pacemakers can be used.[65]

The presence of surgical clips or staples may also affect the area of ablation with larger or unpredictable patterns.

Sedation

Like radiofrequency, MWA is usually an outpatient procedure. The choice of conscious and deep sedation versus general anesthesia is mostly operator-dependent and case-dependent, but most cases can be performed under conscious sedation, as discussed in the technique for RFA procedures.[63]

Technique

Preprocedural preparation, including consultation, consent, and laboratory tests, is generally similar to other ablative modalities. Almost in all cases, CT is used for directing microwave antennas,

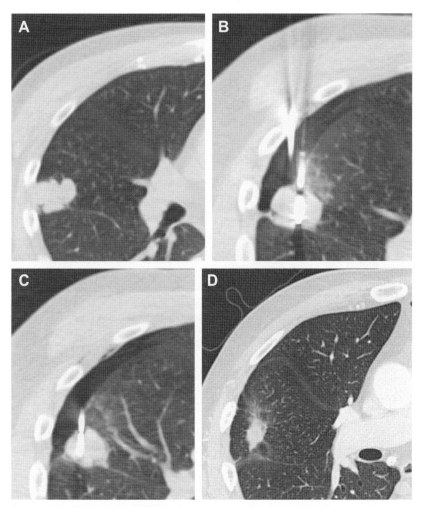

Fig. 10. MWA for peripheral lung tumor. (*A*) Peripheral lobulated right middle lobe mass abutting visceral pleura. (*B, C*) Two microwave antennae were placed within the mass. Small protective pneumothorax was induced, to avoid back burn along the shaft of the antennae. (*D*) 9 months after ablation, CT scan shows continued decrease in size of postablation zone without significant peripheral enhancement.

although the use of ultrasonography for peripheral lesions has been described.[66]

Six microwave systems are commercially available in the United States (Tyco Healthcare Group, Boulder, CO; MicrothermX, BSD Medical, Salt Lake City, UT; Avecure, Medwaves, San Diego, CA; Certus 140, Neuwave, Madison, WI; Amica, Hospital Service, Rome, Italy; Acculis MTA, Microsulis Medical, Hampshire, United Kingdom).[67] Although the principle used to obtain cell death is the same, the technology differs and the operators need to understand the technical parameters dictating the end point of ablation for each system before embarking on cases. In MWA, 3 technical factors affect the ablation zone: the frequency of microwave (MHz), the power of generator (W), and the exposed or active tip (cm) emitting the current.

The microwave technologies use frequencies ranging from 915 MHZ to 2450 MHZ. The generator powers can reach up to 200 W, with higher powers depositing more energy in the tissue. The active tip ranges from 0.6 mm to 40 mm long and 14.5 to 17 G in diameter, with the ablation zone being larger with use of longer active tips. The length of the antenna can vary from 11 to 25 cm and is not related to the active tip or ablation zone. Some vendors use peristaltic pumps to perfuse the outer shaft of the antenna with normal saline to prevent thermal injury along the proximal antenna shaft.[63] Depending on the size of the target lesion and the duration of ablation, the number of antennae can be selected keeping the 3 technical factors in mind. The duration of ablation can range from 2 minutes to 10 minutes and up to 3 antennae can be used simultaneously.

Usually for tumors larger than 2 cm, more than 1 antenna needs to be used.[68] Each vendor provides a technical chart representing the ablation zone, which provides the information mostly obtained through in vivo animal or in vitro gel model experiments (**Fig. 11**). These charts and predicted ablation zones are not specific to lung and can be used as a road map in planning the number of antennae and duration of ablation. When using multiple antennae, it is recommended to place them at least 1 cm apart.

Many operators use the radiologic end points of ablation as a sign of complete ablation. Intermittent scanning during the ablation allows for detection of these signs. In a comparison study between MWA and RFA, similar zones were seen but they were larger with microwave.[60] The zone of low attenuation should engulf the tumor and the intended ablation area, keeping microscopic extent of tumor in mind.[69]

After treatment, the microwave antenna is removed and a CT image is acquired to check for the presence of pneumothorax. Postablation care remains the same as for patients undergoing RFA.

Single Probe Ablations

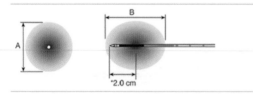

*2.0 cm

Certus^LN Probes (LN15 and LN20) in Bovine Lung - Ex-Vivo

Time	Length (B)	Diameter (A)	Axial Area
140W Power Setting			
5 Minutes	6.0cm	3.3cm	15.6cm²
10 Minutes	6.0cm	3.9cm	19.3cm²
90W Power Setting			
5 Minutes	4.6cm	3.1cm	11.7cm²
10 Minutes	5.4cm	3.5cm	15.8cm²
40W Power Setting			
5 Minutes	1.7cm	0.8cm	1.2cm²
10 Minutes	3.8cm	2.3cm	9.8cm²

Fig. 11. A MWA chart showing the ablation zone obtained from ex vivo MWA of healthy bovine tissue. Larger ablations can be achieved with the use of higher power (W) and longer duration of ablation. (*Courtesy of* NeuWave Medical, Madison, WI; with permission.)

Complications of MWA

Similar to RFA, the most common immediate complication of MWA in the lung is pneumothorax. The incidence of pneumothorax after MWA is approximately 8.5% to 39%, with about one-third of these severe enough to require chest tube placement.[63,68] Of these patients, most can be managed as outpatients and are safely discharged home with a Heimlich valve apparatus and close follow-up every 24 hours for up to 3 days.

Postprocedural pain is experienced commonly, and is usually well managed with analgesics; however, severe pain is less commonly encountered compared with RFA and is usually adequately controlled before discharge.[63,68]

Intraprocedural skin burns have been described with chest wall or peripheral tumors and are considered an occasional complication of MWA therapy, occurring in 3% of patients in 1 series. Such injuries are usually mild; however, third-degree burns have been reported after ablation of superficial lesions, requiring plastic surgery consultation and debridement.[63]

Infrequently, postablation syndrome occurring several days after ablation has been described in 2% of patients and is less commonly seen compared with RFA, especially in the liver, with up to 36% of patients experiencing some degree of postablation syndrome.[63,70] Other uncommon complications of MWA include acute respiratory distress, self-limiting hemoptysis, pulmonary hemorrhage, and empyema, all occurring less than 5% of the time.

No reports of MWA-associated mortality have been documented occurring either intraprocedurally or in the immediate postprocedural period. However, 1 study comprising 50 patients documented a single procedure-related death, occurring more than 8 months after ablation.[63] The cause of mortality was attributed to delayed infection of a postablation cavity.

Imaging Protocol After MWA

The postprocedure imaging follow-up procedure is similar to RFA.

Imaging Appearance After MWA

Immediate postablation CT scans show changes in the appearance of the ablated tumor, showing the effects of thermally induced coagulation necrosis. An area of hazy ground-glass opacity is most commonly observed within and extending from the zone of ablation, penetrated by well-defined antennae tracks.[60] This zone is in turn surrounded by an area of hypodensity, which corresponds to coagulation necrosis. A third layer of ground-glass opacity represents hemorrhage and partially ablated tissue (**Fig. 12**A). The ablation zone shows marked increase within 24 hours after ablation, followed by subsequent volume reduction over 3 to 6 months, at which time the treatment zone is usually smaller than the original tumor.[68]

Cavitary changes were identified in 35 (43%) of 82 treated tumors.[63] Cavitation had a statistically significant inverse relationship to cancer-specific mortality ($P = .02$). This finding is possibly explained by the fact that complete tumor destruction and thermocoagulation lead to more tumor destruction and cavitation (see **Fig. 12**B).

On postcontrast CT scans, no enhancement or a smooth, thin (less than 5 mm) rim of residual enhancement surrounding the ablation zone may be seen up to 6 months after the procedure, representing benign inflammatory granulation tissue. Development of nodular enhancement or enhancement more than 15 HU on nodule densitometry studies is suggestive of local recurrence.[71]

The role of PET-CT in follow-up of patients undergoing MWA has not been clearly documented. It is expected to show similar imaging features to RFA.

Early Recurrence and Local Tumor Progression After MWA

Although not many long-term studies are available, it is expected that the early recurrence and evidence for local tumor progression parallels the data from RFA. Failure of decrease in size of ablation zone at 3 months, progressive volumetric increase during subsequent follow-ups, or presence of nodular hypermetabolic activity on PET is suggestive of ablation failure and early recurrence[68] (**Fig. 13**).

MWA Outcome

Outcome data after microwave therapy for lung cancer are limited. Most data are from combined reports of MWA treatment of lung cancer and metastases. Feng and colleagues[72] reported on MWA of 28 tumors in 20 patients. A response of 50% ablation or more was noted in 13 (46.4%) nodules and a complete response in 3 (10.7%). No significant complications were noted.

Wolf and colleagues[63] reported their results of MWA in 82 lung tumors of 50 patients. Local control at 1 year was seen in 67%. Unlike RFA, the index tumor size of larger than 3 cm did not affect patients' actuarial survival or cancer-specific mortality. However, patients with an index tumor size of larger than 3 cm were significantly more likely to have recurrent disease at the ablation site (residual disease) ($\leq$3 cm vs >3 cm, $P = .01$). At a mean follow-up of 10 months, 26% of the patients had residual disease at the ablation site and another 22% had recurrent disease distant from the ablation site. Kaplan-Meier analysis yielded an actuarial survival of 65%

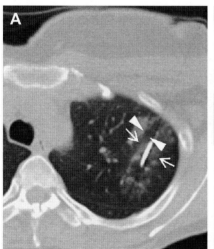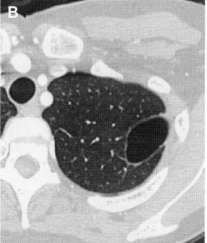

Fig. 12. MWA of 1.2-cm left upper lobe NSCLC. A single antenna was used at 90 W for 5 minutes. (*A*) After 5 minutes, a central zone of hazy ground-glass opacity is seen surrounding the antenna and the nodule (*arrow*). A hypodense rim surrounds the central zone and corresponds to coagulation necrosis (*arrowheads*). The tumor should be engulfed by this rim of hypodensity. The third layer of peripheral ground-glass opacity represents hemorrhage. (*B*) 3 months after ablation, cavitation has replaced the ablation zone and corresponds to complete tumor destruction.

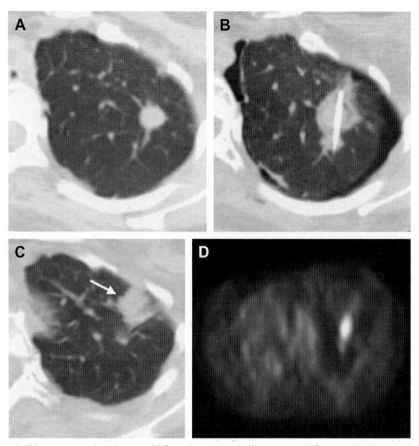

Fig. 13. Left apical lung cancer in 74-year-old female patient. (*A*) A 1.9-cm left upper lobe nodule. (*B*) A single antennae was used, with adequate hypodense rim surrounding the nodule. (*C, D*) CT and PET scans at 9 months after ablation show development of irregular nodule (*arrow*) at the edge of ablation scar and nodular hypermetabolic activity, respectively.

at 1 year, 55% at 2 years, and 45% at 3 years after ablation.

CRYOABLATION
Introduction

Percutaneous cryoablation (PCT) is another thermal-based ablative modality, which has shown renewed attention in the past decade. Unlike other heat-based ablative techniques, cryoablation uses subzero temperatures and development of ice as the mode of cell destruction. The intrasurgical use of cryotherapy for management of prostate and hepatic tumors has been a common practice among surgeons, and interventional pulmonologists have used bronchoscopy-directed cryoprobes since the early 1980s. The unique ability of cryoablation to preserve the collagenous architecture and thereby the integrity of the tracheobronchial tree has been used to perform transbronchial cryoablation of endobronchial tumors without complication.[73–75] With development of techniques to safely deliver cryogas through smaller-caliber probes, it became possible to perform PCT in prostate, liver, kidney, and lung. Wang and colleagues[76] were among the first to describe the use of PCT in the thorax, with early results comparable with the more established RFA.

Mechanism of Action

PCT technology is provided by 2 manufacturers: Endocare (Irvine, CA, a wholly owned subsidiary of HealthTronics) and Galil Medical (Arden Hills, MN). Both base their technology on the Joules-Thompson effect and the use of argon gas as a medium for cryogenesis. The change from the liquid to gaseous state decreases the temperature surrounding the probes to subzero temperatures, leading to cell death. The temperatures are coldest just adjacent to the probe and can reach up to −150°C The various temperature zones are referred to as isotherms, and each manufacturer provides a chart of these isotherms for PCT planning

(Fig. 14). Another cycle during PCT is the thaw cycle, which allows for warming of tissue. During thaw, helium gas is used to raise the temperature to 40°C. Stick cycle uses predominantly helium with a burst of argon gas to maintain the temperature at −10°C A small ice ball is formed around the probe, which sticks the probe to the tissue for stabilization.[76]

Cell death is achieved through direct and indirect mechanisms, causing coagulative necrosis in tissues.[77] Direct mechanism of cell death is through rapid reduction in temperatures less than −40°C, causing intracellular entrapment of water molecules and ice formation; the ice crystals extend to involve the intracellular organelles and cell membrane. This process is lethal to the cells and leads to enzymatic dysfunction and cell membrane disruption. With slower rates of tissue cooling at temperatures ranging to −20°C, there is formation of ice in the extracellular matrix. This situation results in osmosis of water out of the cell and cellular dehydration, inducing a hypertonic stress, which in turn causes damage to the cellular constituents. During the rewarming or thaw cycle, water returns to the intracellular space and causes cellular swelling and lysis. In the second cryoablation cycle, the ice formation is enhanced through an already damaged and dysfunctional cell membrane, hence creating a larger ice ball. This situation is of particular interest at the periphery of the ice ball, allowing for a larger cryozone and tumor ablation.[78]

Indirect mechanisms of cell death include vasoconstriction, occlusion of blood vessel through compression of vessel wall from adjacent swollen cells, and freezing of blood in small vessels, leading to hypoxic tissue injury and coagulation necrosis.[78] Another indirect action of cryoablation is through cryoimmunotherapy. Sabel and colleagues[79] documented that cryoablation in mouse breast cancer models promotes the inflammatory cytokines involved in cell-mediated immunity such as interleukin 12 and interferon-c. It is suggested that higher levels of these cytokines allow for adoptive immunotherapy. However, the cryoimmunology effects in lung cancer are yet to be determined.

Patient Selection

When performing cryotherapy, lesions less than 3 cm are preferred, as is the case for RFA. Tumors larger than 3 cm are at higher risk of recurrence at periphery because of geometry of tumor and may need multiple probes. Another limiting factor in prognosis of patients with tumors larger than 3 cm unrelated to ablative technique is the tumor biology, because there is a high probability of distant metastasis at time of diagnosis.[80] However, if ablation for larger tumors is undertaken, cryoablation is preferred and multiple probes can be used.

For successful cryoablation, the cryozone has to extend beyond the edge of the tumor by approximately 1 cm and should be seen by intermittent scanning, allowing for control of ablation and use of multiple probes. The reason for larger ablation zone is that cell death is not absolutely achieved

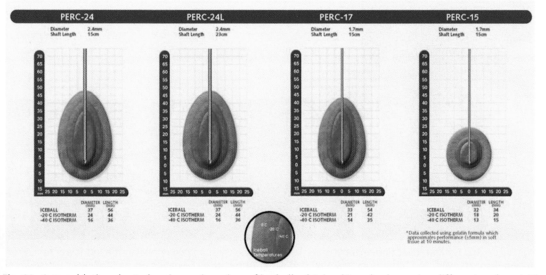

Fig. 14. A cryoablation chart, showing various sizes of ice balls obtained in gel, when using different probes at 10 minutes. Various isotherms are shown using shades of blue. (*Courtesy of* Endocare Inc., Irvine, CA, a wholly-owned subsidary of Health Tronics, Inc.; with permission.)

at the periphery of ice ball and an isotherm of at least −20°Cis required to achieve definite cell death.[81,82] In addition, microscopic extension beyond the visible edge of the tumor should be considered when mapping the ablation, which may extend up to 8 mm for adenocarcinoma.[69]

Cryoablation also benefits from preservation of the collagenous architecture and thereby the structure of the tracheobronchial tree, larger vessels, and muscles, including the diaphragm, remain intact.[73] Central tumors close to major bronchi and large vessels can be safely ablated and the ice ball carves out the edge of the larger vessels (**Fig. 15**). However, like RFA, cryoablation also suffers from a heat/cold sink effect. The placement of a probe adjacent to a vascular structure could result in an inhomogeneous isotherm and increase the risk for recurrence in these areas.

Tumors close to the pleura and chest wall lesions are preferentially treated with cryoablation, because RFA can be painful at these locations (**Fig. 16**).

Patients with pacemakers and other electrical generators can undergo cryoablation, because the mechanism of ablation does not interfere with the electrical circuit.

Absolute contraindications for cryoablation include pneumonia and presence of uncorrectable coagulopathy. Many patients with severe emphysema or pulmonary fibrosis have limited respiratory reserve and may show significant intra-alveolar hemorrhage after the procedure and rapidly progress to respiratory failure, requiring intubation and critical care.

Sedation

Lack of significant pleural pain during cryoablation allows for conscious sedation and use of local anesthesia as the preferred method.[83] For central lesions or larger lesions in which hemorrhage may be expected between the 2 ablative cycles, patients need to be intubated for airway access and clearance if needed. Intubation is also beneficial to obtain single-lung ventilation to decrease heat/cold sink effect.[84]

Technique

PCT is performed under CT guidance to ensure appropriate placement of probes. Experimental models to perform MR-guided PCT are still under investigation. As detailed earlier, the choice of probe gauge and the number of probes is dependent on tumor size and geometry.

Patients should be positioned to obtain adequate trajectory for placement of probes and also allow for patient's movement through the gantry while placing the probes. A coaxial needle is placed up to the pleural surface to provide local anesthesia and direct the probe trajectory. Before placement, the probe should be tested for proper function and absence of leakage. If more than 1 probe is to be used, all the probes should be placed along the expected trajectory up to the

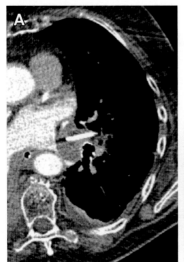
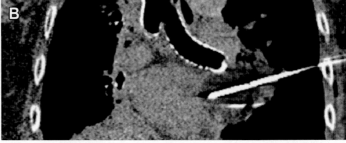

Fig. 15. Central left infrahilar unresectable mass, limited to the chest and compressing the left lower lobe bronchus, pulmonary vein, and left atrium. Planned debulking of tumor by cryoablation was followed by radiation. Two probes were used. (*A*) Axial postcontrast CT scan was performed before final adjustment of the probes. (*B*) Coronal reconstructed CT at 10 minutes through ablation shows the low-density ice ball, carved out by the left atrium, and left lower lobe bronchus.

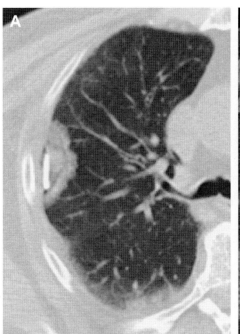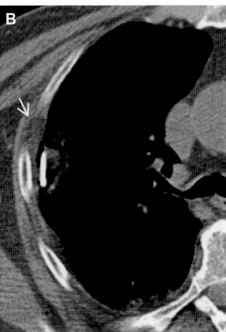

Fig. 16. 82-year-old man with peripheral NSCLC abutting the pleura. Cryoablation was performed with images obtained at 10 minutes through the second cycle. (A) Lung window shows the probe placed at the periphery of the nodule. The hypodensity surrounding the nodule represents the edge of the cryozone, with hemorrhage at the periphery. (B) Soft tissue window shows the hypodense ice ball extending into the chest wall (arrow).

pleural surface. After satisfactory positioning of the first probe, the probe is placed into the stick mode option to ensure that the probe does not move. Thereafter, each probe can be placed sequentially and PCT initiated.

The initial freeze cycle is considered for 10 minutes, followed by 8 minutes of thaw cycle and a final 10 minutes of freeze cycle.[31] However, the double-freeze technique (10–8–10) is not optimum in the lung. The air-filled lung surrounding the tumor may not provide adequate tissue for the initial freeze to extend beyond the few millimeters, thereby limiting the extent of cryonecrosis. To overcome this potential problem, modified triple freeze is suggested, whereby an initial 3 minutes of thaw to allow hemorrhage to take place at the periphery of tumor, is suggested. As pulmonary fluid and hemorrhage fills the alveolar spaces after the first thaw, the thermal conductivity increases 20-fold. This situation may result in more rapid formation of the ice ball on subsequent freeze cycles, thereby also expanding the cytotoxic isotherm for more thorough cell kill throughout the visualized ablation zone. Subsequently, a full cycle of ablation is performed with a 7 and 5 minutes of cryoablation and 7 minutes of thaw between (3 freeze–3 thaw–7 freeze–7 thaw–5 freeze).[82] In our experience, to avoid hemorrhage

between freeze cycles, the duration of thaw cycle can be reduced to 3 minutes. Also, if needed, the final freeze cycle can be extended beyond 5 minutes to confirm desired cryoablation (Fig. 17).

Another issue that warrants special attention is that cryoprobes are of larger caliber (13 G for 2.4 mm probe) than the heat-based counterparts (17 G). Although this may not be a problem for larger tumors, the tumors smaller than 1.5 cm may be difficult to skewer, in particular within a diseased emphysematous lung. It is suggested that 2 probes can be used to be placed on either side of the tumor to perform the ablation.

Once the final freeze cycle is completed, the final thaw cycle is initiated. It may take up to 2 minutes for the temperatures to reach 20°C. The probes can be moved to confirm mobility and separation from the ice ball before extraction. Once removed, the patient should be positioned to keep the ablation site dependent to avoid transbronchial spillage of hemorrhage.

Postprocedural Care

After PCT, patients are observed and monitored for at least 6 hours before discharge. Patients are positioned to keep the target lobe in the dependent position, to avoid transbronchial spillage of

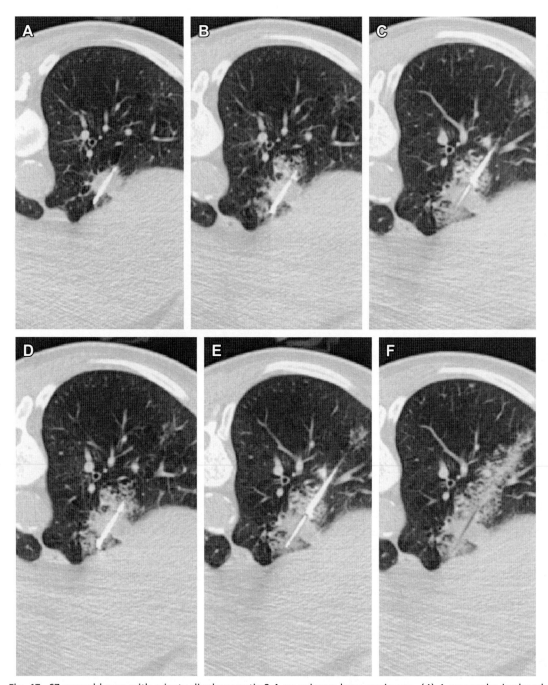

Fig. 17. 67-year-old man with a juxta diaphragmatic 2.4-cm primary lung carcinoma. (*A*) A cryoprobe is placed within the center of the lesion, followed by 3 minutes of freeze. (*B*) At 3 minutes of thaw, a small amount of hemorrhage is present around the tumor. (*C*) A second cycle of cryoablation with 7 minutes of freeze. (*D*) A second cycle of thaw for 3 minutes, allows for minimal hemorrhage between the 2 cycles. (*E*) A third cycle of cryoablation for 7 minutes. (*F*) Postablation image shows probe tract within the ice ball and hemorrhage along the probe tract.

hemorrhage and to promote sealing of the probe tract. Most patients benefit from 3 to 5 days of antiinflammatory therapy. Use of prophylactic and postprocedural broad-spectrum antibiotics is not proved but is encouraged in presence of hemorrhage. Patients are contacted in 24 hours to assess for any complications, and a 48-hour chest radiograph is obtained to evaluate for late complications, in particular pleural effusion and thereafter planned management.

Complications

The main complications associated with PCT include pneumothorax and hemorrhage[76,85,86] (Fig. 18). Wang and colleagues[76] performed more than 200 PCTs on patients with NSCLC and metastatic disease and showed overall complication rate of 12% for pneumothorax. Pleural effusion was seen in 14% of cases, mostly when performed for peripheral tumors. Hemoptysis was common and seen in approximately 62% of patients, although this was self-limited and did not require additional intervention. Relatively more severe complications have been observed by other investigators. In a cohort of 27 patients with NSCLC treated with PCT, Zemlyak and colleagues[86] reported pneumothorax in 10 (37%) and hemoptysis in 6 (22%) patients. In half of patients with radiographic pneumothorax, the size warranted chest tube insertion. Two of the 6 cases of hemoptysis required bronchoscopy.

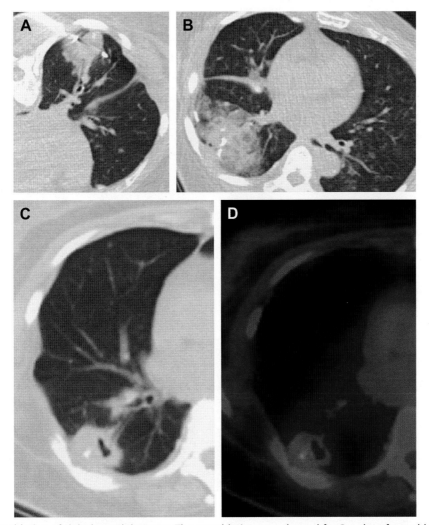

Fig. 18. Cryoablation of right lower lobe mass. The cryoablation was planned for 2 cycles of cryoablation for 10 minutes each, and 8 minutes of thaw between the freeze cycles. (*A*) Two probes were used, but only one is shown. During the ablation, a small area of hemorrhage is seen surrounding the tumor, but the cryozone did not extend beyond the lateral edge of tumor. (*B*) During the thaw cycle, there was evidence of significant hemorrhage surrounding the tumor, with transbronchial spillage of blood in other lobes. Unlike this case, it is suggested that after removal of the probe, patients be turned to make the ablation zone dependent to avoid transbronchial spillage of blood. The second freeze cycle could not be performed. (*C*, *D*) 3 months after cryoablation. CT scan shows small cavitation but persistent peripheral nodular mass, which appears hypermetabolic on the fused PET/CT scan, suggestive of local recurrence.

Kawamura and colleagues[85] had almost the same complications, but there was 1 death from massive hemoptysis. Some of the other less common complications include fever, hypertension, hoarseness of voice from recurrent laryngeal nerve ablation, hemothorax, and subcutaneous emphysema.

Follow-Up Imaging Protocol

No standard clinical protocol for post-PCT follow-up has been developed. CT is most commonly used as the first-line modality, because it is widely available. Contrast-enhanced CT with nodule densitometry may be used in patients with solitary tumors in whom iodinated contrast is not contraindicated.[23] Postprocedure imaging follow-up can be performed using CT at 1 and 3 months, and thereafter every 3 months for 2 years. The use of integrated PET-CT is encouraged at 1, 6 and 12 months, and thereafter every 6 months.

Follow-Up Imaging Appearance

Immediately after the PCT and removal of cryoprobe, a track can be seen within the cryozone (see **Fig. 17F**). The ice ball appears hypodense compared with the original tumor and measures less than 0 HU. A rim of hypodensity surrounding the tumor represents the zone of cryonecrosis, presumably from a combination of the air trapped within the ice and the lower density of ice itself (**Fig. 19**). The ice ball is in turn surrounded by peripheral hyperdensity, representing the thawing edge of cryozone and hemorrhage.[82] If scanned after the ice ball has completely thawed, which

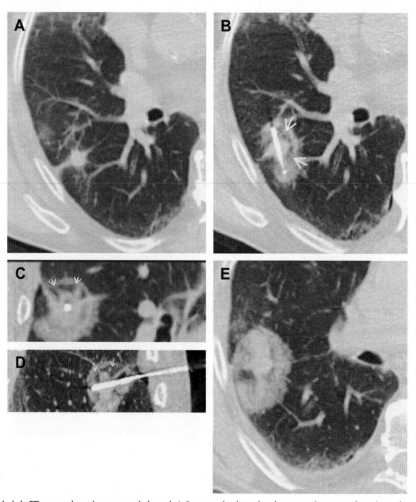

Fig. 19. (*A*) Axial CT scan showing a peripheral 1.8-cm spiculated adenocarcinoma abutting the oblique and horizontal fissure. (*B–D*) Axial, coronal oblique and sagittal oblique views show a cryoprobe through the nodule. 7 minutes through the cryoablation, there is a rim of hypodensity surrounding the tumor, representing the zone of cryonecrosis (*arrows*). The cryozone is in turn surrounded by peripheral denser hemorrhage. (*E*) After removal of the probe, the ice ball thaws and hemorrhage develops.

may take up to 15 minutes, the entire cryozone may appear hemorrhagic and hyperdense.

Not many studies are available to describe the short-term and long-term imaging appearance after PCT. Wang and colleagues showed an area of cavitation larger than the original tumor in 80% of treated areas 1 week after PCT, which persists on the 1-month scan (**Fig. 20**). By 3 months, the cavitation rate had decreased to only 7%, suggesting resorption of nearly all necrotic debris. By 6 months, 86% of the treated areas were stable or smaller than the original tumor. Thereafter the treated area should continue to regress in size and become scarred.

CT-PET shows an area of increased rim uptake surrounding the cryozone or the cavity. The uptake is similar to background mediastinal activity, representing inflammatory granulation tissue at the

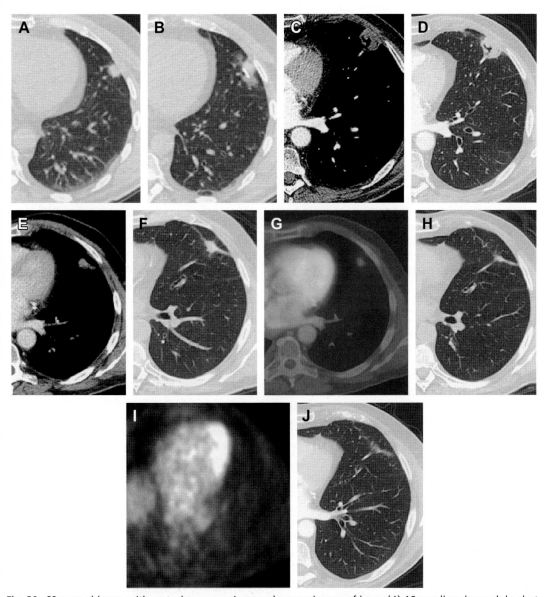

Fig. 20. 69-year-old man with metachronous primary adenocarcinoma of lung. (*A*) 16-mm lingular nodule abutting the pleura. (*B*) A single probe was used and placed adjacent to the nodule. (*C, D*) 1-month postablation, postcontrast axial images show cavitation with no nodular enhancement. (*E–G*) 3 months after ablation, CT images show continued decrease in size of nodular scar without significant enhancement. Fused PET/CT (*G*) shows only mild activity not exceeding mediastinal activity. (*H, I*) 6 months after ablation, CT and PET show continued decrease in size and absence of metabolic activity, respectively. (*J*) 9 months after ablation, there is continued regression in postablation zone scar.

interface of necrotic and viable tissue. With continued regression of the postablation zone, the metabolic activity should decrease and remain at background mediastinal to mild activity.

Early Recurrence and Local Tumor Progression

For early recurrence and local progression of tumor, the imaging findings are extrapolated from the more widely studied RFA data. Both the pattern and appearance of increasing or eccentric contrast enhancement may serve as useful indicators of incomplete tumor ablation or tumor progression within the ablation zone.[87]

CT-PET is preferably used for detection of early recurrence. It is preferred to CT alone because it allows assessment of the entire body and detection of other distant metastatic sites, after ablation.[88] Presence of peripheral ring-shaped hypermetabolic activity surrounding the ablated tumor and larger than the original tumor can be seen immediately after ablation, but the activity should decrease to blood pool levels by 2 months.[50] Although not yet confirmed for cryoablated nodules, CT-PET is superior to CT or CT nodule densitometry in detection of early recurrence. CT-PET also allows for survey of the body for extrathoracic tumor progression or recurrence. Akeboshi and colleagues[89] compared PET with contrast-enhanced CT and found PET to be more sensitive for detecting early local tumor progression.

PCT Outcome

Long-term outcome studies are lacking, but the initial data show promising results. Short-term outcomes after PCT were reported by Kawamura and colleagues,[85] who evaluated the safety and feasibility of cryoablation in a mixed cohort of patients with metastasis and primary lung carcinoma. One-year survival according to the Kaplan-Meier method was 89.4%.

Compared with RFA and sublobar resection, PCT seems to have a comparable outcome. Zamlyak and colleagues[86] presented 64 patients with biopsy-proved stage I NSCLC who were unfit for medical resection and underwent sublobar resections, RFA, and PCT. Median follow-up was 33 months. Three-year survival rates with sublobar resection, RFA, and cryoablation were 87.1%, 87.5%, and 77%, respectively, with no statistically significant difference between groups. The 3-year cancer-specific survival was also comparable between the 3 groups at 90.6%, 87.5%, and 90.2%, respectively.

SUMMARY

Image-guided ablation has recently been introduced as a safe, alternative treatment of localized disease in carefully selected patients with lung cancer. The most commonly used ablative techniques including RFA, MWA, and PCT share common principles of patient selection and follow-up, although each has its own specific merits. Ablative therapies offer the advantages of lung preservation and low morbidity and mortality and provide a viable treatment option for patients who have significant comorbidities. Further longitudinal experience will define their role in the treatment algorithm for lung cancer.

REFERENCES

1. Ginsberg RJ, Rubinstein LV. Randomized trial of lobectomy versus limited resection for T1 N0 non-small cell lung cancer. Lung Cancer Study Group. Ann Thorac Surg 1995;60(3):615–22 [discussion: 622–3].
2. El-Sherif A, Gooding WE, Santos R, et al. Outcomes of sublobar resection versus lobectomy for stage I non-small cell lung cancer: a 13-year analysis. Ann Thorac Surg 2006;82(2):408–15 [discussion: 415–6].
3. Sienel W, Dango S, Kirschbaum A, et al. Sublobar resections in stage IA non-small cell lung cancer: segmentectomies result in significantly better cancer-related survival than wedge resections. Eur J Cardiothorac Surg 2008;33(4):728–34.
4. Bernard A, Ferrand L, Hagry O, et al. Identification of prognostic factors determining risk groups for lung resection. Ann Thorac Surg 2000;70(4):1161–7.
5. Goldberg SN, Gazelle GS, Compton CC, et al. Radiofrequency tissue ablation in the rabbit lung: efficacy and complications. Acad Radiol 1995;2(9):776–84.
6. Goldberg SN, Hahn PF, Halpern EF, et al. Radiofrequency tissue ablation: effect of pharmacologic modulation of blood flow on coagulation diameter. Radiology 1998;209(3):761–7.
7. Steinke K, Haghighi KS, Wulf S, et al. Effect of vessel diameter on the creation of ovine lung radiofrequency lesions in vivo: preliminary results. J Surg Res 2005;124(1):85–91.
8. Goldberg SN, Gazelle GS, Dawson SL, et al. Tissue ablation with radiofrequency: effect of probe size, gauge, duration, and temperature on lesion volume. Acad Radiol 1995;2(5):399–404.
9. Goldberg SN, Gazelle GS, Halpern EF, et al. Radiofrequency tissue ablation: importance of local temperature along the electrode tip exposure in determining lesion shape and size. Acad Radiol 1996;3(3):212–8.
10. Goldberg SN, Gazelle GS, Compton CC, et al. Radio-frequency tissue ablation of VX2 tumor nodules in the rabbit lung. Acad Radiol 1996;3(11):929–35.

11. Nomori H, Imazu Y, Watanabe K, et al. Radiofrequency ablation of pulmonary tumors and normal lung tissue in swine and rabbits. Chest 2005; 127(3):973–7.

12. Oyama Y, Nakamura K, Matsuoka T, et al. Radiofrequency ablated lesion in the normal porcine lung: long-term follow-up with MRI and pathology. Cardiovasc Intervent Radiol 2005;28(3):346–53.

13. Tominaga J, Miyachi H, Takase K, et al. Time-related changes in computed tomographic appearance and pathologic findings after radiofrequency ablation of the rabbit lung: preliminary experimental study. J Vasc Interv Radiol 2005;16(12):1719–26.

14. Yamamoto A, Nakamura K, Matsuoka T, et al. Radiofrequency ablation in a porcine lung model: correlation between CT and histopathologic findings. AJR Am J Roentgenol 2005;185(5):1299–306.

15. Miao Y, Ni Y, Bosmans H, et al. Radiofrequency ablation for eradication of pulmonary tumor in rabbits. J Surg Res 2001;99(2):265–71.

16. Steinke K, Glenn D, King J, et al. Percutaneous pulmonary radiofrequency ablation: difficulty achieving complete ablations in big lung lesions. Br J Radiol 2003;76(910):742–5.

17. Anderson EM, Lees WR, Gillams AR. Early indicators of treatment success after percutaneous radiofrequency of pulmonary tumors. Cardiovasc Intervent Radiol 2009;32(3):478–83.

18. Lanuti M, Sharma A, Digumarthy SR, et al. Radiofrequency ablation for treatment of medically inoperable stage I non-small cell lung cancer. J Thorac Cardiovasc Surg 2009;137(1):160–6.

19. Grieco CA, Simon CJ, Mayo-Smith WW, et al. Percutaneous image-guided thermal ablation and radiation therapy: outcomes of combined treatment for 41 patients with inoperable stage I/II non-small-cell lung cancer. J Vasc Interv Radiol 2006;17(7): 1117–24.

20. Nachiappan AC, Sharma A, Shepard JA, et al. Radiofrequency ablation in the lung complicated by positive airway pressure ventilation. Ann Thorac Surg 2010;89(5):1665–7.

21. Skonieczki BD, Wells C, Wasser EJ, et al. Radiofrequency and microwave tumor ablation in patients with implanted cardiac devices: is it safe? Eur J Radiol 2011;79(3):343–6.

22. Malloy PC, Grassi CJ, Kundu S, et al. Consensus guidelines for periprocedural management of coagulation status and hemostasis risk in percutaneous image-guided interventions. J Vasc Interv Radiol 2009;20(Suppl 7):S240–9.

23. Suh RD, Wallace AB, Sheehan RE, et al. Unresectable pulmonary malignancies: CT-guided percutaneous radiofrequency ablation–preliminary results. Radiology 2003;229(3):821–9.

24. Simon CJ, Dupuy DE, DiPetrillo TA, et al. Pulmonary radiofrequency ablation: long-term safety and efficacy in 153 patients. Radiology 2007;243(1): 268–75.

25. VanSonnenberg E, Shankar S, Morrison PR, et al. Radiofrequency ablation of thoracic lesions: part 2, initial clinical experience–technical and multidisciplinary considerations in 30 patients. AJR Am J Roentgenol 2005;184(2):381–90.

26. Yasui K, Kanazawa S, Sano Y, et al. Thoracic tumors treated with CT-guided radiofrequency ablation: initial experience. Radiology 2004;231(3):850–7.

27. Lee JM, Jin GY, Goldberg SN, et al. Percutaneous radiofrequency ablation for inoperable non-small cell lung cancer and metastases: preliminary report. Radiology 2004;230(1):125–34.

28. Gadaleta C, Mattioli V, Colucci G, et al. Radiofrequency ablation of 40 lung neoplasms: preliminary results. AJR Am J Roentgenol 2004;183(2):361–8.

29. Pouliquen C, Kabbani Y, Saignac P, et al. Radiofrequency ablation of lung tumours with the patient under thoracic epidural anaesthesia. Cardiovasc Intervent Radiol 2011;34(Suppl 2):S178–81.

30. Elliott BA, Curry TB, Atwell TD, et al. Lung isolation, one-lung ventilation, and continuous positive airway pressure with air for radiofrequency ablation of neoplastic pulmonary lesions. Anesth Analg 2006; 103(2):463–4.

31. Sharma A, Moore WH, Lanuti M, et al. How I do it: radiofrequency ablation and cryoablation of lung tumors. J Thorac Imaging 2011;26(2):162–74.

32. Lee EW, Suh RD, Zeidler MR, et al. Radiofrequency ablation of subpleural lung malignancy: reduced pain using an artificially created pneumothorax. Cardiovasc Intervent Radiol 2009;32(4):833–6.

33. Kodama H, Yamakado K, Murashima S, et al. Intractable bronchopleural fistula caused by radiofrequency ablation: endoscopic bronchial occlusion with silicone embolic material. Br J Radiol 2009; 82(983):e225–7.

34. Steinke K, King J, Glenn D, et al. Pulmonary hemorrhage during percutaneous radiofrequency ablation: a more frequent complication than assumed? Interact Cardiovasc Thorac Surg 2003;2(4):462–5.

35. Thornton RH, Solomon SB, Dupuy DE, et al. Phrenic nerve injury resulting from percutaneous ablation of lung malignancy. AJR Am J Roentgenol 2008; 191(2):565–8.

36. Hiraki T, Gobara H, Mimura H, et al. Brachial nerve injury caused by percutaneous radiofrequency ablation of apical lung cancer: a report of four cases. J Vasc Interv Radiol 2010;21(7):1129–33.

37. Sakurai J, Mimura H, Gobara H, et al. Pulmonary artery pseudoaneurysm related to radiofrequency ablation of lung tumor. Cardiovasc Intervent Radiol 2010;33(2):413–6.

38. Yamakado K, Takaki H, Takao M, et al. Massive hemoptysis from pulmonary artery pseudoaneurysm caused by lung radiofrequency ablation: successful

treatment by coil embolization. Cardiovasc Intervent Radiol 2010;33(2):410–2.

39. Jeannin A, Saignac P, Palussiere J, et al. Massive systemic air embolism during percutaneous radiofrequency ablation of a primary lung tumor. Anesth Analg 2009;109(2):484–6.

40. Radvany MG, Allan PF, Frey WC, et al. Pulmonary radiofrequency ablation complicated by subcutaneous emphysema and pneumomediastinum treated with fibrin sealant injection. AJR Am J Roentgenol 2005;185(4):894–8.

41. Herrera LJ, Fernando HC, Perry Y, et al. Radiofrequency ablation of pulmonary malignant tumors in nonsurgical candidates. J Thorac Cardiovasc Surg 2003;125(4):929–37.

42. Hiraki T, Gobara H, Kato K, et al. Bronchiolitis obliterans organizing pneumonia after radiofrequency ablation of lung cancer: report of three cases. J Vasc Interv Radiol 2012;23(1):126–30.

43. Le TX, Andrews RT. Thermal osteonecrosis of the rib after radiofrequency ablation in the thorax. J Vasc Interv Radiol 2008;19(6):940–4.

44. Marchand B, Perol M, De La Roche E, et al. Percutaneous radiofrequency ablation of a lung metastasis: delayed cavitation with no infection. J Comput Assist Tomogr 2002;26(6):1032–4.

45. Steinke K, King J, Glenn D, et al. Radiologic appearance and complications of percutaneous computed tomography-guided radiofrequency-ablated pulmonary metastases from colorectal carcinoma. J Comput Assist Tomogr 2003;27(5):750–7.

46. Suh R, Reckamp K, Zeidler M, et al. Radiofrequency ablation in lung cancer: promising results in safety and efficacy. Oncology (Williston Park) 2005; 19(11 Suppl 4):12–21.

47. Sharma A, Digumarthy SR, Kalra MK, et al. Reversible locoregional lymph node enlargement after radiofrequency ablation of lung tumors. AJR Am J Roentgenol 2010;194(5):1250–6.

48. Wacker FK, Nour SG, Eisenberg R, et al. MRI-guided radiofrequency thermal ablation of normal lung tissue: in vivo study in a rabbit model. AJR Am J Roentgenol 2004;183(3):599–603.

49. Okuma T, Matsuoka T, Yamamoto A, et al. Assessment of early treatment response after CT-guided radiofrequency ablation of unresectable lung tumours by diffusion-weighted MRI: a pilot study. Br J Radiol 2009;82(984):989–94.

50. Okuma T, Matsuoka T, Okamura T, et al. 18F-FDG small-animal PET for monitoring the therapeutic effect of CT-guided radiofrequency ablation on implanted VX2 lung tumors in rabbits. J Nucl Med 2006;47(8):1351–8.

51. Higaki F, Okumura Y, Sato S, et al. Preliminary retrospective investigation of FDG-PET/CT timing in follow-up of ablated lung tumor. Ann Nucl Med 2008;22(3):157–63.

52. Lencioni R, Crocetti L, Cioni R, et al. Response to radiofrequency ablation of pulmonary tumours: a prospective, intention-to-treat, multicentre clinical trial (the RAPTURE study). Lancet Oncol 2008;9(7): 621–8.

53. Beland MD, Wasser EJ, Mayo-Smith WW, et al. Primary non-small cell lung cancer: review of frequency, location, and time of recurrence after radiofrequency ablation. Radiology 2010;254(1): 301–7.

54. Yamagami T, Kato T, Hirota T, et al. Risk factors for occurrence of local tumor progression after percutaneous radiofrequency ablation for lung neoplasms. Diagn Interv Radiol 2007;13(4):199–203.

55. Stauffer PR, Rossetto F, Prakash M, et al. Phantom and animal tissues for modelling the electrical properties of human liver. Int J Hyperthermia 2003;19(1): 89–101.

56. Wright AS, Lee FT Jr, Mahvi DM. Hepatic microwave ablation with multiple antennae results in synergistically larger zones of coagulation necrosis. Ann Surg Oncol 2003;10(3):275–83.

57. Shock SA, Meredith K, Warner TF, et al. Microwave ablation with loop antenna: in vivo porcine liver model. Radiology 2004;231(1):143–9.

58. Skinner MG, Iizuka MN, Kolios MC, et al. A theoretical comparison of energy sources–microwave, ultrasound and laser–for interstitial thermal therapy. Phys Med Biol 1998;43(12):3535–47.

59. Wright AS, Sampson LA, Warner TF, et al. Radiofrequency versus microwave ablation in a hepatic porcine model. Radiology 2005;236(1):132–9.

60. Brace CL, Hinshaw JL, Laeseke PF, et al. Pulmonary thermal ablation: comparison of radiofrequency and microwave devices by using gross pathologic and CT findings in a swine model. Radiology 2009; 251(3):705–11.

61. Simon CJ, Dupuy DE, Mayo-Smith WW. Microwave ablation: principles and applications. Radiographics 2005;25(Suppl 1):S69–83.

62. Griffin JP, Nelson JE, Koch KA, et al. End-of-life care in patients with lung cancer. Chest 2003; 123(Suppl 1):312S–31S.

63. Wolf FJ, Grand DJ, Machan JT, et al. Microwave ablation of lung malignancies: effectiveness, CT findings, and safety in 50 patients. Radiology 2008;247(3):871–9.

64. Grieco CA, Simon CJ, Mayo-Smith WW, et al. Image-guided percutaneous thermal ablation for the palliative treatment of chest wall masses. Am J Clin Oncol 2007;30(4):361–7.

65. Hidalgo A, Guerra JM, Gallego O, et al. Microwave ablation of a sarcoma lung metastasis in a patient with a pacemaker. Radiologia 2011. [Epub ahead of print].

66. He W, Hu XD, Wu DF, et al. Ultrasonography-guided percutaneous microwave ablation of peripheral lung cancer. Clin Imaging 2006;30(4):234–41.

67. Dupuy DE. Image-guided thermal ablation of lung malignancies. Radiology 2011;260(3):633–55.

68. Vogl TJ, Naguib NN, Gruber-Rouh T, et al. Microwave ablation therapy: clinical utility in treatment of pulmonary metastases. Radiology 2011;261(2): 643–51.

69. Giraud P, Antoine M, Larrouy A, et al. Evaluation of microscopic tumor extension in non-small-cell lung cancer for three-dimensional conformal radiotherapy planning. Int J Radiat Oncol Biol Phys 2000;48(4):1015–24.

70. Dodd GD 3rd, Napier D, Schoolfield JD, et al. Percutaneous radiofrequency ablation of hepatic tumors: postablation syndrome. AJR Am J Roentgenol 2005;185(1):51–7.

71. Goldberg SN, Grassi CJ, Cardella JF, et al. Image-guided tumor ablation: standardization of terminology and reporting criteria. J Vasc Interv Radiol 2009;20(Suppl 7):S377–90.

72. Feng W, Liu W, Li C, et al. Percutaneous microwave coagulation therapy for lung cancer. Zhonghua Zhong Liu Za Zhi 2002;24(4):388–90.

73. Littrup PJ, Mody A, Sparschu R, et al. Prostatic cryotherapy: ultrasonographic and pathologic correlation in the canine model. Urology 1994;44(2): 175–83 [discussion: 183–4].

74. Sanderson DR, Neel HB 3rd, Fontana RS. Bronchoscopic cryotherapy. Ann Otol Rhinol Laryngol 1981; 90(4 Pt 1):354–8.

75. Maiwand MO, Homasson JP. Cryotherapy for tracheobronchial disorders. Clin Chest Med 1995; 16(3):427–43.

76. Wang H, Littrup PJ, Duan Y, et al. Thoracic masses treated with percutaneous cryotherapy: initial experience with more than 200 procedures. Radiology 2005;235(1):289–98.

77. Hoffmann NE, Bischof JC. The cryobiology of cryosurgical injury. Urology 2002;60(2 Suppl 1):40–9.

78. Gage AA, Baust J. Mechanisms of tissue injury in cryosurgery. Cryobiology 1998;37(3):171–86.

79. Sabel MS, Nehs MA, Su G, et al. Immunologic response to cryoablation of breast cancer. Breast Cancer Res Treat 2005;90(1):97–104.

80. Thomas P, Doddoli C, Thirion X, et al. Stage I non-small cell lung cancer: a pragmatic approach to prognosis after complete resection. Ann Thorac Surg 2002;73(4):1065–70.

81. Permpongkosol S, Nicol TL, Link RE, et al. Differences in ablation size in porcine kidney, liver, and lung after cryoablation using the same ablation protocol. AJR Am J Roentgenol 2007;188(4): 1028–32.

82. Hinshaw JL, Littrup PJ, Durick N, et al. Optimizing the protocol for pulmonary cryoablation: a comparison of a dual- and triple-freeze protocol. Cardiovasc Intervent Radiol 2010;33(6):1180–5.

83. Allaf ME, Varkarakis IM, Bhayani SB, et al. Pain control requirements for percutaneous ablation of renal tumors: cryoablation versus radiofrequency ablation–initial observations. Radiology 2005; 237(1):366–70.

84. Anai H, Uchida BT, Pavcnik D, et al. Effects of blood flow and/or ventilation restriction on radiofrequency coagulation size in the lung: an experimental study in swine. Cardiovasc Intervent Radiol 2006;29(5): 838–45.

85. Kawamura M, Izumi Y, Tsukada N, et al. Percutaneous cryoablation of small pulmonary malignant tumors under computed tomographic guidance with local anesthesia for nonsurgical candidates. J Thorac Cardiovasc Surg 2006; 131(5):1007–13.

86. Zemlyak A, Moore WH, Bilfinger TV. Comparison of survival after sublobar resections and ablative therapies for stage I non-small cell lung cancer. J Am Coll Surg 2010;211(1):68–72.

87. Bojarski JD, Dupuy DE, Mayo-Smith WW. CT imaging findings of pulmonary neoplasms after treatment with radiofrequency ablation: results in 32 tumors. AJR Am J Roentgenol 2005;185(2): 466–71.

88. Chua TC, Sarkar A, Saxena A, et al. Long-term outcome of image-guided percutaneous radiofrequency ablation of lung metastases: an open-labeled prospective trial of 148 patients. Ann Oncol 2010;21(10):2017–22.

89. Akeboshi M, Yamakado K, Nakatsuka A, et al. Percutaneous radiofrequency ablation of lung neoplasms: initial therapeutic response. J Vasc Interv Radiol 2004;15(5):463–70.

Future Trends in Lung Cancer Diagnosis

Jared D. Christensen, MD[a], Edward F. Patz Jr, MD[a,b],*

KEYWORDS

- Lung cancer • Biomarker • Diagnostics • Computed tomography • Magnetic resonance imaging
- Positron emission tomography

KEY POINTS

- Conventional imaging relies on changes in normal anatomy and morphology for the diagnosis of lung cancer.
- Morphologic data are not specific and do not provide useful information regarding tumor biology or phenotype.
- Advances in conventional imaging techniques have not significantly improved outcomes for lung cancer.
- Incorporating tumor biology with conventional imaging may improve diagnostic accuracy; ^{18}F-fluorodeoxyglucose positron emission tomography is the prototypical example but still has limitations.
- Novel biomarkers and molecular imaging probes may be used for identifying high-risk patients, diagnosis, staging, and treatment stratification.
- The integration of imaging and biomarkers into patient-evaluation strategies will be required to provide an optimized approach to lung cancer diagnostics.

INTRODUCTION

Lung cancer remains the leading cause of cancer mortality in men and women worldwide, accounting for more deaths than colon, breast, and prostate cancers combined. Despite advances in imaging and molecular diagnostics, the majority of individuals have advanced-stage disease at presentation; only 20% of patients present with potentially resectable early-stage disease. The 5-year survival rate remains poor at approximately 16%,[1] and even with targeted therapy, treatment options have failed to significantly reduce mortality. If there are to be improvements in outcome, novel diagnostic and therapeutic strategies are needed.

DIAGNOSTIC APPROACH TO LUNG CANCER

Diagnostic tests in oncology continue to evolve and play an ever-increasing role in the management of

patients with cancer.[2,3] Radiology, pathology, and molecular diagnostics are distinct entities, with specialists and subspecialists who train and practice in each area. Because of the large amount of information generated, it is understandable that these entities remain as separate domains. But in the move toward personalized medicine, where treatment decisions are tailored to the patient, integration of this broad spectrum of diagnostic information will help facilitate more efficient and cost-effective patient evaluation.

It is not easy to create an organized diagnostic approach from a collection of disparate tests without appropriate trials and evidence-based medicine; this is a daunting, expensive mission that requires the cooperation of multiple specialties. Most diagnostic trials assess a specific technology and do not typically evaluate multiple modalities. However, when considering the spectrum of diagnostic issues in oncology, no single strategy

a Department of Radiology, Duke University Medical Center, Box 3808 Erwin Road, Durham, NC 27710, USA;
b Department of Pharmacology and Cancer Biology, Duke University Medical Center, Box 3808 Erwin Road, Durham, NC 27710, USA
* Corresponding author. Department of Radiology, Duke University Medical Center, Box 3808 Erwin Road Durham, NC 27710.
E-mail address: edward.patz@duke.edu

Radiol Clin N Am 50 (2012) 1001–1008
http://dx.doi.org/10.1016/j.rcl.2012.06.002
0033-8389/12/$ – see front matter © 2012 Elsevier Inc. All rights reserved.

addresses all of the clinical questions. A combination of imaging studies, clinical features, pathologic evaluation, and molecular medicine will be essential if a personalized approach is to be realized. This review first describes the current role of conventional imaging and then explores future directions that integrate a variety of diagnostic tests in the evaluation of patients with lung cancer.

CURRENT IMAGING APPROACH TO LUNG CANCER

Radiology has a central role in all aspects of managing patients with lung cancer. It is essential for localizing abnormalities, suggesting the diagnosis, providing clinical staging, following response to treatment, and facilitating surveillance of patients after therapy is complete. While imaging in each of these areas provides a tremendous amount of information, there are still a number of limitations; not all radiographic abnormalities that appear to be lung cancer are cancer, clinical staging is not uniformly accurate, and response criteria, which were designed as a surrogate for outcomes, do not consistently correlate with survival. Such a situation arises because anatomic and morphologic features displayed with conventional imaging techniques do not clearly reflect pathology. Significant advances in patient management will only occur when fundamental properties of tumor biology are incorporated into the development of novel diagnostics tests that address specific clinical issues.

DIAGNOSING LUNG CANCER

One of the primary roles of imaging is to suggest the diagnosis and then identify patients who require further evaluation. Pathologic confirmation is almost always performed before treatment. Conventional multidetector computed tomography (CT) of the chest remains the standard initial imaging study in patients with suspected lung cancer. In an effort to establish a diagnosis, the primary pulmonary abnormality is described on the basis of size; margins (eg, irregular or spiculated); attenuation values, including the presence or absence of calcification, fat, or ground-glass opacities; and growth characteristics as determined by sequential studies.

With continued changes in technology, including improvements in spatial resolution, there has been increased detection and characterization of small lung nodules, particularly the ground-glass component, in an effort to identify early-stage lung cancer. Although guidelines for managing these patients have been invaluable,[4] this imaging-based approach has several disadvantages, including cost of sequential imaging, cumulative radiation exposure to patients, risks of invasive testing, and potential delays in diagnosis. In addition, it is becoming increasingly clear that ground-glass opacities should be considered a separate entity from solid nodules, and new guidelines for managing patients with these abnormalities are currently under development by the Fleischner Society.

Additional techniques have been used in an attempt to provide greater specificity in nodule characterization. Contrast enhancement has been proposed because malignant nodules typically have greater enhancement than benign lesions.[5–9] In one prospective, multicenter trial, researchers found that for nodule enhancement of 15 Hounsfield units (HU) or greater, the sensitivity, specificity, and accuracy for the diagnosis of lung cancer were 98%, 58%, and 77%, respectively.[8] However, this approach has limitations that have precluded widespread adoption. Large nodules may have heterogeneous enhancement patterns that produce sampling errors. Nodules with necrosis may not demonstrate significant enhancement as a result of tumor growth outpacing the blood supply. Furthermore, some benign lesions, such as vascular malformations and inflammatory or infectious nodules, may actively show enhancement. In addition, the technique requires sequential scans, generating an increased patient radiation dose. Yet perhaps the primary reason dynamic contrast-enhanced CT has not dramatically altered lung cancer diagnostics is because the specificity and accuracy of differentiating malignant from benign lung nodules are not statistically significantly improved from those of routine nonenhanced chest CT.[5,8]

More recently, dual-energy CT (DECT) has been suggested as a technique to further characterize lung nodules. DECT provides both enhanced and nonenhanced images with a single contrast-enhanced acquisition, permitting nodule characterization with a smaller radiation dose compared with conventional dynamic contrast-enhanced CT imaging.[10,11] DECT does have limitations. The 80-kVp dataset from which the virtual nonenhanced images are generated typically have more noise than do conventional nonenhanced images, which may be particularly problematic in obese patients.[10–12] The 80-kVp tube also has a smaller field of view (FOV), which excludes the peripheral portion of the thorax in some patients, limiting its use for peripheral nodule assessment. New-generation DECT scanners have enlarged the FOV from 26 to 33 cm, and future scanners may be able to eliminate the smaller FOV altogether. Further studies are needed to determine whether DECT will have a role in diagnosing lung cancer.

Most patients with a pulmonary abnormality greater than 1 cm and clinically suspected lung cancer will undergo an ^{18}F-fluorodeoxyglucose (FDG) positron emission tomography (PET) study. This helps to differentiate benign from malignant nodules and guide patient management. It must be recognized that a small number of early-stage, typically indolent tumors may not have significant FDG uptake and that benign lesions may have increased FDG activity.[13] Despite these limitations, FDG-PET has become an essential tool in the diagnosis and staging of patients with suspected lung cancer.

While FDG-PET provides an alternative approach to conventional anatomic imaging, the lack of FDG specificity has resulted in an effort to develop new, more specific tumor-imaging probes. ^{18}F-Fluorothymidine is a proliferation marker that may be more specific than FDG for non–small cell lung carcinoma (NSCLC) in the assessment of solitary pulmonary nodules and may provide greater accuracy in the evaluation of early treatment response.[14,15] ^{99m}Tc–Annexin V is an apoptosis-imaging agent whose uptake may correlate with overall and progression-free survival.[16,17] ^{18}F-Fluoromisonidazole PET quantifies cellular hypoxia, and may aid in the diagnosis of NSCLC and prediction of treatment response.[18] ^{18}F-Fluoro-α-methyltyrosine is an amino acid analogue that accumulates in tumor cells and is specific to neoplasms. Early data suggest that ^{18}F-fluoro-α-methyltyrosine is less sensitive than FDG for NSCLC diagnosis, but is promising in monitoring treatment response and predicting prognosis.[19,20] ^{99m}Tc-Ethylene dicysteine glucosamine is a single-photon emission CT agent that has higher spatial resolution than PET, is lower in cost, and is more widely available. Preliminary data indicate a 100% concordance between ^{99m}Tc-ethylene dicysteine glucosamine and FDG for NSCLC.[21]

Magnetic resonance (MR) imaging is currently not indicated for the routine assessment of patients with lung cancer, but has been reserved for the assessment of superior sulcus tumors and cases whereby local invasion is suspected. MR imaging has poor spatial resolution of the lung parenchyma in comparison with CT and does not provide the same metabolic information as PET. As with CT, lung nodule vascularity and perfusion can be assessed with dynamic contrast-enhanced MR imaging. Zou and colleagues[22] found that MR enhancement for benign solitary pulmonary nodules was significantly less than that for other abnormalities. Furthermore, unlike dynamic contrast-enhanced CT, malignant nodules could be differentiated from inflammatory nodules based on quantitative washout kinetics. Notwithstanding, the technique is limited to those patients who can undergo MR imaging and receive contrast media.

Diffusion-weighted (DW) MR imaging has been proposed as an alternative MR technique for the characterization of indeterminate pulmonary nodules. DW imaging provides tissue contrast based on the diffusion of water molecules among tissues between the extracellular and intracellular spaces. Apparent diffusion coefficients are generated, which can be mapped as an image. Preliminary studies suggested DW imaging is comparable to FDG-PET for characterization of malignant pulmonary nodules and may be superior to FDG-PET for mediastinal nodal staging,[23,24] although additional studies are required to demonstrate its true clinical utility.

ASSESSING LYMPH NODE METASTASIS FOR LUNG CANCER STAGING

The International Staging System for lung cancer is an anatomic approach based on features of the tumor, location of involved lymph nodes, and the presence of metastases.[25] Tumor size and location are identified on conventional imaging; however, the presence of local invasion (eg, into the chest wall, diaphragm, or vascular structures) can be more problematic. Imaging of mediastinal lymph nodes rely on either size (eg, CT and endoscopic ultrasonography) or metabolic properties (PET) to infer tumor involvement, although these techniques are not uniformly sensitive or specific.

In general, the positive predictive value of CT for mediastinal lymph node metastasis ($\sim$50%) is worse than that for FDG-PET (80%–90%). Nevertheless, approximately 5% of patients with negative mediastinal nodes by CT and FDG-PET criteria will have positive nodal disease at resection, while 21% of patients with mediastinal nodes positive by CT and negative by FDG-PET are positive at surgery.[26] Therefore, patients without mediastinal lymphadenopathy by CT and an FDG-PET–negative mediastinum may proceed directly to surgery. Patients with enlarged lymph nodes on CT require pathologic confirmation of disease regardless of FDG-PET findings, as do patients with any FDG-PET–positive mediastinal finding regardless of node size. However, some have advocated that mediastinoscopy should be performed in all patients who are potential candidates for surgical resection to prevent futile thoracotomies in those with false-negative imaging and to permit curative treatment in those with false-positive imaging.[27] In addition to nodal characterization, both CT and PET can identify unsuspected soft tissue, bony, or visceral metastasis. Although current imaging techniques have limitations, their data provide an essential road map for further evaluation and help determine patient management.[28,29]

ASSESSING RESPONSE TO TREATMENT AND SURVEILLANCE FOR RECURRENT LUNG CANCER

Besides being used for diagnosis and staging of lung cancer, imaging is the primary tool used to determine response to therapy and for surveillance once treatment is complete. Response is currently determined in large part by changes in tumor size as dictated by the Response Evaluation Criteria In Solid Tumors as well as changes in standardized uptake value (SUV) on FDG-PET. However, these techniques have limitations, as tumors are heterogeneous lesions composed of numerous different cell types. One recent study found no correlation between tumor cellular composition, lesion size, or FDG activity.[30] Decreases in tumor size or SUV may represent a decrease in inflammatory tissue or other components and not necessarily a decrease in tumor burden.[31] Likewise, early changes in tumor size as a measure of treatment response do not correlate with survival.[32]

Some studies suggest that changes in SUV in early-stage patients have prognostic value, with most tumors responding to therapy demonstrating a 20% to 40% decrease in SUV early in treatment.[33] These findings have formed the basis for PET Response Criteria in Solid Tumors guidelines currently under development. However, other studies in patients receiving neoadjuvant therapy suggest that FDG uptake cannot reliably be used as a marker of treatment response, as decreases in SUV may not represent a decrease in tumor burden.[31,34] Further studies are needed to validate the use of FDG-PET in assessing therapeutic response.

Preliminary studies using MR imaging and apparent diffusion coefficients for monitoring treatment response in NSCLC have been reported,[35] but whether diffusion MR imaging is superior to existing imaging modalities remains to be seen.

BIOMARKERS AND MOLECULAR DIAGNOSTICS IN LUNG CANCER

Biomarkers are objective measures of a normal biological or pathologic process. In a broad sense, conventional imaging features such as size, morphology, and growth rates are biomarkers of disease. However, as discussed earlier, these findings are not specific and do not provide prognostic information regarding current or future biological behavior of a lesion. Novel strategies are needed to improve both diagnosis and prognostic ability.

Improved cancer detection has been a primary initiative in the "war against cancer" ever since the National Cancer Institute was created in 1971. Imaging has a fundamental role in this effort, as it often provides the first evidence of cancer. Radiology also presents a unique perspective on tumors, as it noninvasively reveals anatomic and morphologic features, growth rates, and, eventually, patterns of metastasis. However, cancer is a heterogeneous disease and represents a complex, ever-changing relationship between transformed tumor cells and the host.[30,36,37] It has become clear that multiple different strategies will be needed for the development of clinical diagnostics. Rather than diminishing the impact of any technology, this realization serves to recognize the power of integrating modalities.

As discussed earlier, evaluation of patients with cancer can fundamentally be divided into 3 areas: early detection, diagnosis and staging, and response to therapy. Each of these areas has its own set of issues. For early detection programs, a key initial problem is how to best define a high-risk group. In the absence of a clear targeted at-risk population, the utility of screening may be problematic. The prevalence of disease is often low and there are too many false-positive and incidental findings requiring further evaluation. Developing cost-effective biomarkers to identify the "highest risk" of the high-risk patients and determine who needs an imaging study would be more efficient than imaging everyone.

The next area for cancer evaluation is diagnosis and staging. Once a patient is identified as being in the highest-risk category, CT could then be used to localize an abnormality. In the case of lung cancer, many individuals have an indeterminate pulmonary nodule but very few have cancer.[38,39] Almost all require additional imaging or an invasive procedure to distinguish a benign from a malignant lesion. The current Fleischner Society guidelines for the management of a pulmonary nodule suggest stratifying patients into high-risk and low-risk categories based on age, smoking history, and nodule size, which then determines whether intervention or sequential imaging studies are recommended.[4] A potential alternative solution would be to develop a set of specific biomarkers that, in conjunction with imaging, could diagnose cancer. Theoretically this could be done by analyzing biospecimens or imaging with novel molecular imaging probes or a combination of modalities.[40,41] These markers would help determine which patients have lung cancer and which patients require no further evaluation. Biomarkers could then assist in staging tumors, with a more informative, phenotypic description of tumors replacing the primarily size-based classification scheme for clinical staging currently in use.[25]

Finally, once a diagnosis of cancer is made, therapy needs to be optimized and response assessed. Unfortunately, many cancers that have an identical radiographic and histologic appearance have very different phenotypes. Although prognostic and predictive markers have traditionally been outside the purview of imaging, they are an essential part of the diagnostic evaluation. In this scenario, novel imaging or specimen biomarkers could be developed to suggest appropriate therapy, or no therapy at all in the case of indolent tumors. Studies of patients with surgically resectable lung cancer have identified genes that may aid diagnosis and predict which patients will benefit from adjuvant therapy.[42] In patients with NSCLC, tumor mutations in epidermal growth factor receptor (EGFR), KRAS, and anaplastic lymphoma kinase (ALK) are mutually exclusive, and the presence of one mutation can influence response to targeted therapy.[43] Testing for these mutations to direct treatment is therefore gaining acceptance, but continued studies are necessary to validate the use of these markers.

BIOMARKER DISCOVERY

Biomarkers should be relevant to a specific clinical question and represent evidence of a particular normal biological or pathologic state. While there has been a concerted effort to introduce novel biomarkers, very few have been translated into clinical practice. This is due to numerous obstacles, including lack of reproducibility of discovery platforms, unavailability or poor integrity of specimens, difficulties in assay development and bioinformatics, and regulatory issues.[44] The paucity of clinically useful biomarkers may be related to limitations in technology to comprehensively evaluate a biospecimen, although finding consistent protein or genetic differences between heterogeneous tumor and normal tissue is a difficult proposition. Current discovery platforms typically assess only a small percentage of the most abundant proteins, and low-abundance proteins are not adequately interrogated. In addition, it is not trivial to examine posttranslational modifications or mutated proteins. One must also consider that differentially expressed markers in tumor cells may not be of sufficient abundance to cause significant changes in systemic levels. For example, the proteins macrophage migratory inhibitor factor and cyclophilin A are significantly overexpressed in lung cancer relative to normal lung, but serum levels in patients with tumors are no different compared with age-, gender-, and smoking history–matched controls without cancer.[45,46]

Statistical analysis and study design for biomarker discovery also present a significant and complex problem. Many specimen biomarker studies in cancer have explored transcript expression, genome-wide associations, and protein profiling.[45,47–49] These studies typically generate high-dimensional data sets (ie, they have a large number of features), yet the relative number of subject specimens is small. Data analysis depends on creative statistical solutions, which may be fragile and susceptible to noise and overfitting of data.[50,51] Once discovery is complete, validating biomarkers is not a trivial issue. Independent, well-annotated sets of specimens with a sufficient number of cases are difficult to obtain; this creates a problem of determining the clinical utility of a biomarker, as case-to-control ratios do not always reflect the true prevalence in the population.

From an imaging perspective, there are clear limitations in studies that report only gross anatomy and morphology. However, radiology usually looks to technology, not biology, for a solution. The field prioritizes advances in instrumentation, rather than seeking solutions based on pathology. However, more recent efforts in molecular imaging have attempted to incorporate biological properties into imaging studies.[52–55] This has not been a simple proposition, and aside from FDG-PET, most molecular imaging initiatives have yet to be adopted into clinical practice.[56]

Ultimately, there is the fundamental issue of economics and resources. Unfortunately, the diagnostic space has not received the attention of the investment community, which traditionally focused on therapeutics. The margin on new diagnostics, including assays for specimen biomarkers or imaging probes, is low. Most diagnostic trials are supported by an industry that manufactures imaging equipment, with little or no impetus to include biospecimens. The majority of specimens currently collected are part of therapeutic trials, which are guided by a different hypothesis and focus in comparison with diagnostic trials. Most biomarker discovery is intended to facilitate drug development, with little intent to develop clinical cancer diagnostics.

INTEGRATION OF DETECTION, DIAGNOSIS, AND TREATMENT

Ultimately, unification of lung cancer detection, diagnosis, and treatment could be envisioned.

With a combination of imaging, biomarkers, and clinical data, high-risk individuals could be identified, the diagnosis of malignancy established, and a tumor profile would determine the optimal therapeutic strategy. In this ideal scenario, following patients for response would not be required because outcomes could be predicted at presentation.

Although the concept of integration seems logical, the path to implementation is a long, complex, and expensive process. Coordinating multi-disciplinary activities in a multi-institutional trial requires extraordinary planning and constant monitoring. Study design, standardization of imaging protocols, agreement of radiologic interpretation and reporting, collection and collation of relevant clinical data, standardization of specimen collection, processing, handling and storage, and quality assurance concerns are just the beginning.[44] Patient enrollment, retention, and follow-up are not trivial, and all trials must be approved by institutional review boards and comply with Health Insurance Portability and Accountability Act regulations.

SUMMARY

Cancer diagnostics has entered a new phase of development with advances in imaging, pathology, and molecular medicine. It is fueled by improvements in technology, bioinformatics, and an increased understanding of tumor biology. To translate these advances into clinical practice, a concerted multidisciplinary effort by both basic science and clinical researchers is required. The diagnostic community must collate these data and present a coherent, clinically useful strategy. This integrated approach generates several opportunities, including the potential for more rational health care, but also creates challenges such as trial validation to ensure that new strategies are indeed successful. Ultimately, before a more personalized approach to medicine can be achieved, these trials will need to confirm that integration of diagnostic results will be cost effective, change patient management, and improve outcomes.

REFERENCES

1. Jemal A, Siegel R, Xu J, et al. Cancer statistics, 2010. CA Cancer J Clin 2010;60:277–300.
2. Dinan MA, Curtis LH, Hammill BG, et al. Changes in the use and costs of diagnostic imaging among Medicare beneficiaries with cancer, 1999-2006. JAMA 2010;303:1625–31.
3. Song Y, Skinner J, Bynum J, et al. Regional variations in diagnostic practices. N Engl J Med 2010;363:45–53.
4. MacMahon H, Austin JH, Gamsu G, et al. Guidelines for management of small pulmonary nodules detected on CT scans: a statement from the Fleischner Society. Radiology 2005;237:395–400.
5. Yamashita K, Matsunobe S, Tsuda T, et al. Solitary pulmonary nodule: preliminary study of evaluation with incremental dynamic CT. Radiology 1995;194:399–405.
6. Littleton JT, Durizch ML, Moeller G, et al. Pulmonary masses: contrast enhancement. Radiology 1990;177:861–71.
7. Zhang M, Kono M. Solitary pulmonary nodules: evaluation of blood flow patterns with dynamic CT. Radiology 1997;205:471–8.
8. Swensen SJ, Viggiano RW, Midthun DE, et al. Lung nodule enhancement at CT: multicenter study. Radiology 2000;241:73–80.
9. Li Y, Yang ZG, Chen TW, et al. Whole tumour perfusion of peripheral lung carcinoma: evaluation with first-pass CT perfusion imaging at 64-detector row CT. Clin Radiol 2008;63:629–35.
10. Johnson TR, Krauss B, Sedlmair M, et al. Material differentiation by dual energy CT: initial experience. Eur Radiol 2007;17:1510–7.
11. Pontana F, Faivre JB, Remy-Jardin M, et al. Lung perfusion with dual-energy multidetector-row CT (MDCT): feasibility for the evaluation of acute pulmonary embolism in 117 consecutive patients. Acad Radiol 2008;15:1494–504.
12. Chae EJ, Song JW, Seo JB, et al. Clinical utility of dual-energy CT in the evaluation of solitary pulmonary nodules: initial experience. Radiology 2008;249:671–81.
13. Marom EM, Sarvis S, Herndon JE, et al. T1 lung cancers: sensitivity of diagnosis with fluorodeoxyglucose PET. Radiology 2002;223:453–9.
14. Yuka Y, Yoshihior N, Shinya I, et al. 3′-Deoxy-3′-^{18}F-fluorothymidine as a proliferation imaging tracer for diagnosis of lung tumors: comparison with 2-deoxy-2-^{18}F-fluoro-D-glucose. J Comput Assist Tomogr 2008;32:432–7.
15. Kahraman D, Scheffler M, Zander T, et al. Quantitative analysis of response to treatment with erlotinib in advanced non-small cell lung cancer using ^{18}F-FDG and 3′-deoxy-3′-^{18}F-fluorothymidine PET. J Nucl Med 2011;52(12):1871–7 [Epub 2011 Nov 7].
16. Kartachova M, van Zandwijk N, Burgers S, et al. Prognostic significance of ^{99m}Tc HYNIC-Rh-annexin V scintigraphy during platinum-based chemotherapy in advanced lung cancer. J Clin Oncol 2007;25:2534–9.
17. Kartachova MS, Valdes Olmos RA, Haas RL, et al. ^{99m}Tc-HYNIC-Rh-annexin-V scintigraphy: visual and quantitative evaluation of early treatment-induced apoptosis to predict treatment outcome. Nucl Med Commun 2008;29:39–44.

18. Eschmann SM, Paulsen F, Reimhold M, et al. Prognostic impact of hypoxia imaging with ^{18}F-misonidazole PET in non-small cell lung cancer and head and neck cancer before radiotherapy. J Nucl Med 2005; 46:253–60.

19. Kaira K, Oriuchi N, Shimizu K, et al. ^{18}F-FMT uptake seen within primary cancer on PET helps predict outcome of non-small cell lung cancer. J Nucl Med 2009;50:1770–6.

20. Kaira K, Oriuchi N, Yanagitani N, et al. Assessment of therapy response in lung cancer with ^{18}F-α-methyl tyrosine PET. Am J Roentgenol 2010;195:1204–11.

21. Schecter NR, Erwin WD, Yang DJ, et al. Radiation dosimetry and biodistribution of ^{99m}Tc-ethylene dicysteine-deoxyglucose in patients with non-small-cell lung cancer. Eur J Nucl Med Mol Imaging 2009;36:1583–91.

22. Zou Y, Zhang M, Wang Q, et al. Quantitative investigation of solitary pulmonary nodules: dynamic contrast-enhanced MRI and histopathologic analysis. Am J Roentgenol 2008;191:252–9.

23. Chen W, Jian W, Li H, et al. Whole-body diffusion-weighted imaging vs. FDG-PET for the detection of non-small-cell lung cancer. How do they measure up? Magn Reson Imaging 2010;28:613–20.

24. Nomori H, Mori T, Ikeda K, et al. Diffusion-weighted magnetic resonance imaging can be used in place of positron emission tomography for N staging of non–small cell lung cancer with fewer false-positive results. J Thorac Cardiovasc Surg 2008;135:816–22.

25. Rami-Porta R, Crowley JJ, Goldstraw P. The revised TNM staging system for lung cancer. Ann Thorac Cardiovasc Surg 2009;15:4–9.

26. DeLangen AJ, Raijmakers P, Riphagen I, et al. The size of mediastinal lymph nodes and its relation with metastatic involvement: a meta-analysis. Eur J Cardiothorac Surg 2006;29:26–9.

27. Catarino PA, Goldstraw P. The future in diagnosis and staging of lung cancer. Respiration 2006;73:717–32.

28. Dwamena BA, Sonnad SS, Angobaldo JO, et al. Metastases from non-small-cell lung cancer: mediastinal staging in the 1990s: meta-analytic comparison of PET and CT. Radiology 1999;213:530–6.

29. Toloza EM, Harpole L, McCrory DC. Noninvasive staging of non-small cell lung cancer: a review of the current evidence. Chest 2003;123:137S–46S.

30. Christensen JD, Colby TV, Patz EF Jr. Correlation of [18F]-2-fluoro-deoxy-d-glucose positron emission tomography standard uptake values with the cellular composition of stage I nonsmall cell lung cancer. Cancer 2010;116:4095–102.

31. Tanvetyanon T, Eikman EA, Sommers E, et al. Computed tomography response, but not positron emission tomography scan response, predicts survival after neoadjuvant chemotherapy for resectable non-small-cell lung cancer. J Clin Oncol 2008; 26:4610–6.

32. Birchard KR, Hoang JK, Herndon JE, et al. Early changes in tumor size in patients treated for advanced stage NSCLC do not correlate with survival: are current response criteria meaningful? Cancer 2009;115:581–6.

33. Wahl RL, Jacene H, Kasamon Y, et al. From RECIST to PERCIST: evolving considerations for PET response criteria in solid tumors. J Nucl Med 2009; 50:122S–50S.

34. Bertino EM, Confer P, Colonna JE, et al. Pulmonary neuroendocrine/carcinoid tumors: a review article. Cancer 2009;115:4434–41.

35. Yabuuchi H, Hatakenaka M, Takayama K, et al. Non-small cell lung cancer: detection of early response to chemotherapy by using contrast-enhanced dynamic and diffusion-weighted MR imaging. Radiology 2011;261:598–604.

36. Tan TT, Coussens LM. Humoral immunity, inflammation and cancer. Curr Opin Immunol 2007;19:209–16.

37. Amornsiripanitch N, Hong S, Campa MJ, et al. Complement factor H autoantibodies are associated with early stage NSCLC. Clin Cancer Res 2010;16: 3226–31.

38. Swensen SJ, Jett JR, Hartman TE, et al. CT screening for lung cancer: five-year prospective experience. Radiology 2005;235:259–65.

39. The National Lung Screening Trial Research Team, Aberle DR, Adams AM, Berg CD, et al. Reduced lung-cancer mortality with low-dose computed tomographic screening. N Engl J Med 2011;365: 395–409.

40. Patz EF Jr, Campa MJ, Gottlin EB, et al. Panel of serum biomarkers for the diagnosis of lung cancer. J Clin Oncol 2007;25:5578–83.

41. Gottlin EB, Xiangrong G, Pegram C, et al. Isolation of novel EGFR directed VHH domains with diagnostic or therapeutic potential. J Biomol Screen 2009;14: 77–85.

42. Olaussen KA, Dunant A, Fouret P, et al. DNA repair by ERCC1 in non–small-cell lung cancer and cisplatin-based adjuvant chemotherapy. N Engl J Med 2006;355:983–91.

43. Keedy VL, Temin S, Somerfield MR, et al. American Society of Clinical Oncology provisional clinical opinion: epidermal growth factor receptor (EGFR) mutation testing for patients with advanced non-small-cell lung cancer considering first-line EGFR tyrosine kinase inhibitor therapy. J Clin Oncol 2011;29:2121–7.

44. Khleif SN, Doroshow JH, Hait WN. AACR-FDA-NCI Cancer Biomarkers Collaborative consensus report: advancing the use of biomarkers in cancer drug development. Clin Cancer Res 2010;16:3299–318.

45. Campa MJ, Wang MZ, Howard B, et al. Protein expression profiling identifies macrophage migration inhibitory factor and cyclophilin A as potential molecular targets in non-small cell lung cancer. Cancer Res 2003;63:1652–6.

46. Howard BA, Zheng Z, Campa MJ, et al. Translating biomarkers into clinical practice: prognostic implications of cyclophilin A and macrophage migratory inhibitory factor identified from protein expression profiles in non-small cell lung cancer. Lung Cancer 2004;46:313–23.

47. Beane J, Spira A, Lenburg ME. Clinical impact of high-throughput gene expression studies in lung cancer. J Thorac Oncol 2009;4:109–18.

48. Wrage M, Ruosaari S, Eijk PP, et al. Genomic profiles associated with early micrometastasis in lung cancer: relevance of 4q deletion. Clin Cancer Res 2009;15:1566–74.

49. Li Y, Sheu CC, Ye Y, et al. Genetic variants and risk of lung cancer in never smokers: a genome-wide association study. Lancet Oncol 2010;11:321–30.

50. Baggerly KA, Morris JS, Edmonson SR, et al. Signal in noise: evaluating reported reproducibility of serum proteomic tests for ovarian cancer. J Natl Cancer Inst 2005;97:307–9.

51. Morris JS, Baggerly KA, Gutstein HB, et al. Statistical contributions to proteomic research. Methods Mol Biol 2010;641:143–66.

52. Lee JH, Huh YM, Jun YW, et al. Artificially engineered magnetic nanoparticles for ultra-sensitive molecular imaging. Nat Med 2006;13:95–9.

53. Huang L, Gainkam L, Caveliers V, et al. SPECT imaging with ^{99m}Tc-labeled EGFR-specific nanobody for in vivo monitoring of EGFR expression. Mol Imaging Biol 2008;10:167–75.

54. Wang F, Fang W, Zhang MR, et al. Evaluation of chemotherapy response in VX2 rabbit lung cancer with ^{18}F-labeled C2A domain of synaptotagmin I. J Nucl Med 2011;52:592–9.

55. Zander T, Hofmann A, Staratschek-Jox A, et al. Blood-based gene expression signatures in non-small cell lung cancer. Clin Cancer Res 2011; 17(10):3360–7 [Epub 2011 May 10].

56. Hansell DM, Boiselle PM, Goldin J, et al. Thoracic imaging. Respirology 2010;15:393–400.

Index

Note: Page numbers of article titles are in **boldface** type.

Radiol Clin N Am 50 (2012) 1009–1014
http://dx.doi.org/10.1016/S0033-8389(12)00146-7
0033-8389/12/$ – see front matter © 2012 Elsevier Inc. All rights reserved.